NVQs in Nursing and Residential Care Homes

Also of interest:

Nursing in Care Homes
Second Edition
Linda Nazarko
978-0632-05226-4

Dementia Care: A Practical Photographic Guide
James Grealy, Helen McMullen and Julia Grealy
978-1405-13428-6

Knowledge to Care: A Handbook for Care Assistants
Second Edition
Edited by Angela Dustagheer, Joan Hardy and Christine McMahon
978-14051-1111-9

Enabling Independence: A Guide for Rehabilitation Workers
Hazel MacKey and Susan Noncarrow
978-14051-3028-8

NVQs in Nursing and Residential Care Homes

Third Edition

Linda Nazarko
MSc, PGDip, BSc (Hons), RN, OBE, FRCN

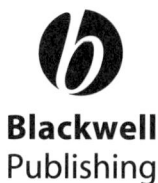

Blackwell
Publishing

© 1996, 2000, 2007 by Linda Nazarko

Blackwell Publishing editorial offices:
Blackwell Publishing Ltd, 9600 Garsington Road, Oxford OX4 2DQ, UK
Tel: +44 (0)1865 776868
Blackwell Publishing Inc., 350 Main Street, Malden, MA 02148-5020, USA
Tel: +1 781 388 8250
Blackwell Publishing Asia Pty Ltd, 550 Swanston Street, Carlton, Victoria 3053, Australia
Tel: +61 (0)3 8359 1011

The right of the Author to be identified as the Author of this Work has been asserted in accordance with the Copyright, Designs and Patents Act 1988.

All rights reserved. No part of this publication may be reproduced, stored in a retrieval system, or transmitted, in any form or by any means, electronic, mechanical, photocopying, recording or otherwise, except as permitted by the UK Copyright, Designs and Patents Act 1988, without the prior permission of the publisher.

First published 2007 by Blackwell Publishing Ltd

ISBN-13: 978-1-4051-5743-8

Library of Congress Cataloging-in-Publication Data

Nazarko, Linda.
 NVQs in nursing and residential care homes / Linda Nazarko. – 3rd ed.
     p. ; cm.
 ISBN-13: 978-1-4051-5743-8 (pbk. : alk. paper)
  1. Nursing–Standards–Great Britain.   2. Vocational qualifications–Great Britain.
 3. National Vocational qualifications–Great Britain.   I. Title.   II. Title: National vocational qualifications in nursing and residential care homes.
  [DNLM: 1. Nursing–standards.   2. Nursing Care–standards.   3. Residential Facilities–standards.
      WY 16 N335n 2007]

RT120.L64N394 2007
610.7302′18–dc22
2006039313

A catalogue record for this title is available from the British Library

Set in 10/12 pt Sabon
by Graphicraft Limited, Hong Kong
Printed and bound in Singapore
by Fabulous Printers Pte Ltd

The publisher's policy is to use permanent paper from mills that operate a sustainable forestry policy, and which has been manufactured from pulp processed using acid-free and elementary chlorine-free practices. Furthermore, the publisher ensures that the text paper and cover board used have met acceptable environmental accreditation standards.

For further information on Blackwell Publishing, visit our website:
www.blackwellnursing.com

Contents

Preface xi
Acknowledgements xiii
How to use this book xv

1 Communication, Relationships and Record Keeping 1

Importance of effective communication 3
Barriers to communicating with older people 3
Effective communication 3
Communication within the home 4
Improving your communication skills 5
How physical disabilities can affect the ability
   to communicate 5
Communication and stroke 6
Helping people to communicate after stroke 8
Parkinson's disease 8
How deafness affects the individual's ability
   to communicate 9
Causes of hearing loss 10
Hearing aids 11
Encouraging and helping people to use their hearing aids 11
Communicating with people who do not have hearing aids 12
Communicating with older people who are confused 13
Causes of confusion 13
Communicating with people who do not speak English 16
Living without language 16
Developing relationships 18
Record keeping 19
Admission records 19
Access to medical and nursing records 23
Confidentiality 24
Communicating with relatives 24
Answering the telephone 25
Keeping records of residents' money 26
Summary 27
Portfolio preparation 27
Further information 28

	Notes	30
	Further reading	30
2	**Health and Safety**	**31**
	Identifying risks and hazards	33
	Risk evaluation	34
	Safety and security within the home	37
	Health and safety laws	38
	Training	44
	Accident prevention	46
	How accidents affect older people	48
	Discovering who is at risk of having accidents	49
	Balancing risks and quality of life	50
	Recording accidents	51
	Protecting residents from infection	52
	Medical emergencies	56
	Summary	61
	Portfolio preparation	61
	Further information	62
	Notes	63
	Further reading	63
3	**Developing Your Knowledge and Practice**	**65**
	How well do you carry out activities at work?	67
	The learning organisation	67
	The need to develop knowledge and practice	67
	Developing your knowledge and practice	68
	Encouraging others to provide feedback on your work	71
	Informal networks	72
	How your values influence your practice	73
	Listening	74
	Reflective practice	75
	Strategies for reflection	75
	Learning from our mistakes	77
	Identifying your learning needs	78
	Choosing suitable training	80
	What are learning styles?	80
	Using your new skills and knowledge in practice	81
	Staying safe and legal	82
	Using your skills and knowledge appropriately	82
	Evaluating how your skills and knowledge have improved your practice	83
	Key points	83
	Portfolio preparation	83
	Notes	84

4 Care, Protection and Well-being of the Older Person 85

Importance of choosing how we live our lives 87
Human needs for well-being 87
Treating people as individuals 89
Enabling people to fulfil their potential 90
Elder abuse 92
What systems exist to protect vulnerable adults? 98
What to do if abuse occurs 103
Preventing abuse 104
Caring for older people who are confused 104
Caring for people with dementia 107
Conclusion 110
Key points 110
Portfolio preparation 110
Further information 111
Notes 112
Further reading 114

5 Care Planning 115

Why use care plans? 117
The principles of planning care 118
Setting goals and planning care 120
Delivering care 121
Evaluating care 121
Common care planning problems 122
National minimum standards on care planning 122
Information recorded on a care plan 124
Contributing to care planning 128
Conclusion 129
Key points 129
Portfolio preparation 129
Notes 130
Further reading 130

6 Recreational Activities 131

Enabling older people to identify activities and interests 133
Benefit of activities and interests 134
What happens when people stop engaging in activities? 135
Encouraging individual activities and interests 137
Types of activities 138
Pets 144
Key points 146
Portfolio preparation 146
Further information 147
Further reading 148

7 Food and Drink — 149

Importance of fluids — 151
Why older people become dehydrated — 151
Helping and encouraging older people to drink — 154
Recording fluid intake and output — 156
Importance of a healthy diet — 157
What is a healthy diet? — 157
Special diets — 162
Why some older people have difficulty eating — 166
Serving food and making mealtimes a pleasure — 168
Enabling people to choose — 169
Key points — 170
Portfolio preparation — 171
Further information — 171
Further reading — 172

8 Mobility — 173

Benefits of remaining mobile — 175
How illness affects ability to move around — 175
Dangers of immobility — 183
Helping older people to move around — 184
Wheelchairs — 187
Exercise and passive movement — 189
Journeys and visits — 189
Summary — 190
Key points — 191
Portfolio preparation — 191
Further information — 192

9 Pressure Area Care — 195

What is a pressure sore? — 197
Why do pressure sores develop? — 197
Who is at risk? — 198
Where do pressure sores occur? — 203
Pressure sore grading — 204
Preventing pressure sores — 212
Treating pressure sores — 219
Summary — 220
Key points — 220
Portfolio preparation — 221
Further information — 221
Further reading — 222

10 Personal Care and Hygiene — 223

Understanding elimination	225
How ageing affects the urinary system	227
Examining and testing urine	230
Bowel function	231
Enabling older people to use the toilet	238
Enabling individuals to maintain personal hygiene	241
Bathing	242
Skin care	249
Mouth care	250
Nail care	252
Hair care	253
Shaving	255
Cosmetics	256
Key points	256
Portfolio preparation	256
Notes	257
Further reading	257

11 Continence — 259

Continence problems	261
Continence assessments	262
Causes of incontinence	262
Caring for people who are incontinent	270
Bowel function	279
Key points	282
Portfolio preparation	282
Further information	283
Further reading	284

12 Moving and Handling — 285

Legal issues	287
Manual handling regulations	287
Responsibilities of the employer	288
Pregnant staff	289
The Health and Safety Executive	290
Employee responsibilities	290
Care plans	292
Training	292
Equipment	294
Preparing for moving and handling	299
Summary	300
Key points	301
Portfolio preparation	301

	Further information	302
	Further reading	302
13	**Equality, Diversity, Rights and Responsibilities**	**303**
	Older people and society	305
	Older people and their families	306
	The legal rights of a person living in a home	306
	Rights to healthcare and services	307
	Right to confidentiality	308
	Right to dignity and respect	309
	Right to choose	309
	Right to culturally sensitive care	310
	Right to worship	310
	Summary	311
	Key points	311
	Portfolio preparation	311
	Further reading	312
14	**Negotiating Specific Environments**	**313**
	Why older people need support	315
	Preparing for admission	315
	Admission to the home	316
	Supporting the individual after admission	317
	Hospital admission	318
	Outpatient visits	321
	Rehabilitation	322
	Respite care	322
	Summary	323
	Key points	323
	Portfolio preparation	324
Glossary		325
Index		329

Preface

Welcome to the third edition of *NVQs in Nursing and Residential Care Homes*. Older people living in care homes have complex care needs and if we are to meet these needs we need to understand normal ageing and the changes that can occur because of illness. We need the ability to enable the individual to enjoy life despite the limitations of any long-standing condition. We need knowledge to enable the older person to do what he or she is able to do and to provide care that is sensitive and supportive.

The care assistant's role is vitally important within a care home. Enthusiastic, knowledgeable care assistants can make a huge difference to the lives of the older people they care for. In the past, the skills and knowledge of the experienced care assistant were not always recognised. The introduction of National Vocational Qualifications changed that. NVQ qualifications enable care assistants to gain a qualification that demonstrates to employers their level of skills.

Care assistants studying for NVQ qualification work through a closely monitored programme, which increases their level of knowledge and enables them to gain credit for practical skills. Care assistants, even those with years of practical experience, learn a great deal when gaining NVQ qualifications. This enables them to understand the problems older people face and equips them with the skills required to care for older people sensitively. This is good news for older people in homes, who benefit from higher-quality care.

This book is written specifically for care assistants working in nursing and residential care homes who are studying for NVQ level 2 qualifications. There have been many changes in care homes since the last edition. Government has now formally recognised the value of NVQ qualifications and half of all care assistants working in a care home *must* have a qualification at NVQ level 2 or above. Those who do not have NVQ qualifications must undertake a comprehensive structured induction programme that can be built on if the person wishes to obtain an NVQ qualification in the future.

Many staff who work as care assistants do not have formal educational qualifications. Obtaining an NVQ qualification provides you with a formal qualification and makes you more attractive to employers. Increasingly employers are paying NVQ-qualified staff a premium in recognition of their qualification. An NVQ also provides you with the requirements to enter nurse education programmes leading to qualification as a registered nurse.

This book aims to provide care assistants and NVQ assessors with information and advice to help them meet the challenges of caring for older people in a rapidly changing environment. It provides information on the normal ageing process and how illness can affect the older person. It aims to help you to work with the older person to help the individual enjoy life.

Since the first edition was published I have had many letters from readers and have had the opportunity to meet many of you on my travels. Many of you have found the book useful, not only in completing NVQ level 2 studies but also in NVQ level 3 studies. Readers come from a range of backgrounds: many NVQ assessors use the book to work through the NVQ syllabus with students; care assistants who are not planning to study for NVQs, at least for now, use the book as a reference; and managers of nursing and residential homes buy the book and use it for training and teaching care assistants.

The future for NVQ students has never been brighter. I hope that you enjoy this book and find that it fulfils its aims. The feedback you have provided has been very helpful. I have done my best to use your comments to improve this edition. If you have any comments to make, please get in touch.

Linda Nazarko
March 2007

Acknowledgements

I would like to thank everyone who contributed to this book. I would like to thank David Miller, Chief Executive of Pentlow Nursing and Care Group, and Kath Parkinson of Springhill Nursing Home for the wonderful positive pictures they supplied of older people living in nursing homes. I would also like to thank the staff who posed for pictures and the older people and their families who allowed me to publish their photographs.

I would also like to thank the following for permission to use the following copyright material:

Figures 1.0 and 7.0 Springhill Care Home, Figure 1.1 Blackwell Publishing Ltd., Figure 2.2 Kirton Healthcare, Figure 2.3 The National Osteoporosis Society, Figure 3.1 The McGraw-Hills Companies, Figure 4.1 American Psychological Association, Table 5.1 and Box 10.2 BMJ Publishing Group Ltd., Figures 6.3 and 10.6 Summerdown Nursing Home, Figures 7.2 and 7.3 Katharine Unwin, Table 9.2 Branden and Bergstrom, Prevention Plus, Figure 9.7 Judy Waterlow, www.judy-waterlow.co.uk, Figures 9.8–9.12 Talley Group Limited, Figures 10.1 and 10.3 Coloplast Ltd, Figure 10.4 Taylor & Francis Ltd. www.tandf.co/gastro, Figures 11.3 and 11.4 Pfizer, Figures 12.2–12.4 Arjo UK, Figures 3.0, 4.0, 5.0, 6.0, 6.1, 6.2, 7.4, 8.0, 12.0, 14.0 the staff and residents at Pentlow Nursing and Care Group.

I would also like to thank Katharine Unwin and Heather Addison for their meticulous editing and their help.

And last but not least, thanks to Sam and Rachael, my children.

With love to my husband Ed whose enthusiasm, support and endless cups of coffee enable me to continue to write.

How to use this book

What is an NVQ?

An NVQ is a National Vocational Qualification. It aims to recognise a person's skills, knowledge and understanding in the workplace. NVQs are based on national occupational standards that describe the level and breadth of performance expected of individuals working in health and social care. The national occupational standards were devised by government-approved bodies in England, Scotland, Wales and Northern Ireland. NVQs were introduced in 1988 and were last revised in 2005.

In order to obtain an NVQ level 2 qualification in health and social care you must complete six NVQ units. An NVQ consists of mandatory units that you must complete and optional units. The mandatory units are referred to as core units. Normally you must complete two core units and can choose four further units from either the core or optional units to complete the NVQ. This is the route that most candidates choose, especially if they plan a career in health or nursing. If you have plans to develop a career in social care and perhaps become a social worker in the future, you should plan your NVQ differently. The Social Care Council recommend that candidates planning a career in social care complete the four core units and then choose two units from the range of optional units. If the four core units are combined with the two optional units then the qualification will be recognised by the Social Care Council.

Each unit contains:

- A summary: this is a summary of the content, the elements of the unit and the values that underpin the unit
- Key words and concepts, and scope
- Performance criteria: the tasks and activities in which you must demonstrate your performance
- Knowledge and understanding: what you need to know and understand
- Evidence requirement: this specifies the type and level of evidence needed to show competence.

Each unit is divided into elements. There are usually two or three elements to each unit. The elements are then divided into performance criteria.

How do I obtain an NVQ?

In order to obtain an NVQ you must register at an *approved assessment centre*. This may be a further education college, a private training organisation or your workplace. All of these organisations can be approved as assessment centres. The assessment centre will register you for an NVQ and allocate you an assessor.

When you are registered as an NVQ candidate you will normally be allocated a tutor or trainer. NVQs are structured in different ways and sometimes learning is based at your place of work. Sometimes the learning is based at the assessment centre and you are allocated a certain number of study days while completing your NVQ. The tutor provides opportunities for learning, and enables you to practise what you have learnt in a realistic protected environment or, where this is not appropriate, in a simulated environment. The tutor also provides ongoing mentorship and feedback. You must show that you are able to put the learning into practice.

All registered NVQ candidates are allocated an assessor. The assessor must have completed an assessor's course and be approved by the assessment centre to assess candidates. Assessors may be based in the workplace or they may come into the workplace to assess competency.

Expert witnesses, who are approved by the assessment centre, may also be used to verify your competency in certain circumstances.

Witness testimony from senior staff may also be used as part of the evidence to verify your competency; however, most of the evidence is normally gained from assessment by the assessor.

The assessment centre will explain how the evidence will be logged. This is normally kept in a portfolio. The portfolio may be a large folder or it may be a 'paperless portfolio' stored electronically. Your assessment centre will guide you. The portfolio will be verified by an internal verifier from the assessment centre who checks that it contains the appropriate evidence for each unit. When the evidence is internally verified it is passed to an external verifier and if satisfactory the NVQ is awarded.

How can this book help?

Reading this book as a whole will enable you to gain a greater understanding of the physical and psychological aspects of ageing. It will enable you to understand the reasons why some older people have difficulties with some aspects of daily living and require support. Each chapter relates to a unit of the NVQ level 2 course in health and social care. Candidates studying a particular unit will find most of the information required for that unit in a particular chapter of the book. A list of units and the relevant chapters is provided on pages xvii–xviii.

Type of unit	Name	Content	Chapter
Core/Mandatory	HSC21	Communication, relationships and record keeping	1
Core/Mandatory	HSC21a	Work with individuals and others to identify the best forms of communication	1
Core/Mandatory	HSC21b	Listen and respond to individuals' questions and concerns	1
Core/Mandatory	HSC21c	Communicate with individuals	1
Core/Mandatory	HSC21d	Access and update records and reports	1
Core/Mandatory	HSC22	Support the health and safety of yourself and individuals	2
Core/Mandatory	HSC22a	Carry out health and safety checks before you begin work activities	2
Core/Mandatory	HSC22b	Ensure your actions support health and safety in the place where you work	2
Core/Mandatory	HSC22c	Take action to deal with emergencies	2
Core/Mandatory	HSC23	Develop your knowledge and practice	3
Core/Mandatory	HSC23a	Evaluate your work	3
Core/Mandatory	HSC23b	Use new and improved skills and knowledge in your work	3
Core/Mandatory	HSC24	Ensure your own actions support the care, protection and well-being of individuals	4
Core/Mandatory	HSC24a	Relate to and support individuals in the way they choose	4
Core/Mandatory	HSC24b	Treat people with respect and dignity	4
Core/Mandatory	HSC24c	Assist in the protection of individuals	4
Optional	HSC25	Carry out and provide feedback on specific plan of care activities	5
Optional	HSC25a	Carry out specific plan of care activities	5
Optional	HSC25b	Provide feedback on specific plan of care activities	5
Optional	HSC25c	Contribute to revisions of specific plan of care activities	5
Optional	HSC210	Support individuals to access and participate in recreational activities	6
Optional	HSC210a	Support individuals to identify their recreational interests and preferences	6
Optional	HSC210b	Encourage and support individuals to participate in recreational activities	6
Optional	HSC210c	Encourage and support individuals to review the value of the recreational activities	6
Optional	HSC213	Provide food and drink for individuals	7
Optional	HSC213a	Support individuals to communicate what they want to eat and drink	7
Optional	HSC213b	Prepare and serve food and drink	7
Optional	HSC213c	Clear away when individuals have finished eating and drinking	7

Type of unit	Name	Content	Chapter
Optional	HSC214	Help individuals to eat and drink	7
Optional	HSC214a	Make preparations to support individuals to eat and drink	7
Optional	HSC214b	Support individuals to get ready to eat and drink	7
Optional	HSC214c	Help individuals consume food and drink	7
Optional	HSC215	Help individuals to keep mobile	8
Optional	HSC215a	Support individuals to keep mobile	8
Optional	HSC215b	Observe any changes in the individual's mobility and provide feedback to the appropriate people	8
Optional	HSC217	Undertake agreed pressure area care	9
Optional	HSC217a	Prepare to carry out pressure area care	9
Optional	HSC217b	Carry out pressure area care	9
Optional	HSC218	Support individuals with their personal care needs	10
Optional	HSC218a	Support individuals to go to the toilet	10
Optional	HSC218b	Enable individuals to maintain their personal hygiene	10
Optional	HSC218c	Support individuals in personal grooming and dressing	10
Optional	HSC219	Support individuals to manage continence	11
Optional	HSC219a	Support individuals to maintain continence	11
Optional	HSC219b	Support individuals to use equipment to manage continence	11
Optional	HSC223	Contribute to moving and handling individuals	12
Optional	HSC223a	Prepare individuals, environments and equipment for moving and handling	12
Optional	HSC223b	Enable individuals to move from one position to another	12
Optional	HSC234	Ensure your own actions support the equality, diversity, rights and responsibilities of individuals	13
Optional	HSC234a	Respect the rights and interests of individuals	13
Optional	HSC234b	Treat everyone equally and in ways that respect diversities and differences	13
Optional	HSC234c	Act in ways that promote individuals' confidence in you and your organisation	13
Optional	HSC235	Enable individuals to negotiate specific environments	14
Optional	HSC235a	Support individuals to assess their ability to negotiate specific environments	14
Optional	HSC235b	Support individuals to negotiate specific environments	14
Optional	HSC235c	Observe and contribute to the evaluation of programmes	14

Chapter One
Communication, Relationships and Record Keeping

HSC21
Communicate with and complete records for individuals

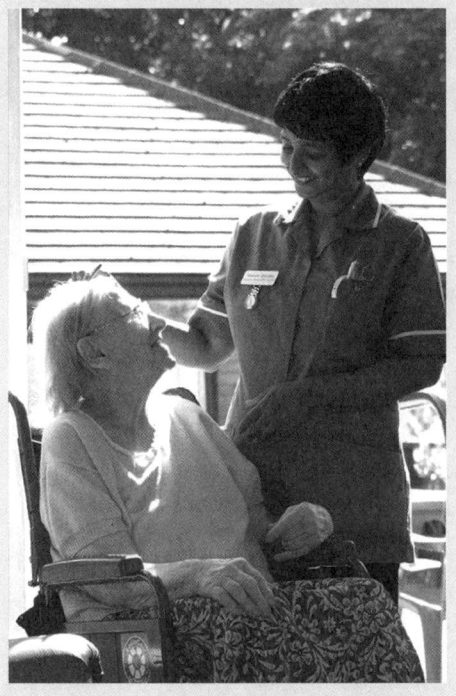

This unit consists of four elements:
HSC21a Work with individuals and others to identify the best forms of communication
HSC21b Listen and respond to individuals' questions and concerns
HSC21c Communicate with individuals
HSC21d Access and update records and reports

This chapter

- Provides information and guidance to enable you to communicate effectively
- Explains how physical disabilities can cause communication problems
- Discusses how stroke may affect a person's ability to communicate
- Discusses how Parkinson's disease may affect a person's ability to communicate
- Discusses how hearing problems affect the ability to communicate
- Explains how to help older people use hearing aids
- Explains how confusion and dementia can cause communication problems
- Discusses ways of communicating with people who are unable to speak
- Enables you to improve your ability to communicate effectively
- Explains your responsibilities in maintaining confidentiality
- Explains your responsibilities in recording information

Importance of effective communication

The ability to understand others and to make ourselves understood is a skill we often take for granted. In some circumstances, perhaps when on holiday abroad, we have difficulty in communicating with others. Ending up with the wrong meal, being directed to the wrong place or being thought a little crazy by the locals is often part of the fun of being on holiday. Sometimes, though, difficulty in communication can be maddening.

Older people living in care homes often have difficulty communicating with staff. Recent research found that 78% of people living in care have at least one type of mental impairment. Over half of all people resident in care homes have a neurological disease (a disease of the nervous system) such as stroke, Parkinson's disease or dementia.[1] People who have problems communicating react in different ways.

Some can become frustrated, angry and aggressive, while others can become withdrawn and depressed. Your ability to enable people to communicate their needs is crucially important and makes a real difference to the older person's quality of life. When you are aware of the reasons why a person has difficulty communicating you can develop your skills and learn how to use these to remove the barriers to communication and enable the person to be heard.

Barriers to communicating with older people

Older people are admitted to care homes because it is no longer possible to provide the care required at home. Most people living in care homes are in their 80s or 90s. Most older people, even of this age, continue to live at home. Over 90% of people who enter care homes have long-standing medical conditions and require high levels of care.

Some individuals are physically frail but very alert. Some are physically well but confused. Others are both physically and mentally frail. Most older people do not wish to leave their own homes and live in 'a home'. Older people admitted to homes often feel anxious and upset because of the move. They may become withdrawn and unwilling to communicate. It is important to spend time getting to know the person and encouraging the individual to express their feelings.

Some individuals may find communication difficult because of physical problems such as hearing difficulties. Some people may not speak English, others may have lost the ability to speak English because of ill health and may only be able to communicate in their first language.

Effective communication

Communication is not simply about the ability to speak and understand speech. We use all five senses to communicate and receive information:

1   Visual – seeing
2   Auditory – hearing
3   Olfactory – smelling
4   Kinaesthetic – feeling
5   Gustatory – tasting

We receive input from all five senses. If you walk in the garden, your skin will sense temperature. Your vestibular system will sense whether the ground is uneven or not. Your olfactory system will allow you to enjoy the scent of the flowers and your auditory system will enable you to hear the birds sing. Your brain integrates all these sensory stimuli and you respond. If it is freezing cold, the garden is like a mud bath and the birds are dive bombing your washing, you will probably retreat indoors. If it is warm and pleasant, you will probably remain in the garden. You make these decisions because of information received from a fully functioning sensory system. Older people often have sensory difficulties that make communication difficult. The older person with poor vision will find it hard to see the expression on your face. She may think you are being serious when you are joking. The person with poor hearing may not hear the joke in your voice. The person with a poor sense of smell may not be aware of what is for lunch because, unlike you, she cannot smell the joint roasting.

Good communication is about finding out who the person is. It is about finding out what the person's values and hopes are. We do this in our everyday lives. When we meet people socially for the first time we ask gentle probing questions: 'What do you do?' 'Is Sam your only child?' We probe gently to find out about the person. We make allowances for people and compensate gently for any limitations they have. Sometimes in homes we don't really get to know about the lives and achievements of the people we care for.

Communication within the home

Care homes are busy places. Residents require more care than ever before and there is always something to do. Sometimes it can be difficult to make time to get to know people and to talk to them. Sometimes an individual relates better to some members of staff and those people really know the individual as a person; but the other staff do not. The way work is organised within a home can make communication easy or difficult. Many homes have now introduced a key worker scheme. This means that the individual is looked after by a small number of people. Key worker schemes are popular with staff and residents. They help make care personal and help improve quality. Key worker schemes depend on effective communication. When communication is poor, the quality of care suffers.

Life histories

Some people living in homes work with their key worker or another member of staff to make a life history. Some individuals like to make a picture collage. This can include pictures of the person in different stages of life together with family, friends and loved ones. Others like to make a book about their life. You can buy a book, fill in details, and add pictures or make your own. Some people like to paint or create a tapestry. Life histories give you information about a person and enable you to strike up a conversation and get to know the person. Life histories are particularly helpful when working with people who have dementia. They enable you to see the whole person and not just the person as she is now. They enable you to make sense of some of the things the person says and to understand her values.

Improving your communication skills

We communicate in a range of ways. The most powerful means of communication is non-verbal. You know exactly what mood your partner is in by the way he or she enters the house. A slammed car door, a coat thrown off and a rigid facial expression speak volumes.

Be aware of how residents will interpret your body language. Many people who find it difficult to communicate become very sensitive to body language. It is all very well saying that you have plenty of time but if you are standing up and glancing at the door every few minutes your body language is contradicting your words and residents will notice. You can use body language to reinforce your words. When you say you are unhurried, look unhurried. When you are listening look at the person, lean forward, use touch to reinforce your words.

How physical disabilities can affect the ability to communicate

Physical disabilities can affect the individual's ability to communicate in a number of ways. Strokes can affect the ability to understand speech and to speak. Parkinson's disease can cause individuals to have difficulty forming words, and speech can sound slurred. People who are deaf may be unable to hear clearly, even when wearing a hearing aid. Non-digital hearing aids amplify all sound and background noise can make it difficult to hear clearly. Non-digital hearing aids can also distort speech sounds, making it difficult to understand.

Communication and stroke

Imagine for a moment that you have had a severe stroke: you have no feeling in half of your body, you have difficulty understanding what is said, and it is difficult to explain what you mean. This is how stroke affects many older people living in care homes. Stroke and the communication problems that often accompany it can make people despair. We can enable people to communicate after stroke if we understand the difficulties they face. Strokes can cause communication problems if they affect the speech centre in the brain (Fig. 1.1). Sometimes the person cannot understand what we are saying – it is as if we were speaking a foreign language. The person cannot receive and make sense of the messages we send them in our speech; this is known as *receptive dysphasia*.

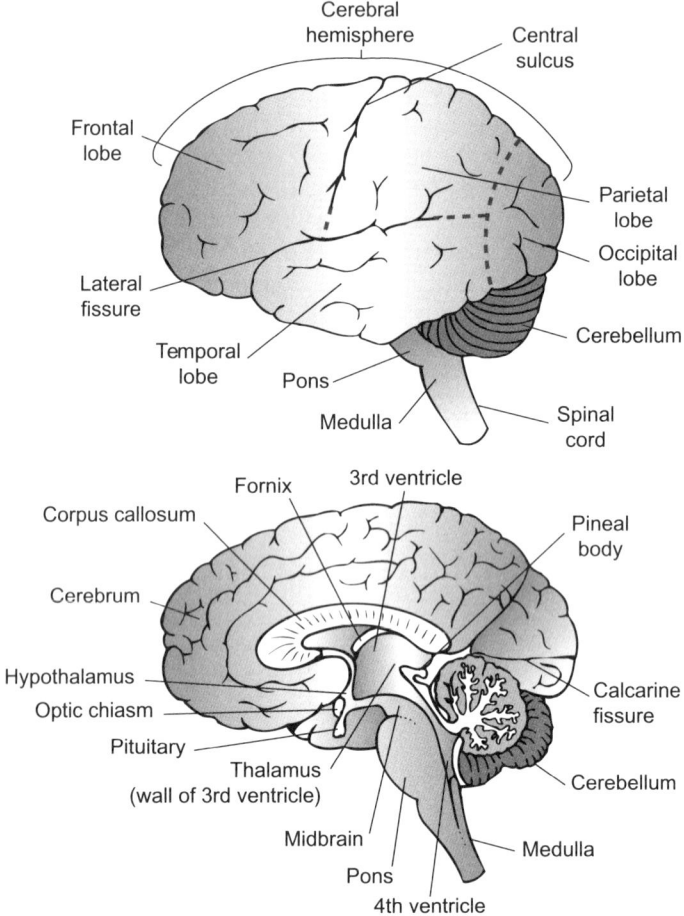

Figure 1.1 The brain.[2]

There are degrees of dysphasia. People with mild dysphasia understand most of what is being said. Tiredness, background noise, people speaking too quickly or more than one person speaking at once affect the ability to understand. People with moderate dysphasia find it more difficult to follow conversations: long and complicated sentences are difficult to follow; some words are only partly understood. The individual may have difficulty concentrating and may be able to understand the start of a conversation but become confused if the conversation is too long. People with severe dysphasia may have difficulty in understanding even single words. Many people who suffer from dysphasia after a stroke find that their condition gradually improves over weeks and months. People who are suffering from receptive dysphasia rely on tone of voice, movement and gestures to help fill in the words that they do not understand. Ensuring that short-sighted people are wearing their glasses helps them to see and interpret expressions and gestures.

Some individuals understand every word and gesture but cannot find the right words to communicate. This is known as *expressive dysphasia*. Individuals mix up words and may say 'yes' instead of 'no' or 'plate' instead of 'cup'. Some individuals have difficulty in finding the correct word and use a similar word instead. This difficulty in finding the correct word is known as *anomia* and is part of a general difficulty in expressing what they want to say.

Strokes can affect the muscles of the throat, tongue, lips and face. This can lead to difficulty swallowing after a stroke. Many older people wear dentures and these are kept in place partly by the muscles in the mouth. If these muscles are affected, dentures can slip around or be almost impossible to wear. Poor muscle control and difficulty with dentures can make it difficult for individuals to form words. This difficulty in articulating is known as *dysarthria*.

Some individuals lose the ability to speak. This is known as *aphasia*. The person who is unable to speak may understand your every word but be unable to reply.

Reading and writing

Strokes can affect vision. The person may have restricted vision. People who needed reading or distance glasses may need an eye test and new glasses to maximise their vision after a stroke.

Sometimes words make no sense to an individual; this may improve in the weeks and months after a stroke.

Strokes can paralyse limbs and can cause individuals to lose the ability to write. Some older people can learn to write with a non-affected hand. Speech and language therapists can assess individuals with such problems and can help them to regain skills.

Helping people to communicate after stroke

It is important to realise that many people can recover most if not all speech following a stroke. Recovery is dependent on the site and severity of the stroke, therapy from speech therapists, the individual's motivation and the help and encouragement you offer. Your role is to assist the person to recover whenever possible. When further recovery is not possible your role is to enable the person to communicate effectively. The suggestions outlined in Box 1.1 will help you to enable the person to communicate after stroke.

> **Box 1.1 Communicating with a person who has had a stroke**
>
> - Speak slowly
> - Use simple clear language
> - Use short sentences
> - Only ask one question at a time
> - Only give one piece of information at a time
> - Use gestures
> - Encourage the individual to use gestures
> - Encourage the individual to speak
> - Ensure that the individual who requires glasses is wearing them
> - Ensure that the individual who requires a hearing aid is wearing it
> - Listen carefully and be patient

Parkinson's disease

Parkinson's disease is a progressive neurological disease. It is caused by a reduction in dopamine. Dopamine enables nerve cells to transmit messages to each other. An individual suffering from Parkinson's disease has difficulty in moving because of the disease. The disease also affects the ability to move the muscles in the mouth and tongue that are used to form words. Individuals suffering from Parkinson's disease often have difficulty in speaking clearly and their words can become slurred.

The disease is now treated with a number of drugs that help replace the dopamine shortage that causes the disease. At first, the individual with Parkinson's disease appears to have fully recovered because of the medication. As the disease progresses, greater amounts of medication are required. Individuals in the early stages of Parkinson's disease are normally able to live at home. It is only in the later stages of the disease that they are admitted to care homes. At this stage, many older people with

Parkinson's disease are taking large amounts of medication to control the disease. These drugs work for shorter and shorter periods and in the final stages of the disease some of these drugs may be given as often as every three hours while the individual is awake.

Individuals who have Parkinson's disease may be able to speak clearly if they have recently had some medication but as the medication begins to wear off they may have great difficulty in forming words. People with Parkinson's disease often speak very quietly; this is called *hypophonia*. Sometimes the drugs given to control Parkinson's disease can cause the individual to hallucinate or become confused. An estimated 25% of people with severe Parkinson's disease also develop dementia. Box 1.2 outlines ways to help people with Parkinson's disease to communicate.

> **Box 1.2** Communicating with a person who has Parkinson's disease
>
> - Speak slowly and clearly
> - Give the individual time to speak
> - Be aware that ability to speak will vary
> - Eliminate background noise and listen carefully
> - Check that you have understood what has been said
> - Encourage the individual to speak

How deafness affects the individual's ability to communicate

Hearing loss is often referred to as the 'hidden handicap'. It is very common. Approximately 7.5 million people in the UK have some degree of hearing loss. It is estimated that 4 million people would benefit from hearing aids but only 2.5 million actually have one. A significant number of people who have hearing aids don't actually use them. Hearing deteriorates as people age and, by the age of 70, approximately 60% of people have some hearing loss. This figure rises to 90% by the age of 90 years.

Most people living in care homes are in their 80s and 90s and most of them will suffer from some hearing loss. This affects the ability to communicate with staff and with others living in the home. Unfortunately, some people who meet deaf people automatically dismiss them as stupid. Older people with hearing loss state that others are inclined to 'talk over them' and that people who are deaf 'tend to be left out of conversations'. Other people are 'inclined to think that deaf people are not with it'.

Many older people with hearing loss find communicating with others extremely frustrating. If they feel that people are ignoring them, talking over them or treating them as though they were senile, they may simply give up trying to communicate. As one lady with hearing loss stated: 'If they make no effort why should I bother?' Care assistants who understand the causes and effects of deafness will be able to communicate more effectively with older people with hearing loss, and can encourage them to communicate and take part in the daily life of the home.

Causes of hearing loss

Wax

The commonest cause of hearing loss is wax in the ears. Even older people who suffer from deafness find that their hearing is improved if a build-up of wax in the ear is removed. Older people who appear to be deaf should have their ears checked by a doctor or nurse who will use an instrument known as an auroscope to check for the presence of wax in the ear.

Normally any wax in the ear is softened by putting drops in one or both ears three times daily for up to five days. Care assistants in residential homes may be asked to put these drops in an older person's ears. This may clear wax from the ears. If there is still some remaining wax then the ears may be syringed by a registered nurse.

If the person still has difficulty hearing the general practitioner (GP) will arrange a hearing test at the local hospital. Hearing tests are known as audiograms and cannot be carried out if ears are full of wax.

Conductive deafness

Conductive deafness is caused by damage or obstruction to the structure of the ear. Wax in the ear, by blocking the ear, can cause conductive deafness, and hearing is restored when the wax is removed. A heavy cold can cause the ears to become blocked and can cause temporary conductive deafness. An ear infection, which if untreated can persist for months or years, can cause conductive deafness. A perforated eardrum can cause deafness; a repair of the perforation can restore hearing.

Sensorineural deafness

Although sensorineural deafness is the most common deafness in older people, there is no treatment available. As adults age the nerve that connects the ear to the brain, the auditory nerve, becomes less sensitive to noise, and the ability to hear is reduced. Hearing is lost first at higher frequencies. This means that older people with hearing difficulties can hear low-pitched noise quite well but have difficulty with higher-pitched sounds. Women tend to speak at a higher pitch than men and many older people find it more difficult to follow a woman's speech than that of a man. The only available treatment for sensorineural deafness is to make sounds louder so that the individual can hear. Hearing aids are used to amplify sounds so that people with sensorineural deafness can hear.

Hearing aids

If an older person has difficulty hearing, their GP writes a letter to the ear, nose and throat specialist at the local hospital. The person visits the hospital as an outpatient and their hearing is tested. The type of deafness and causes are identified. If the individual is suffering from sensorineural deafness, arrangements are normally made for a hearing aid to be supplied.

Hearing aids consist of two main parts. The earpiece, which is made of clear plastic, fits into the ear. Each earpiece is made especially for the individual. A mould of the ear is taken and the earpiece is made to fit snugly into the ear. A tube connects the earpiece to the amplifier section of the aid. The amplifier section is normally known as the 'body' of the aid. There are several different strengths of amplification to suit the level of deafness. The body is mass produced. Most older people who are supplied with NHS hearing aids are supplied with an aid that fits behind the ear. People who are extremely deaf may be supplied with a different type of aid that has an earpiece attached to a long cord. The body of the aid is the size of a pocket calculator and is clipped onto the chest over clothing.

The design of hearing aids remained unchanged for almost 40 years but now digital hearing aids are becoming available on the NHS. These hearing aids do not simply make things louder, they also aim to mimic natural hearing by using digital technology.

Encouraging and helping people to use their hearing aids

Many older people who have been supplied with hearing aids no longer use them. This is known as 'fruit bowl syndrome' because older people often leave their unused hearing aids in fruit bowls. In one survey of nursing and residential homes, half of the older people who had hearing aids did not wear them. The reasons given were that they found them difficult to put in and adjust or that the aids no longer worked.

Older people living in homes often find it difficult to perform tasks that require fine muscle control. They find it difficult to do up small buttons and similar tasks. This may be because of illness. Arthritis can leave fingers stiff; Parkinson's disease can cause a tremor. In most cases, older people do not ask care assistants for help: 'They have enough to do.' Earpieces must be fitted firmly into the ear if the aid is to work. Aids must be turned on and turned to the correct setting. The setting varies from individual to individual and environment to environment but is set at the level that enables the older person to hear easily. Batteries must be changed regularly. These simple tasks take only a few minutes but enable older people to communicate. This saves time spent trying to communicate and reduces frustration; it also makes a real difference to the person's quality of life.

Helping people with hearing aids to hear

Many people, including some registered nurses, think that if an older person has a hearing aid they can hear normally. Unfortunately, this is not the case. A hearing aid works by amplifying all sound and aids can easily distort hearing. Care assistants communicating with older people who have hearing loss, including those who wear hearing aids, should use special techniques to make it easier for individuals to understand them. Box 1.3 outlines ways to enable people with hearing difficulties to communicate:

> **Box 1.3** Communicating with a person who has hearing loss
>
> - Cut down on background noise. Close the door if it is noisy outside. Close the window to reduce the roar of traffic.
> - Move near to the person.
> - Speak a little more loudly than usual – but do not shout. Shouting can appear threatening. It also distorts the voice, raising the pitch and making it more difficult for the person to hear.
> - Always face the person.
> - Speak directly to the person.
> - Do not attempt to have conversations with more than one person at the same time. The deaf person will have difficulty following this.
> - Do not cover your mouth while speaking.
> - Speak slowly and clearly.
> - If you have not been understood, rephrase the sentence using different words with similar meanings.
> - Check that the individual has understood.
> - Use gestures.
> - Offer to write things down.

Communicating with people who do not have hearing aids

Hearing aids can only help people who have some hearing. Some people are totally deaf and are not helped by hearing aids. In this situation care assistants must find other ways to communicate. Many profoundly deaf older people have learnt to lip-read. Using the techniques above will enable people who lip-read to work out what you are saying.

Some older people do not have hearing aids because they are waiting for an appointment for one to be fitted. In these circumstances, the care assistant can write things down for the older person. It can be helpful to supply a notebook and pen, which the older person carries. You can then write down messages and the older person can reply. Remember to write clearly. If the person's eyesight is poor, writing in large letters can help.

Communicating with older people who are confused

Communicating with older people who are confused is perhaps one of the greatest challenges that care assistants face. It is difficult and some care assistants feel that it is not worth trying because they will be unable to 'get through' to the individual. Often a little time and patience will pay dividends and will enable you to communicate with the confused older person. This enables you to meet the person's needs. People who have their needs met are more likely to be relaxed, settled and happy within the home. It is important to be aware of the causes of confusion as this will affect how you can communicate with the individual.

Causes of confusion

There is always a reason for confusion. Sometimes staff make incorrect assumptions about confusion: 'It's just her age, what do you expect at 92?' There are two major causes of confusion: an acute illness, or the individual is suffering from a neurological disease such as senile dementia.

Older people who have suddenly become confused are usually ill. People who have a chest infection or a urine infection often become confused. Care assistants often know individual residents better than senior staff do because they spend more time with them. They can often observe a cough or notice that an older person is going to the toilet more frequently. They should inform nursing staff, so that the person can undergo investigations and treatment.

Medication can cause confusion. Care assistants, because they spend a great deal of time with residents, are often the first to notice any side effects caused by medication. In residential care homes, care assistants will be aware of any changes of medication because they are usually responsible for giving out medication. In nursing homes, medication is given out by registered nurses. Care assistants, though, are often aware that medication has been changed. Care assistants who notice that an individual has become confused should inform a registered nurse in a nursing home, or the manager or a senior member of staff in a residential home.

Sometimes confusion creeps up slowly but staff should always check that there is no treatable physical cause before accepting confusion. Certain diseases such as diabetes, Parkinson's disease, thyroid disease and kidney disease can cause confusion. The registered nurse or doctor should be informed if an older person is becoming confused.

Dementia and confusion

Dementia is fairly common in older people. Dementia is not a disease but a label used to describe a cluster of symptoms. It is estimated that 25% of people over the age of 85 suffer from dementing illness. The commonest cause of dementia is Alzheimer's disease. This is a progressive illness. At first individuals become forgetful and muddled but eventually they become completely disorientated and unable to care for themselves. Individuals suffering from dementia are normally able to carry on living at home in the early stages of the disease. When the disease becomes more advanced the person may be admitted to a residential or nursing home. Normally individuals admitted to nursing homes are suffering from a more advanced stage of dementia than those in residential homes. Dementia is a progressive neurological disease that eventually leads to death.

Memory loss

Memory is lost in dementia. Short-term memory is most affected. The individual suffering from dementia may not be able to remember what he or she ate at lunchtime but can remember the events of long ago very clearly. It is important that the care assistant bears this in mind. An older person with Alzheimer's disease can often remember the names of close friends and family but forgets the care assistants' names. He or she may have to be shown the way back to the bedroom each time because short-term memory is so poor. People with Alzheimer's disease can become very bewildered because they cannot remember where they are. The care assistant has an important role to play in gently reminding the older person of his or her whereabouts.

Wandering, shouting and screaming

Some older people with Alzheimer's disease appear to wander around without a purpose. They may shout out and scream. This is very distressing for care assistants and other patients. It is important to find out if there are reasons for the person's behaviour:

Is the person in pain? Pain killers may help.
Is the person constipated? Treatment will help.

Is the individual hungry? Perhaps that walk to the kitchen is to get a snack.
Is the person bored? Spending time doing something with the patient will help.
Does the individual want to go for a walk? Imagine how you would feel after a
few weeks sitting around in the home if you were used to being active.

Making sense of an individual's behaviour

Often confused people will do things that upset other residents, but if we take time to find out the reasons for the behaviour, we can improve the situation. An elderly confused lady was upsetting all the other patients because she was constantly taking their handbags and hiding them in her locker. She had no family or visitors. The care assistant looking after her brought in a spare handbag from home and put a comb, some lipstick, tissues and a few biscuits in the bag. The lady stopped taking other people's bags because she had one of her own. Care assistants can, by taking time to talk to and listen to the older person, help them enjoy a good quality of life within the home. Care assistants should communicate their findings to more senior staff within homes so that these can be recorded and all staff are aware of information which improves care.

Communicating with confused people

People with Alzheimer's disease and other forms of dementia have major difficulties communicating. You need to use all your skills to enable you to communicate (see Box 1.4). Communicating with people with dementia is hard work and cannot be rushed. If you do not have enough time to spend, then wait until later.

Box 1.4 Communicating with a person who is confused

- Find a quiet place.
- Eliminate distractions.
- Take time to communicate. Sit down and relax.
- Speak slowly and clearly.
- Use only one idea in each sentence.
- Use plain language.
- Check that the person has understood. If not, repeat the information in a slightly different way.
- Use short sentences.
- Do not give too many choices in one sentence.
- Ask the person's family and friends what methods of communication they have found most effective.

If you suspect that there are other barriers to communication, such as deafness or poor eyesight, inform a registered nurse within the nursing home, or your manager or a senior member of staff in the residential home. Then the individual can be helped, perhaps by having a hearing aid or new glasses.

Communicating with people who do not speak English

Some older people have come to the UK from abroad and have never learnt to speak English. Many other older people have learnt to speak English but because of a neurological condition such as a stroke or dementia have lost the ability to communicate in English. Many people understand more of a language than they can speak.

The older person's family can help you to discover how much the person understands. Care assistants can rule a piece of paper into two columns and write words in English on one side; the older person's family and friends can write these words in the person's own language in the other column and this can be used to help communicate. A scrapbook full of pictures with the words written in English and the person's own language can help. Using a picture board, such as those used by stroke patients, can also help with communication.

Beware of using gestures. Before you use gestures check with the person's family that the gestures you use have the same meaning in that person's culture. If gestures are the same then use them. If gestures differ slightly, make a note of this.

When it is important that staff and patient communicate accurately, perhaps when the person is feeling unwell or is attending an outpatient's appointment, ask if a member of the family can act as an interpreter. Finally, don't forget that facial expressions and touch are very important aids to understanding. Face the person so that you can be seen clearly and use touch to reinforce your words. It is important to sit down if the individual is seated. Getting down to the same level makes communication friendlier, less threatening and easier.

Living without language

We develop the ability to speak as babies. We learn by hearing our voices and those of our families. Some people who are born deaf do not learn to speak. Most people you will meet in nursing and residential homes will have lost their speech because of illness. Some people lose the ability to speak, known as aphasia. Loss of speech can occur suddenly when a person has a stroke, or slowly as dementia progresses. Some people who are no longer able to speak can use aids to enable them to communicate; others are no longer able to use aids. It is very important that you discover as much as possible about the person's remaining abilities. This enables you to work out ways of communicating.

Speech and language therapists

Speech and language therapists specialise in enabling people with communication problems to communicate. If you are caring for a person with communication problems who has not been assessed by a speech and language therapist, suggest that a therapist is called. Speech and language therapists have an open referral system. This means that anyone, including the person with the problem, a relative or a care assistant, can request a visit.

The speech and language therapist visits and carries out an assessment of the person's abilities. If the person is frail, nervous or has profound problems communicating, the therapist may visit several times to complete the assessment. When the assessment is completed, the therapist will have worked out the person's problems and developed ways to enable communication to take place. The therapist will provide staff with information and suggestions based on the person's ability to communicate.

Aids to communication

Some people, although unable to speak, understand speech well. Cards with a single word or a commonly used phrase can help in such circumstances. Computers have the potential to revolutionise the lives of people with an intact intellect who lose the ability to speak. The person can type with their fingers; or, if the person is unable to use their hands, even a pencil between the teeth enables the person to type words. There are now systems that allow the person to blow a certain number of times for each letter. Research is being carried out on the use of eye movements to communicate. In the future, we will see computers used more to enable people to communicate.

Some people who are unable to speak also have difficulty reading. If the problem is poor vision, this is often easily corrected by using glasses. Sometimes cataracts clouding the vision are the problem. Cataracts can now be easily treated on a day surgery basis. Sometimes, though, the problem is that the person can no longer make sense of written words. In such cases pictures can be used. In the past staff used to look through catalogues and magazines and pick out pictures. These were glued onto cards and used to help people communicate. Often the pictures were small or difficult to obtain. Now computers can be used to prepare communication aids. Most care homes now have computers, and Clipart packages, once an expensive luxury, are now available for a few pounds. Non-copyright images can also be downloaded from the internet. These can be used to produce large clear pictures. The pictures can be printed onto card and given to residents who have communication problems. If you do not have access to a computer at home or at work, one of your colleagues or a relative may be able to help.

Using non-verbal communication

Assessment gives you the information you need to develop ways to communicate. If the person is unable to read there is no point in writing things down. If the person is unable to see there is no point in providing pictures. If the person is unable to hear there is no point in speaking. The challenge then is to develop ways to enable you to communicate and to enable the person to communicate with you.

The speech and language therapist will be able to advise you of ways to communicate. Often touch is an important way of communicating and of reinforcing our words. Touch is very powerful. One research project a few years ago demonstrates this. The researcher left money on top of a telephone box and waited for someone to enter the booth. When the person came out the researcher asked if they had found her money. She touched half of the people on the arm as she asked her question. People who were touched were much more likely to return the money than those who were not. Touching someone gently on the arm is one way of breaking through the communication barriers that exist.

Developing relationships

The ability to communicate is so important to the development of relationships. Communication enables you to find out who the person is and how the person reacts. Relatives and friends can help you find out about the person who has communication problems. Often, if these problems are longstanding, relatives and friends have developed ways to communicate. Develop relationships with the relatives and friends of those you care for and work with them to improve communication skills.

Maintaining relationships

Sometimes a person you are caring for loses the ability to communicate because of an illness such as stroke. The person may be able to understand everything you say but because she is unable to reply you no longer make the effort to communicate. This can be soul-destroying. Don't assume that lack of response means lack of understanding. Continue to communicate and observe how the person responds. You may have to use some of the tips outlined earlier in the chapter to enable you to maintain communication.

Record keeping

Current legislation requires homes to maintain certain records and sets out how homes should be run. Legislation differs in England, Wales, Scotland and Northern Ireland. In all the countries homes are required to keep admission records, records of accidents and a daily record of patient treatment. Let's look at what records should be kept and how these are updated.

Preadmission assessments

People are normally assessed by care home staff before admission. An example of a patient assessment sheet is given in Fig. 1.2. Assessments are normally carried out by a senior member of staff. The person assessing will visit the older person, who may be living at home or in a residential home (if nursing home admission is being considered) or may be in hospital. The aims of assessment are to meet the older person and to check that the home can meet the individual's care needs. If the manager of a residential home discovers that the older person has nursing needs, the manager may suggest that a nursing home is more appropriate. Under current legislation, residential homes should provide the type of care that would be given by a caring relative at home. The aim of preadmission assessment is to ensure that the home can meet the person's care needs and that the person is happy to enter the home.

The assessment gives both the older person and the member of staff the opportunity to meet and discuss the home. If possible, the older person should visit the home. If the person is recovering from an illness in hospital, this is not always possible and relatives or friends may visit on the person's behalf. Next time someone from your home is visiting an older person to carry out an assessment, ask if you can accompany them. This will give you an opportunity to watch an assessment and get to know the older person before admission. The information obtained at assessment (Fig. 1.2) enables the assessor to begin to plan care.

Admission records

Homes are required to keep a register of all residents admitted to the home. This should include details of the person's name, address, place admitted from (for example, a local hospital), GP's name, the address and telephone numbers of the next of kin, name of person arranging the

Admission Details

Surname:	Name & contact details of GP:	Previous medical history:
First names:		
Date of admission:	Name & contact details of social worker:	
Wishes to be called:		
Date of birth:	Name & contact details of other therapists:	
Place of birth:		
Marital status:		
Details religious practice:		
Previous occupation:		
Admitted from:	Baseline observations:	
	TPR/BP:	
Home address:	Urinalysis:	Activities and interests:
	Other:	
☎	Life history:	
Next of kin contact 1:		
Name:		
Relationship:		Wishes in the event of illness:
Address:		
☎ Home:		
☎		
Next of kin contact 2:		
Name:		
Relationship:		
Address:		
☎		

Name: Date of Birth: GP: Primary Nurse: Room No:

Assessment of Activities of Daily Living

Vision	Walking and moving around	Dressing
Wears glasses? Yes☐ No☐	Fully mobile without aids? Yes☐ No☐	Able to dress unassisted? Yes☐ No☐
Last sight test:	Aids required e.g. zimmer frame, stick:	Assistance required:
Any visual impairment?	Able to walk unassisted? Yes☐ No☐	**Passing urine**
Hearing	If no, state help required:	Results of routine urinalysis:
Any hearing impairment? Yes☐ No☐	If unable walk unaided, trigger physio assessment	Continent of urine? Yes☐ No☐
Uses hearing aid? Yes☐ No☐	History of falls? Yes☐ No☐	Trigger continence assessment.
	If yes, trigger falls assessment & liaise with GP & physio	**Bowel care**
Speech and communication	Able to move around freely in bed? Yes☐ No☐	Normal bowel habit e.g. daily, once every two or three days:
Any difficulty communicating? Yes ☐ No☐	If no, trigger Braden pressure sore risk assessment	Any history of bowel problems? Yes☐ No☐
If yes, what can we do to help?	**Mental health**	Constipated? Yes☐ No☐
	AMT =	Are laxatives taken regularly? Yes☐ No☐
Yes = Trigger communication assessment	Depressed? Yes☐ No☐	If yes, trigger bowel assessment
Eating and drinking	If yes, trigger assessment	**Sleeping**
Weight:	**Washing and grooming**	Normal times of rising and retiring:
Height:	Able to bathe unaided? Yes☐ No☐	Any problems sleeping? Yes☐ No☐
BMI =	If no, specify assistance required	If yes, what helps promote sleep?
If BMI = <20, trigger nutritional assessment	Prefers to bathe or shower?	Night sedation? Yes☐ No☐
Any difficulty with chewing? Yes☐ No☐	How often?	If yes, trigger sleep assessment
If difficulty with chewing, trigger oral assessment	Able to comb hair unassisted? Yes☐ No☐	**Pain**
Any difficulty with swallowing? Yes☐ No☐	Able to shave independently? Yes☐ No☐	Is pain present? Yes☐ No☐
If difficulty swallowing, trigger swallowing assessment	Assistance required:	Is this controlled? Yes☐ No☐
	Mouthcare	If no, trigger pain assessment
Special dietary needs	Natural teeth present? Yes ☐ No☐	**Special needs**
Special diet required? Yes☐ No☐	Any pain or problems?	E.g. wound care: please indicate:
If yes, give details:	Dentures, please state if full or partial	
Caterers informed of special dietary needs? Yes☐ No☐	Able to care for teeth unassisted? Yes☐ No☐	
Able to eat independently? Yes☐ No☐	Assistance required:	
If assistance required, give details:		

Assessment completed by   Date of assessment:

Figure 1.2 Admission details/Assessment of activities of daily living.

admission, details of funding and the date of admission. The date of discharge or death should be entered when the patient leaves the home. If the person dies the time and cause of death must be entered.

The admission register may be filled in by a receptionist, a care assistant or a registered nurse. Ask if your home has a policy on who can complete the admission register. These records must be retained by law for one year after the last entry. Many homes retain these records for seven years after the last entry for legal reasons.

Daily statements of person's health

Homes are required by law to keep a daily statement of patients' health. One record of the patient's health must be entered every 24 hours by law. In practice, most homes write in the patient's records at least twice in 24 hours. One record is normally made by the day staff and one by the night staff. The daily statement of person's health is normally referred to as a progress report (see Case Study 1.1, p. 24).

Care plans

The Care Standards Act (2000) requires homes to maintain care plans. Homes are required to assess the level of care that a person requires and to keep a written record (care plan) of how those needs are met. You'll find details of how to plan and manage care in Chapter 5.

Further records stored in the home

People living in homes have other records. When the older person is admitted to the home, a letter is normally sent from the person's GP if the person was admitted from their own home. If the person was admitted from hospital, a discharge summary will have been sent to the home. If the person's GP has asked other professionals, such as a physiotherapist, speech therapist or clinical nurse specialist, to treat the patient, a referral letter will be written. Details of outpatient visits or hospital inpatient treatment while the person is living in the home will also need to be stored. Old care plans, medication charts and other papers will require storage. In many homes, each resident has a folder containing all records. Many GPs also write notes about the treatment they prescribe and keep them in this folder. Although GPs keep separate records detailing patient treatment, they may also keep notes at the home. GPs prefer to do this in case the patient needs to be seen by another doctor in an emergency. These records are normally stored in a locked cupboard or filing cabinet in the home, to protect confidentiality.

Computerised records

Some homes are now using computers to plan and manage care and to keep records. If computerised records are used in your home, you will receive training to enable you to use the system. Some homes use electronic mail (e-mail) to send information from one home to another. If the home you work in uses e-mail, you can ask how to use this.

Facsimile transmissions

Sending information by a facsimile is now commonplace. If there is a fax machine in your home find out the policy for communicating information received in faxes and how faxed information is filed.

Access to medical and nursing records

Individuals now have a legal right to have access to their health records under the Access to Medical Records Act which became law in 1990. The patient writes to the doctor who is providing care, normally the older person's GP in homes, and requests copies of all records.

Care homes are inspected by registered inspectors employed by the Commission of Social Care Inspection (CSCI). Inspectors have the power to ask to see day-to-day records relating to care. They do not have the right to see medical records unless the inspector is a qualified medical practitioner. Government have now announced plans to merge CSCI and the Healthcare Commission (the body responsible for regulating and inspecting the NHS). This is not likely to change inspectors' rights to view records.

Recording information

Your workplace will have policies and procedures on storage and access to resident records and you must adhere to these. The Nursing and Midwifery Council (NMC) standards on record keeping emphasise the importance of record keeping. They state that the ultimate aim of record keeping is the promotion of quality care. The care assistant has an important role to play in promoting quality care. You may have a wealth of information that enables you to provide individualised quality care to a resident. It is important to record this information so that other members of staff can offer high quality care when you are not on duty.

Any information that you record must be signed and dated. You must keep records up to date because people's needs change. Records must be clear and sufficiently detailed to enable other staff to follow them. Case Study 1.1 provides an example of a progress report.

> **Case Study 1.1**
>
> Mrs Smith now has her new hearing aid. She is finding it much easier to communicate. Please help her to put it in her ear in the morning and make sure that it is set to volume level 3.
>   Mrs Smith can remove the hearing aid but needs help to switch it off at night.

Confidentiality

Staff who work with older people learn a great deal about those they care for. All staff must ensure that information that they discover in the course of their work remains confidential. Most care assistants are very aware of how essential it is to maintain confidentiality at all times; however, staff can inadvertently betray confidentiality. This may occur in the following situations:

- Discussing the patient's condition with another member of staff within earshot of other residents or relatives
- In conversation outside of work, perhaps at the bus stop, on a train or in a restaurant or pub, where this conversation may be overheard by others
- By using the patient's name in NVQ evidence gathering – normally initials are used to maintain confidentiality
- By leaving patient records lying around – the nursing notes or other records may be left where other residents have access to them
- By disclosing information about the person's condition to relatives and friends without their consent.

It is important that care assistants are always aware of the need to maintain confidentiality, as the relationship between care assistant and patient is built on trust. Betraying that trust may destroy the caring relationship.

Breaking confidentiality

In certain circumstances you may be forced to break confidentiality, for example, if the person tells you that she is being abused. You have a duty to report this so that the person can be protected. Details of adult protection procedures can be found in Chapter 4.

Communicating with relatives

Many relatives will approach care assistants, even junior members of staff who have not been working in the home for very long, and ask how the older person is. It is important that you find out the home's policy on giving information to relatives. Care assistants who have worked in some hospitals or homes before may have been told to refer all queries to registered nurses. Individual care homes will have different policies. Sometimes the enquiry is partly a way of starting a conversation and only a general answer is required. For example, Mrs Jenkins' daughter might say:

'Hello, Julie, I've come to see Mum. How is she today?'

In this case, the care assistant would reply:

'Well, she's just had her hair done and she's been looking forward to your visit.'

In other cases the relative might be asking for more specific information, but the care assistant can deal with this; for example, Mrs Franklin's daughter asks:

'How did Mum get on at the optician's when she had her eyes tested?'

The care assistant might reply:

'The optician said she needs new glasses so she's chosen the frames and they should be ready on Tuesday.'

In other cases the care assistant may not have the information or may not be able to answer the relative's questions fully and should ask the registered nurse or the home's manager to speak to the relative. For example, Mrs Davis' daughter asks:

'How did Mum get on down at the hospital when she saw the specialist about her arthritic hip?'

The care assistant might reply:

'I think the specialist spoke to Sister James about her hip. If you hold on I'll just see if I can find her and she can have a word with you.'

In each of these examples the care assistant has given the relative as much information and help as possible. The care assistant has shown the relative that she is aware of the patient's treatment but is not getting out of her depth and attempting to give information which she does not completely understand.

Answering the telephone

In many homes, a senior member of staff answers the telephone whenever possible and deals with telephone queries. When the person in charge is busy, other staff often answer the telephone. It is important to state the name of the home and your name when answering, for example 'High Trees Nursing Home, Penny Jones speaking,' or 'care assistant Jones speaking'. This helps maintain the home's professional image.

Always find out who is calling, and if the person is asking to speak to the person in charge ask the nature of their call. If the nurse in charge of the nursing home is attending to a resident who is ill and she is aware that the call is from the representative of a company selling cleaning products, she can give you a message to tell them to call back at a more convenient time.

Many relatives and friends telephone to ask how residents are. This is often just a general enquiry, for example:

> 'This is Mrs Gibson. How is my mum, Mrs Kelly, today?'
> 'She's fine; all her birthday cards have arrived and she's opening them now.'
> 'Can you tell her we'll pick her up at 1 o'clock and take her out to lunch?'

If Mrs Kelly was unwell, the care assistant would fetch the person in charge who could speak to the relative. Many homes have a policy about who should answer the telephone, who should give certain information and under what circumstances this information is given. Many homes do not tell relatives over the telephone that a person has died, unless the older person has been ill and the death is expected. Find out policies in your home on relaying information over the telephone. If you are unsure of what to say in certain circumstances ask a more senior member of staff to take the call.

Keeping records of residents' money

Homes are obliged to keep a record of any money that they look after for older people. In many homes residents ask staff to buy things for them at the shops. Whenever possible older people should be encouraged to accompany staff to the shops and given the opportunity to select and buy things themselves. When staff buy things for residents a receipt and a full record of the money spent should be kept. This protects residents from financial abuse and protects staff from any accusations of theft.

Keeping records of other items left for safekeeping

Staff may be asked to keep other items for the patient. A record of this should be kept. This may be a note in the person's progress notes or it may be written in a book kept for this purpose, normally known as a property or valuables book. Care assistants should be careful about recording items. All that glitters is not gold and all white stones that sparkle are not diamonds. You should record 'one yellow metal ring with a white stone' not 'gold ring with diamond solitaire'.

Residents who retain valuable items

Some older people wear valuable items and do not wish to leave them in the home's safe. They have every right to continue to wear valuable items of jewellery. Imagine how you would feel if your treasured engagement ring or locket was taken away and locked in a safe in case you lost it. If the older person is wearing rings or has brought jewellery into the home a note of this should be made.

Many homes state that they cannot take responsibility for items that have been lost unless a robbery has taken place. In some homes, residents can take out an insurance policy to insure against losing valuables.

It is important that relatives and staff communicate well. Staff in countless homes have spent hours searching for 'lost' rings only to discover later that relatives have taken them to jewellers to have them adjusted because they no longer fit. In the home where I worked, several staff spent hours searching for a ring that a forgetful resident had misplaced. It was eventually retrieved from the dustbag of the vacuum cleaner. Later we discovered that the ring we thought we were searching for, which had been in the older person's family for over 100 years, had in fact been replaced with a copy by the patient's family with her consent. The resident had forgotten to tell us and so had the relatives.

Summary

Effective communication is vital if you are to provide high quality care. You need to have the ability to communicate with residents who may have communication difficulties because of age-related changes or illness. You need to be able to communicate effectively with the older person's family and friends. You also need to be able to communicate effectively with colleagues and to complete records.

This unit aims to assess your ability to communicate effectively, to record information, to maintain confidentiality, and to receive, transmit, store and retrieve information.

Portfolio preparation

Your assessor will use a variety of methods to assess how effectively you communicate and maintain records. The most popular methods of assessing a student's communication skills are direct observation and questioning. Your assessor may wish you to prepare written work when it is not possible to assess your skills in the workplace. Direct observation of communicating with a person who is unable to speak may not be possible if all the people in the home are able to speak.

Before beginning this module, discuss assessment strategies with your assessor. Most of this unit can be assessed using direct observation. You may be asked to provide the following types of evidence:

Products: This might include a copy of patient records that you have completed. Remember to delete the resident's name to preserve confidentiality.

Witness testimony: a statement from a senior member of staff.

Your assessor will also use other methods to help you gain evidence for this unit. These may include:

- Verbal questioning
- Written questions.

Written work can be used to assess your understanding of communication or record keeping or to supplement the evidence gained by direct observation and questioning. Discuss portfolio preparation with your assessor before beginning any written work. Some suggestions for portfolio work are:

- Explain the ways we communicate. What difficulties do you face when communicating? How do you overcome these problems?
- Write a short case history about a person you have cared for. This should be one to two sides of A4 paper. Outline the communication difficulties and how these were overcome.
- Write one page of A4 paper about the importance of communication in care settings.
- Explain who has the ability to access care records and under what circumstances.

Further information

Alzheimer's Society
Gordon House
10 Greencoat Place
London SW1P 1PH
Telephone: 020 7306 0606
E-mail: enquiries@alzheimers.org.uk
Website: http://www.alzheimers.org.uk

The Alzheimer's Society provides information about Alzheimer's to people with dementia, carers and professionals. Their website contains information on dementia including many downloadable booklets.

Speakability
1 Royal Street
London SE1 7LL
Telephone: 020 7261 9572
Helpline: 0808 808 9572
E-mail: speakability@speakability.org.uk
Website: http://www.speakability.org.uk

This charity provides information to dysphasic people, carers and professionals. It produces a number of information sheets. These are all available to download. The site has a wealth of information on dysphasia.

Parkinson's Disease Society
215 Vauxhall Bridge Road
London SW1V 1EJ
Telephone: 020 7931 8080
Helpline: 0808 800 0303
Website: http://www.parkinsons.org.uk

The Parkinson's Disease Society produces an enormous range of information on communication and other aspects of Parkinson's disease. You can obtain these easily by downloading from their website or by writing and enclosing a stamped self-addressed envelope.

Hearing Concern
95 Gray's Inn Road
London WC1X 8TX
Telephone: 020 7440 98718
Website: http://www.hearingconcern.org.uk

This organisation operates a scheme known as the sympathetic hearing scheme, which aims to make people more aware of hearing difficulties. The organisation produces leaflets, and a video that can be hired and enables you to understand what speech sounds like to hearing aid wearers. The association is run by people who are hard of hearing. It has a network of volunteers and may be able to provide a volunteer speaker to visit the nursing or residential home where you work, or your college, to speak to a group of care assistants. The association also produces a magazine four times a year.

Sign Community (The British Deaf Association: BDA)
British Deaf Association (London and South East)
69 Wilson Street
London, EC2A 2BB
E-mail: london@signcommunity.org.uk
Videophone IP: 81.138.165.105
Textphone: 020 7588 3529
Telephone: 020 7588 3520
Website: http://www.signcommunity.org.uk

This charity has offices in all of the UK countries and in the English regions. It produces a monthly newsletter as well as information sheets and leaflets. You'll find information and downloadable leaflets on their website.

Royal National Institute for Deaf People (RNID)
19–23 Featherstone Street
London EC1Y 8SL
Telephone: 020 7296 8000
Website: http://www.rnid.org.uk

The RNID produces a guide to local and national services for deaf people, plus a range of useful leaflets including *The ear and how it works* and *Understanding deafness*. These can all be downloaded from their website.

Notes

1. Bowman C, Whistler J & Ellerby M (2004) A national census of care home residents. *Age and Ageing* 33:6: 529–530.
2. Bray J, Cragg PA, Macknight A, Mills R (1999) *Lecture Notes on Human Physiology*, 4th edition. Blackwell Publishing, Oxford.

Further reading

These books may be available in your local or college library.

Grealy J, McMullen H & Grealy J (2005) *Dementia Care: A Practical, Photographic Guide*. Blackwell Publishing, Oxford.

Hutton C (2005) *After a Stroke: 300 Tips for Making Life Easier*. Demos Medical Publishing, New York.

Counsel and Care (1993) *Sound Barriers: A study of the needs of older people with hearing loss living in residential care and nursing homes*. Available from the charity Counsel and Care, Twyman House, 16 Bonny Street, London NW1 9PG. Telephone: 020 7485 1550.

Parr S, Byng S, Gilpin S & Ireland C (1998) *Talking about Aphasia*. Open University Press, Buckingham. This book is based on interviews with people who have had strokes. It explains what it is like to lose the ability to communicate.

Access to Health Records Act 1990. The Stationery Office, London. Your local college may have a copy of this Act in the library. If not you can visit the reference library at your local library, read the Act and take photocopies if you wish.

Chapter Two

Health and Safety
HSC22
Support the health and safety of yourself and individuals

This unit consists of three elements:
HSC22a Carry out health and safety checks before you begin work activities
HSC22b Ensure your actions support health and safety in the place where you work
HSC22c Take action to deal with emergencies

Details on moving and handling individuals safely can be found in Chapter 12. The aim of this chapter is to outline how you can contribute to maintaining the health and safety not only of older people but also of visitors and colleagues within the home.

This chapter

- Provides information and guidance on identifying people at risk of accidents and accident prevention
- Provides information and guidance on safety and security within the home
- Explains health and safety legislation – employer and employee responsibilities
- Provides information on recording and learning from accidents
- Discusses how to balance risk of accidents against quality of life
- Provides information on restraint and its risks
- Provides information on what to do if a fire occurs
- Provides information on what to do if a resident is missing
- Explains action to be taken when medical emergencies occur

Identifying risks and hazards

All environments have hazards and these hazards place people in that environment at risk of injury. People living in care homes are more vulnerable to hazards than other people because of ageing and poor general health. It is important that you can identify hazards and wherever possible act to remove these hazards.

A hazard is the potential to cause harm or damage.

> Hazard identification is the systematic consideration of all the equipment, processes, activities etc. associated with your work and that of others in the home, that may cause anyone personal injury or ill health or that may cause damage to property.[1]

Hazards can potentially harm residents, staff, relatives and other visitors. Table 2.1 gives details of possible hazards that residents may face.

As you can see from Table 2.1, residents are at risk not only from staff practice but also from the actions of other residents and relatives. One resident may wet the toilet floor, exposing other residents to the risk of falls or injuries. A relative may bring in medication for her mother's pain

Table 2.1 Some potential hazards to residents.

Hazard	Cause	Consequence
Abuse	Staff, relatives, residents	Physical and psychological harm
Alteration of room layout	Staff, relatives, residents	Physical and psychological harm
Changes in floor level	Design home	Falls, injury
Chemicals left out	Staff	Skin damage, ingestion
Fire	Equipment, staff, residents, relatives	Physical and psychological harm
Floors strewn with obstacles	Staff, residents, relatives	Falls, loss of mobility
Hot water, exposed piping, radiators	Design, management	Injury or death
Inappropriate care	Staff, relatives	Loss of independence, neglect
Inadequate or absent lights	Poor maintenance, design	Falls, injury
Manual handling techniques	Staff, relatives	Falls, dislocations, injury
Medication	Staff, GPs, relatives	Adverse reactions, illness
Poorly maintained furniture	Staff, management	Falls, injuries
Poorly maintained equipment, e.g. wheelchairs with flat tyres, broken brakes	Staff, management, outside agencies	Falls, injuries
Stairs	Design, management, inspectors	Falls, injuries
Wet floors	Staff, residents, relatives	Falls, injuries

Table 2.2 Some potential hazards to staff.

Hazard	Cause	Consequence
Abuse	Residents, relatives, manager, staff	Physical and psychological harm
Alteration of room layout	Residents, relatives, staff	Physical
Biological hazards	Contact with body fluids, infected material	Hepatitis and blood-borne infection
Changes in floor level	Design of home	Falls, injury
Chemicals	Working practice, poor ventilation	Skin damage, inhalation
Fire	Equipment, staff, residents, relatives	Physical and psychological harm
Floors strewn with obstacles	Staff, residents, relatives	Falls, loss of mobility
Inappropriate staff care	Manager, inspectors	Stress, illness
Inadequate or absent lights	Poor maintenance, design	Falls, accident, injury
Manual handling techniques	Inadequate equipment, space, training, inadequate staffing	Injury, stress, burnout
Needle-stick injury	Poor practice, inadequate facilities	Infection, illness, injury
Poorly maintained furniture	Staff, management	Injuries
Poorly maintained equipment, e.g. wheelchairs with flat tyres, broken brakes	Staff, management, outside agencies	Injuries
Stairs	Design, management, inspectors	Falls, injuries
Wet floors	Staff, residents, relatives	Falls, injuries

and give it to her, exposing the resident to many risks such as side effects. The home is also hazardous to staff. Table 2.2 outlines some of the risks to which staff are exposed in the workplace.

As you can see from these tables, if a home isn't safe for staff, it isn't safe for residents. Residents can be put at risk by other residents as well as staff. Staff can be put at risk by thoughtless or overworked colleagues who fail to report hazards. Staff can be put at risk by managers who fail to take health and safety seriously. Managers can be placed in impossible situations by staff who think health and safety is solely a management responsibility. Health and safety in the workplace must be a team effort.

Risk evaluation

When you have identified hazards the next step is to determine the level of risk. Is the level of risk high, medium, or low? Figure 2.1 illustrates the risk assessment process.

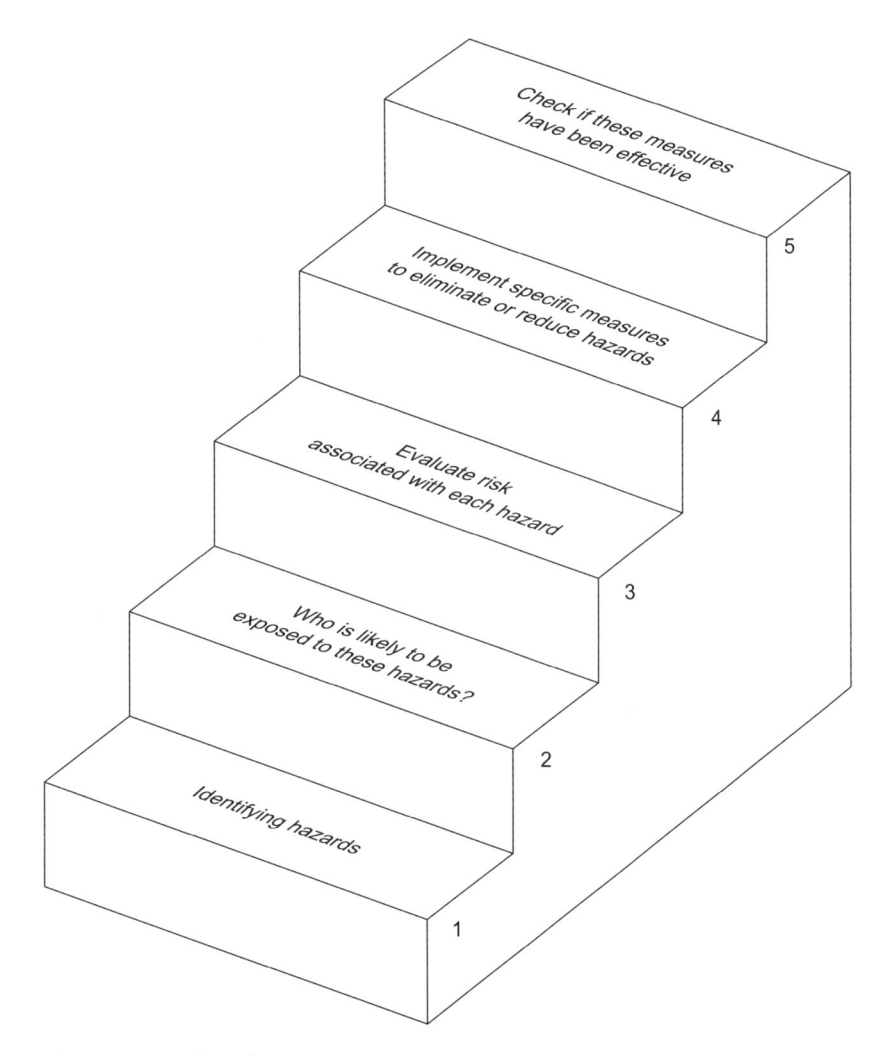

Figure 2.1 The risk assessment process.

Steps (from bottom to top):
1. Identifying hazards
2. Who is likely to be exposed to these hazards?
3. Evaluate risk associated with each hazard
4. Implement specific measures to eliminate or reduce hazards
5. Check if these measures have been effective

Staff carrying out risk assessment can feel overwhelmed. You might identify twenty or thirty potential hazards in one area such as the kitchen. Where do you start? How do you begin to prioritise?

Risk ratings

Assessing the level of risk as high, medium or low enables you to begin to prioritise. Is the chef likely to burn his hand on a saucepan? The difficulty with this approach is that although something might be very likely to happen the consequences might not be very serious. Assessing the risk and the

Table 2.3 Risk rating.

Risk likelihood	Consequence severity	Risk rating
High = 3	Death or major injury = 3	3 × 3 = 9
Medium = 2	Minor injury = 2	2 × 2 = 4
Low = 1	No injury = 1	1 × 1 = 2

Table 2.4 Risk scale.

Risk rating	Potential consequences	Priority
3 × 3 = 9	Highest risk, most serious consequences	Urgent, highest possible priority
3 × 2 = 6	High risk, serious consequences	High priority
2 × 2 = 4	Medium risk, less serious consequences	Medium priority
1 × 3 = 3	Low risk, most serious consequences	Medium priority because of the severity of consequences
2 × 1 = 2	Medium risk, less serious consequences	Medium priority
1 × 1 = 1	Low risk, less serious consequences	Low priority, but do not ignore

severity makes it easier for you to determine priorities. Table 2.3 shows how this works.

Using this method enables you to draw up a risk scale, illustrated in Table 2.4.

Using a risk scale gives you the ability to determine what you need to deal with today and how to prioritise all the other risks within the home. You can then draw up a table to enable you to go through the home identifying risks and determining priorities.

Control measures

Identifying and measuring risk gives you the ability to begin to manage that risk. You must deal with high risk, severe consequence risk urgently. Control measures aim, wherever possible, to eliminate risk. If elimination is not possible then introduce measures to control risk. This can avoid incidents such as the one which caused the death of an older woman, described in Case Study 2.1.[2]

You can use the information on risk identification and risk management in two ways. You can use it to increase your general awareness of risks so

Case Study 2.1

A Buckinghamshire care home and its director were fined a total of £17,000 at Reading Crown Court on 29 April for breaching health and safety legislation.

Whitefields Care Homes Ltd, Station House, 11 Masons Avenue, Harrow, Middlesex – owners and operators of Beaconsfield House Nursing Home, Ledborough Lane, Beaconsfield, Buckinghamshire – was fined £10,000 plus £5,569.18 costs for breaching Section 3(1) of the Health and Safety at Work, etc. Act 1974 (HSWA) in failing to ensure the health and safety of persons not in its employment.

Mr Bipin Bhagani, a director of Whitefields Care Homes Ltd, was also fined £7,500 and £15,000 costs for breaching Section 37(1) of the HSWA, in that the offence was committed with his consent or connivance, in relation to the same incident. This fine was the fourth highest imposed on a director in recent years for a breach under Section 37(1).

The Health and Safety Executive (HSE) prosecution followed an incident on 7 February 2001 in which an 85-year-old resident, Mrs Violet Frith, sustained serious burns to her legs while she was sleeping in her bed at Beaconsfield House Nursing Home. The burns arose from contact with the hot surface of a radiator, which was located next to the bed. Mrs Frith contracted a wound infection and died on 4 March 2001.

The case was heard before Reading Crown Court, Old Shire Hall, The Forbury, Reading, on Tuesday 29 April 2003. The company and the director entered guilty pleas to the charges.

After the hearing, HSE investigating inspector Stephen Hartley said: 'This sad incident could have been easily prevented. Care homes and hospitals should be well aware of the risk that hot radiators and pipework present to vulnerable, elderly people . . . This case serves to remind Directors of the need to ensure that their organisations manage risks to health and safety effectively.'

---

that when you come on duty you are aware of how certain aspects of the environment can be hazardous to the older person. If you are asked to help assess risk formally, you can use the tools given above.

Safety and security within the home

Employers and managers are required to assess risks and act to reduce the risk of accidents occurring. Staff are required to comply with the health and safety policy in the home. Accidents are less likely to occur if every member of staff is aware of how accidents can occur and works to reduce the risk of accidents occurring. More details about this are given later in the chapter.

Older people living in homes and staff working within homes can be vulnerable to attack. There have been cases where intruders have entered homes and robbed and attacked staff and residents. In some cases, people have been seriously injured. In the past, many homes left the front entrance to the home 'on the latch' so that visitors could enter without having to be let in. Now the majority of homes have the front door closed and visitors must ring the doorbell. Some homes now use a combination lock. Staff (and sometimes regular visitors) are given a four-digit combination and punch in the numbers to enter the home. These measures increase the safety and security of the people in the home. Staff are also more aware of who is in the building and this is important if a fire occurs.

Some homes still leave a side entrance open during daylight hours. At night, it is the policy in most homes that doors are locked and ground-floor windows (apart from fanlights) are closed. Check what policies your home has for ensuring security.

Who can enter the home

Nursing and residential homes are the homes of older people; they are not public places and there is no automatic right of entry for the public. In practice people who have a purpose in visiting the home, such as relatives and friends of patients and people who have come to deliver goods or services, are allowed free entry to the home. If a person living in the home does not wish to see someone (perhaps a neighbour), the neighbour has no right to enter the home. Certain people have the legal right to enter the home, and they are listed in Table 2.5.

Although these groups of people have the legal right to enter the home, you should check the person's identification before allowing entry.

Health and safety laws

There are several laws governing health and safety in the workplace. These include:

- Common law
- Health and Safety at Work Act 1974
- Management of Health and Safety at Work Regulations 1992, amended 1994
- Control of Substances Hazardous to Health 1988, known as COSHH
- Reporting of Injury, Disease and Dangerous Occurrences Regulations 1995, known as Riddor
- Manual Handling Operations Regulations 1992
- Fire Safety Regulations 1997.

Table 2.5 Persons who have a legal right to enter a care home.

Organisation/Person	Reason
CSCI inspectors	To carry out announced and unannounced inspections.
Electricity board	To read meter if it is indoors.
Gas board	To read meter if it is indoors, to check for gas leaks.
Water board	To read meter if it is indoors, to check for water leaks.
Fire brigade	To familiarise themselves with the layout of the home. This enables them to evacuate everyone quickly and safely if a fire occurs.
Health and safety officers	To ensure that health and safety standards are met.
Environmental health officers	To ensure that food handling and storage are satisfactory and that policies on waste disposal are satisfactory.
Pharmacists employed by the PCT	To ensure that medicines are stored and administered correctly.
Police	To investigate crime.

Common law

Common law has evolved over the last 1000 years and is unwritten. Under common law, each of us has a 'duty of care'. Employers, statutory bodies and professionals who breach this duty may be sued for negligence. The introduction of 'no win, no fee' cases means that people are now more likely to sue. In negligence claims the person suing must prove: that the company/person had a general duty of care to prevent foreseeable injuries; that the failure to prevent injury was negligent; and that this failure caused the injury. Case Study 2.2 illustrates how negligence claims can work.

Health and Safety at Work Act 1974

The Health and Safety at Work Act was introduced in 1974. The Act is a piece of criminal law. People who fail to comply with the Act can be prosecuted and fined or jailed if found guilty. The Act is the main piece of UK health and safety legislation and outlines broad principles concerning health and safety. Other more recent legislation is more specific. Employers and employees have responsibilities under the Act.

> **Case Study 2.2**
>
> A resident's bath oil was spilt on a vinyl 'non-slip' floor. The care assistant bathing the resident accompanied the resident to her room. She did not mop up the bath oil, as she was busy; anyway, it was the last bath of the morning. Soon the domestic would come to clean the bathroom.
>
> Unfortunately, the domestic did not come soon enough. The resident's elderly visitor, noting that the bath oil had not been brought back from the bathroom, went to fetch it. She slipped on the floor and fractured her femur. She sued the home for negligence.
>
> Her solicitor argued that the home was negligent in failing to prevent a foreseeable accident. The nursing home settled out of court on legal advice. People whose actions have contributed to their injury may be found 'contributory negligent' and any damages awarded may be reduced.

Employers' responsibilities

Employers must ensure the health and safety of employees at work and other people on the premises. Those who employ more than five people must prepare, review and revise a written health and safety policy. This should acknowledge and comply with legislation. Employers must display a certificate of employer's liability insurance. Employers must display the poster 'Health and Safety Law – what you should know' or distribute leaflets giving this information. Employers must ensure that employees receive adequate and appropriate information, instruction and training to carry out their work safely.

Employees' responsibilities

Employees must comply with legislation and ensure that their actions do not adversely affect others. Employees are entitled to sue their employers if they have been injured in the course of their work.

Self-employed people (such as the window cleaner) must comply with legislation and ensure that their actions do not adversely affect others. Manufacturers and suppliers must ensure that their products are safe when used properly. They must provide health and safety information about their products.

Management of Health and Safety at Work Regulations

The Management of Health and Safety at Work Regulations 1992 were amended in 1994 by the Management of Health and Safety at Work (Amendment) Regulations. These regulations require employers to carry out risk assessments. The key points of the Regulations are as follows.

Employers are required to:

- Assess risks associated with the business to determine how to eliminate or minimise those risks.
- Take action to eliminate or minimise risk.
- Appoint 'competent persons' to help meet the requirements. This can be the manager or a member of staff. If no one within the home has the skills then consultants can be used.
- Ensure that temporary staff (including agency staff) are informed of any health and safety information and/or the skills necessary to do their job.
- Consider the capabilities of each individual to do their work safely.

The aim of the legislation is to ensure that the employer takes care to ensure the health and safety of employees and people living in or entering the home, such as by taking precautions to reduce accidents. This means that if an employer is aware of some problem that may cause an accident, steps should be taken to prevent accidents occurring. If the employer knows that a carpet is frayed and could cause someone to trip, but does not act, a breach of the Act has occurred. There have been cases where employers have been prosecuted for failing to clear snow from paths because accidents have occurred.

Employers who have more than five employees are required to have a policy statement. This details the employer's responsibilities and the staff's responsibilities. The policy statement may give details about special precautions to be taken to prevent accidents; for example, it may be policy for domestic staff to leave signs saying 'Caution wet floor' on floors that they have just mopped. The policy statement may also give detailed instructions about the safekeeping of items such as cleaning materials and medicines. It will also instruct all employees about action they should take if they become aware of a hazard or a breach of the health and safety policy.

Employers have a duty to provide equipment to prevent accidents. This means that employers should provide a range of equipment, from rubber gloves and overalls for domestics required to clean toilets, to hoists for staff required to move residents.

Employees are required to: adhere to the instructions, policies and procedures laid down by their employer; and report any shortcomings in the employer's arrangements; for example, if there are instructions that Mrs X is to be moved using the hoist but the hoist is broken.

Staff working within the home have duties and responsibilities to work in ways that reduce the risk of accidents and make the home as safe as possible.

Control of Substances Hazardous to Health 1988 (COSHH)

COSHH regulations distinguish between the hazards and risks of substances commonly used in the home. The manager's responsibilities under COSHH are to:

- Identify hazardous items. Some common kitchen hazards are bleach, disinfectant, descaler and dishwasher powder.
- Identify how these items could affect health. Ensure that potentially harmful substances such as bleach are labelled. Maintain a file of chemicals used and action to be taken in case of splashing or swallowing. Your suppliers can provide this information.
- Devise secure storage systems. Ensure that potentially hazardous substances are stored under lock and key. Beware the bottle of bleach under the sink or staff leaving cleaning trolleys where they are easily accessible.
- Train staff. National Required Standards recommend induction courses and three study days for all staff including ancillary staff.

Reporting of Injury, Disease and Dangerous Occurrences Regulations 1995 (Riddor)

Riddor legislation is not specific to care environments. It was, in fact, drafted with the building industry in mind. Under Riddor, employers, or designated managers, must report the following occurrences to their local Health and Safety Executive.[3]

Death or major injury of a member of staff, the public or a subcontractor

In the case of death or major injury requiring hospitalisation, the manager must telephone the HSE and details will be taken. This should be followed up with a completed accident report on form F2508 within ten days of the occurrence. Relevant reportable injuries are:

- Fracture other than to the fingers, thumbs or toes
- Amputation
- Dislocation of the shoulder, hips, knee or spine
- Acute illness requiring medical treatment where there is reason to believe that this resulted from exposure to a biological agent or its toxins or infected material.

Over three-day injury

If an accident occurs, including an assault, connected with work and the employee or contractor is unable to work for three days or more then a completed accident report form must be sent to the HSE. This three-day period includes non-working days. If a member of staff injures her back and has one day off, unless she reports that she is taking her days off as usual, the manager should report the incident to the HSE.

Disease

If a doctor informs a manager that an employee is suffering from a reportable work-related disease, the manager must send a completed disease report form (F2508A) to the HSE. Relevant examples are:

- Skin diseases such as occupational dermatitis. Current HSE opinion is that this includes latex allergy and hand dermatitis.
- Infections such as hepatitis, tuberculosis, legionellosis and MRSA.

Dangerous occurrences

This near-miss clause compels managers to report occurrences that could have but did not cause serious injury. If a wall collapsed and narrowly missed hitting someone, this should be reported. The HSE should be telephoned and a completed form (F2508B) should be completed within ten days. Relevant examples are:

- Unintended collapse of a wall or floor in a place of work
- A chandelier falling from the ceiling
- Explosion or fire causing suspension of normal work for over 24 hours
- Collapse of load-bearing parts of lifts.

Records

Employers must keep records of any injury, reportable disease or dangerous occurrence. They can comply with legislation by keeping copies of the report forms in a file, recording details on computer or maintaining a written log.

New and expectant mothers

The workplace can damage the health of mothers and their unborn children. Research shows that working long hours, working shifts, heavy physical labour and stress can affect pregnancy. The 1994 amendment regulations recognise that new and expectant mothers are particularly vulnerable in the workplace. Employers must carry out specific risk assessment that includes the risks to expectant mothers, new mothers and mothers who are breastfeeding. The Health and Safety Executive produces guidance. Staff must inform employers when they become pregnant, are breastfeeding or have recently given birth. This enables the employer to meet legal requirements.

Documentation

The approach to record keeping which courts of law adopt tends to be 'if it is not recorded it has not been done'. Record keeping enables the home to demonstrate that staff have worked safely. Further information on record keeping is given in Chapter 1.

Training

Employers are required to provide adequate training of staff to prevent accidents. In care homes, this means for example that staff who are required to move residents should have regular instruction and updating in moving and handling; further details are given in Chapter 12. The Care Standards Act and national minimum standards state that all staff must have health and safety training as part of their induction. Employers have a duty to ensure that staff are aware of what action they must take in case of fire or accident or if a resident goes missing.

Hazardous materials

Many cleaning materials are very toxic. Bleach and toilet cleaners can damage the skin and cause serious injury if drunk. Other cleaning materials may not appear dangerous but can cause accidents; for example, spilt washing-up liquid can cause a fall. In some smaller homes, care assistants may be responsible for cleaning as well as caring. Staff should ensure that all cleaning materials are kept locked away. It may be convenient to have the toilet cleaner by the side of the toilet but this could cause serious harm to a confused patient. Larger homes normally employ domestic staff but you may find cleaning materials left about. You have a duty to remove these from patient areas to prevent the possibility of injury.

Medications

In nursing homes, medicines are stored in a locked cabinet and only registered nurses have access to the drugs cupboard or trolley. Medicines that are being returned to the pharmacy are often stored in the treatment room. Creams and lotions are also stored in the treatment room. Treatment rooms should be locked if there are hazardous materials such as medication, creams or lotions in unlocked containers. You should make sure you always lock treatment room doors after leaving. In some homes some residents keep their own medicines and take them when prescribed. If the older person leaves her medicine lying around there is a danger that a confused patient might take these medicines. If you are worried about such a situation, consult your manager.

Fire training

Every person working in the home should be aware of what to do in case of fire. Each person working in the home should be given training in this and should attend a fire drill every six months. It is important that you are aware of where each fire exit is and what to do in case of fire. Normally when the fire alarm goes off all staff report to a fire assembly point. Find out where the fire assembly point is in your home. It is usually by the main panel of the fire alarm. The fire alarm in homes normally has one large panel and a number of smaller panels. The home is divided into zones and the rooms and areas covered by each zone will be indicated on the fire panel; for example, zone 1 might be the lounge, kitchen and laundry. If a fire has occurred in zone 1, staff would check in which part of this area the fire had occurred. If the fire alarm has been triggered in the kitchen by burning toast the action taken would be different from that required if the deep-fat fryer were in flames.

Find out if your home has written guidance on what action is to be taken in case of fire. Many homes have this guidance framed and hung on the wall next to fire alarm panels.

Fire exits

All fire exits in the home should be clearly marked and should be kept clear at all times. It is easy though for busy staff to allow fire exits to become blocked. A delivery of stationery or goods may be left blocking a fire exit as staff intend to put things away later. Relatives can easily place a chair in front of the fire exit in the lounge and then leave without putting it back. Homes are for living in but it is important that carers are aware that blocked exits cause delay in evacuating the home if a fire breaks out. At times, staff must exercise great tact in ensuring that residents and their families are not offended, but that exits are kept clear.

Accident policy

The aim of all accident policies is to prevent accidents occurring whenever possible. It is not possible to make any home completely safe and this will be discussed later in the chapter. You can contribute to safety within the home by reporting anything that is likely to cause an accident and by taking action, wherever possible, to prevent accidents occurring.

Missing resident

The home should have a policy on action to be taken if a resident goes missing. If the person tends to go out unaccompanied, suggest that the individual carry identification in case of accident. A note tucked into a wallet or purse saying 'Mrs Doris Swan is a resident of Eastways Residential Home. In case of accident please telephone . . .' will help ensure that the home is contacted if an accident occurs.

If the person tends to wander and may have left the home in a confused state, the home should have a policy for dealing with this. Normally such a policy involves both calling the police and staff searching for the older person. It is possible for the individual to get some distance from the home very quickly. An older person dressed in ordinary clothes will not attract attention. Many bus drivers do not ask to see bus passes when a person is obviously above retirement age. The police will find it difficult to locate a lady of 83 with white hair and glasses wearing a flowered dress! Many homes now take photographs of residents. A photograph is often attached to the medication chart to enable temporary staff to identify residents. In some homes, photographs of patients are put on their bedroom doors. This helps residents, visitors and staff to find a person's room. If the person goes missing and the police have a recent photograph, their job becomes easier.

Accident prevention

You can contribute to safety within the home by reporting anything that is likely to cause an accident, and by acting wherever possible to prevent accidents occurring. Let's explore some of the factors we identified earlier in more detail.

Environmental hazards

A wet floor can be slippery and can cause a fall. A toilet that is dark because the light bulb does not work and has not been replaced can make it difficult for the older person to see where she is going and can cause her to fall. A building that is poorly maintained can lead to accidents.

Equipment that is not working properly can also cause accidents. If you discover that the brakes on a wheelchair are not working, remove the wheelchair and report the problem so that repairs can be organised quickly. Homes should have a spare wheelchair that can be used to transport residents who are ill, or can be used temporarily by a patient whose wheelchair is unsafe.

Objects left carelessly on the floor may not be noticed by older people, who can fall over. Remove any hazards, wherever possible, and inform the person in charge of the home at once. Inadequate seating can lead to some disabled people falling out of chairs. Some older people living in nursing homes are very disabled and are unable to sit in ordinary armchairs. It is now possible to buy chairs specially designed to enable these people to sit comfortably in chairs that will support them. An example of one of these is given in Fig. 2.2a. Specially designed chairs provide support for disabled older people but do not restrain or restrict the person in any way (Fig. 2.2b).

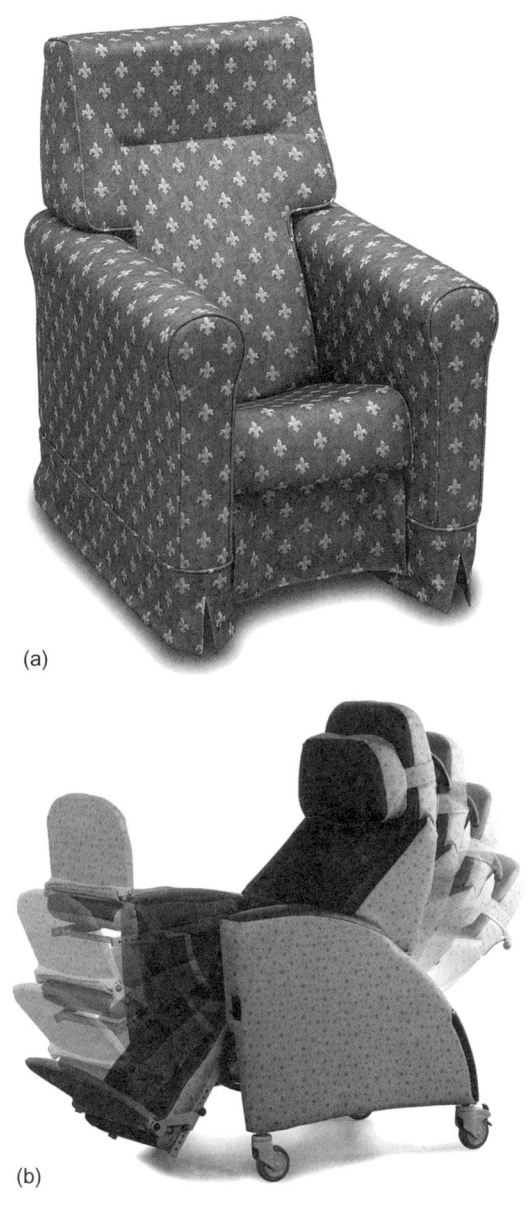

Figure 2.2 A specially designed chair (a) gives support; (b) does not restrict or restrain.

Unsuitable footwear

Unsuitable footwear can make it difficult to walk and can lead to accidents. Many older people, especially those who do not walk much, find that their feet swell. This can make it difficult to find shoes that fit properly. Some older people have bunions, and arthritis can cause foot deformities. These problems can make it difficult for older people to find shoes that fit properly.

Wide-fitting shoes that can be adjusted when feet swell are now available by mail order from two companies (details can be found at the end of the chapter). If it is not possible to buy suitable shoes from these companies, special shoes can be made for the person.

The person's general practitioner (GP) writes to the surgical fitter (known as an orthotist) and asks for shoes to be made for the person. The orthotist visits, measures the person's feet, and discusses which type and colour of shoes or boots the person would prefer. These are made specially and the orthotist returns to fit them when they are ready. Some older people, particularly those who have suffered from strokes, require a calliper to provide support. These are supplied by the orthotist. Sometimes special shoes are made and the calliper is designed to fit into the heel of the shoe. Sometimes the older person's own shoes can be adapted so that the calliper will fit.

People who suffer from arthritis of the knee may find that one of their knees tends to 'give'. A knee support, supplied by the orthotist, can prevent this. People who have broken a leg may have one leg shorter than the other because of surgery. Special shoes can be made to correct this and enable the older person to walk normally.

If the older person has been supplied with special footwear or an aid such as a calliper, you may need to help them put it on. Older people who have suitable footwear are less likely to have accidents.

Clothing

Clothing can cause accidents. Many older women prefer full-length nightdresses and dressing gowns. If these are too long, the individual can trip over and fall. Gentlemen can also trip on pyjama legs if they are too long.

How accidents affect older people

Accidents can have serious consequences. The older person can lose confidence because of a fall and this can cause them to walk less and to become weaker. Sometimes the older person who falls fractures a bone; if she puts out a hand to save herself the wrist may fracture, known as a Colles fracture. The thigh bone (femur) may also become fractured as a result of a fall, affecting either the shaft of the femur or the neck of the femur near the hip joint, a common form of hip fracture in the older person.

Older people often suffer from a condition known as osteoporosis, which causes the bones to become thinner, weaker and more easily broken.

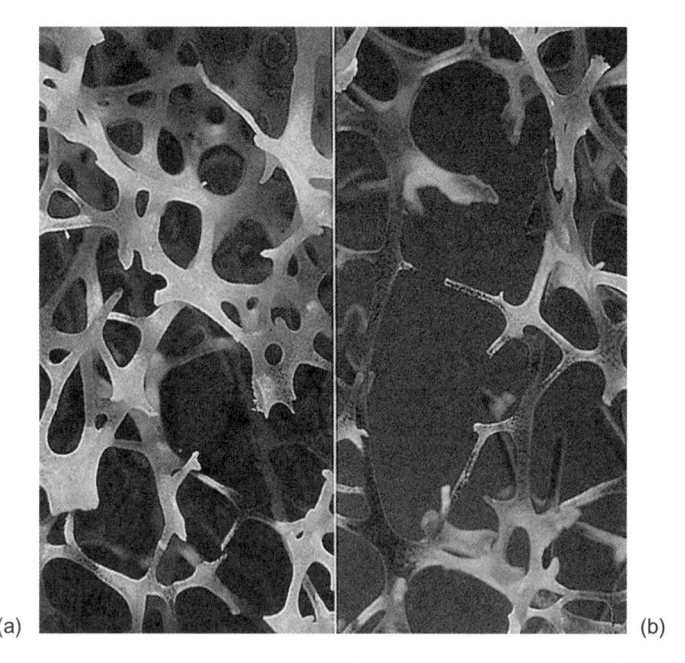

Figure 2.3 (a) Normal bone structure; (b) osteoporotic bone.

Figure 2.3 shows (a) a section of healthy bone and (b) bone which has been weakened by osteoporosis.

Discovering who is at risk of having accidents

People living in homes have a wide range of abilities. Some have few problems in walking while others require aids and help to move around. Some residents are alert while others are not. Some individuals see well while others have very poor vision. Some of the people living in your home will be much more likely to have accidents than others.

Homes aim to enable older people to live their lives as they would wish if they were at home. The aim of care within homes should be to reduce the risk of accidents and to protect individuals who are at risk of having accidents. Most homes now assess residents to discover who is most at risk of having an accident. If the person is at risk this is noted in the care plan along with action to be taken to reduce risks. Many primary care trusts now have falls prevention services and if a person has suffered multiple falls you should ask for advice on falls prevention from the falls service. It is important to realise that no home can be made totally safe and that no one can guarantee that accidents will not happen.

Balancing risks and quality of life

Living is about taking risks. We all take risks every day of our lives. We risk crossing the road where there are no traffic lights; we take risks every time we step into a car or onto a bus, or take part in sports. Yet if we stayed at home and took no risks life would not be worth living. When we take risks we weigh up the risk and decide on the possible gains and losses from taking that risk.

In homes, staff must balance the duty of care and the possibility of trying so hard to avoid accidents that we risk making the older person's life a misery by preventing her from living life to the full. The care assistant who leaves a confused resident alone and unsupervised in the bath, knowing that she is not capable of calling for help, would be failing in her duty of care. Another individual recovering from illness might ask you to sit with her while she bathes because she is feeling nervous. Another individual might wish to bathe in private and may ask you to leave after she has been helped into the bath. It is important to treat people as individuals; older people are just like us, only older. Some older people who are recovering from illness are determined to 'get back on their feet'. In the process of regaining mobility and strength, the person may sometimes fall. Staff should respect the individual's wishes and offer support, help and encouragement.

Restraint

It is illegal to restrain anyone without their consent. It is also illegal to restrain any person on another person's instructions. In some homes, you may see different types of restraint used, including bed rails, tables and lockers.

Bed rails

Bed rails or cot-sides were used routinely in hospitals until a few years ago. Some hospitals had policies that stated that all individuals over a certain age were to have bed rails fitted to their beds to prevent falls. We now know that bed rails can lead to serious injury and they are only used in special circumstances. Bed rails prevent individuals getting up and this can lead to incontinence. When bed rails are used some older people become depressed and upset, and this can affect their mental and physical health and lead to them becoming weaker and sicker. Some people climb over bed rails and can fall. There have been reports of people who caught an arm or leg in the bed rail, struggled to get free and broke a limb. The bed rail, which is designed to prevent accidents, can actually cause them. Bed rails should only be used in very specific circumstances after a full risk assessment has been carried out.

Tables, chairs and lockers

These can be used intentionally or unintentionally to barricade the person into bed, making it difficult or impossible for them to get out. This can lead to distress and may cause rather than prevent accidents.

Preventing the older person falling out of bed

Staff often worry that if a person falls the staff will be blamed and everyone will think the person has been neglected. Homes that have risk assessment policies will have these documented and patients, staff, relatives and registration officers will be aware of these policies. Older people do not normally fall out of bed and many staff worry unnecessarily about them doing so.

You can reduce the risk of accidents at night by:

- Making sure that the patient can reach the call bell
- Assuring the person that staff are there to help and that they should not hesitate to ring if help is required
- Answering bells promptly
- Making sure the person does not feel rushed or a 'nuisance'
- Leaving a light on so that if the person wishes to get up in the night, she can see
- Leaving the room tidy and not leaving any obstacles which could cause a fall
- Leaving any aids such as a walking frame and shoes where the person can reach them.

Recording accidents

All accidents that occur in the home must be recorded in an accident book. The type of record kept varies from area to area. There are no national guidelines stating how these records should be kept. In practice accident records that satisfy the local inspection team are kept. In some areas, a form is issued in triplicate: one form is kept in the patient's notes, another in an accident folder and another is placed in the care plan. In other areas, all accidents are recorded in a bound book. Find out the policy for recording accidents in your home.

Learning from accidents

Some accidents that occur could, with hindsight, have been prevented. In other cases, perhaps involving faulty equipment or poor handling techniques, accidents may recur if action is not taken. In some homes senior staff discuss and review accidents so that, wherever possible, lessons can be learnt and further accidents prevented.

Protecting residents from infection

Infection control is a most important aspect of healthcare. People requiring care in hospitals, care homes, clinics, doctors' surgeries and in their own homes may have infections or may be at risk of picking up infection from other people. Staff and visitors are also at risk of infection. Until recently, training and education on infection control has concentrated on professional staff rather than healthcare assistants and support staff. Now there is a greater awareness that support staff have a very important role to play in the prevention of infection.

What is infection control?

'A managed environment, which minimises the risk of infection to patients, staff and visitors.'

What infection risks exist in healthcare?

In healthcare settings people with infections are cared for and people who are ill are vulnerable to infection from other people including staff and visitors. Bacteria, fungi, viruses and parasites can cause infections.

Bacteria are single-celled organisms. They live on or in just about every material and environment on Earth, from soil to water to air, in your home, in the cold Arctic ice and the hot vents of volcanoes. Each square centimetre of your skin, on average, hosts about 100 000 bacteria. A single teaspoon of topsoil contains more than a billion (1 000 000 000) bacteria.

Bacteria normally do us no harm but in certain circumstances some bacteria can cause serious illness and even death. In many cases antibiotics can destroy bacteria. Overuse of antibiotics can cause bacteria to become resistant to antibiotics and this is a growing problem in healthcare.

Fungi are organisms that produce spores. Some fungi such as mushrooms are edible. Some provide numerous drugs (such as penicillin and other antibiotics). Some, such as yeast, are used to make bread and beer.

Fungi also cause a number of diseases: in humans, fungi cause ringworm, athlete's foot and several more serious diseases. Because fungi are chemically and genetically more similar to animals than to other organisms, this makes fungal diseases very difficult to treat.

Viruses are much smaller than bacteria. They can cause minor problems such as cold sores and flu, and also major, life-threatening infections. Antibiotics do not kill viruses. A few new drugs can kill some viruses.

Parasites are organisms that obtain nourishment and protection from other living organisms, known as **hosts**. They may be transmitted from animals to humans, from humans to humans, or from humans to animals. Parasites are significant causes of food-borne and waterborne disease. These organisms live and reproduce within the tissues and organs of infected human and animal hosts, and are often excreted in faeces.

They may be transmitted from host to host through consumption of contaminated food and water, or by putting anything into your mouth that has touched the stool (faeces) of an infected person or animal.

Parasites are of different types and range in size from tiny, single-celled, microscopic organisms (**protozoa**) to larger, multicellular worms (**helminths**) that may be seen without a microscope. Some common parasites are head lice, threadworms, scabies and tapeworms.

How does infection spread?

The spread of infection within healthcare requires three elements (see Fig. 2.4):

1. A source of infecting organisms (bacteria, viruses, fungi)
2. A susceptible host
3. A route of transmission of the organism from one person/site to another.

Source of infection

The source may be patients, staff or visitors. The source may be a person who has signs of infection, or he or she may be colonised and show no signs of infection. The person may become infected by bacteria that normally live on the person and cause no harm. The source may be objects within the environment that have become contaminated. These may be equipment and sometimes medicines.

Host (patient)

The person's resistance to pathogenic (harmful) micro-organisms can vary greatly. Some people may be immune to or able to resist infection; others may simply be colonised and become carriers with no symptoms. Some will develop a clinical disease.

Source → Vulnerable host → Route transmission → Infection spread

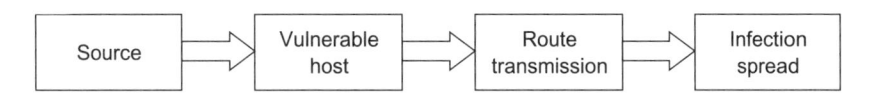

Figure 2.4 The route for the spread of infection.

Transmission

Micro-organisms can be transmitted by a variety of routes and the same micro-organism may be transmitted by more than one route. For example, the virus that causes chickenpox can spread in the air or by direct contact.

There are four main routes of transmission:

- Contact
- Droplet/airborne
- Infected food or drink
- Vectors.

Contact transmission

This is the most important and most frequent means of transmission of infection. People can be infected by:

- **Direct contact:** involves direct physical transfer of the micro-organism from one site to another, e.g. from patient to patient or different sites on the same patient. Most frequently this is done via the hands of healthcare staff or the patients themselves. MRSA is normally spread by direct contact. The nurse or care worker may touch a dressing that is infected with MRSA. The MRSA lives on the warm moist hands and is transmitted to the next vulnerable host who may have a wound or catheter.
- **Indirect contact:** this involves contact with a contaminated object such as bed linen, instruments, equipment and dressings.

Airborne/droplet transmission

- **Droplet transmission:** by large droplets during coughing, sneezing, talking and during procedures which may generate droplets such as suctioning and bronchoscopy. The droplets are propelled only a short distance through the air. The rotavirus that causes winter vomiting is transmitted in this way. Droplets from vomit or loose stool can infect people who are some distance away.
- **Airborne transmission:** caused by dispersal of smaller micro-organisms, e.g. viruses, or airborne dust particles containing the infectious agent. These organisms can be widely dispersed by air currents before being inhaled or deposited on the susceptible host, or, in the case of dust particles, onto horizontal surfaces, equipment and so on.

Food and water transmission

This occurs via contaminated food or water supplies. Organisms can be introduced via the food chain, e.g. salmonella in eggs or by inappropriate handling of contaminated raw food or inadequate cooking. Water provides an ideal breeding ground for some micro-organisms, which can then be infected, if the water supply has not been appropriately treated.

Vector-borne transmission

This occurs when vectors such as flies, mosquitoes, rats and other pests transmit infection. This route of transmission is rare in the UK.

Breaking the chain of infection

Direct contact

The single most important measure in preventing direct contact infection is hand washing. You should also wear gloves whenever there is any possibility of direct contact with infected blood, body fluids or contaminated material. It is important to wash your hands before and after removing gloves. This prevents contaminating the gloves and your hands.

Indirect contact

To prevent infection from beds, equipment and the environment, keep the environment clean and tidy. Wash and disinfect equipment such as beds and commodes between patients. Ensure that spills are mopped up and treated. Ensure that the healthcare environment is clean.

Food and water

To prevent infection by food and drink, ensure that you maintain good handwashing habits, especially after using the toilet. Do not come to work if you are suffering from diarrhoea or vomiting. If you have a cut or infection on your hands cover this with a clean waterproof dressing. Adhere strictly to food hygiene regulations.

Airborne

In healthcare settings we can prevent the spread of infection by the airborne route through vaccination programmes. Pneumonia and flu vaccinations reduce the risk of infection in older people. We can segregate people with airborne infections from others who are at risk. People who have infectious pulmonary tuberculosis will require barrier nursing in hospital. Hospital wards and care homes may stop admissions if they experience an outbreak of infection such as rotavirus (winter vomiting).

Vector

While most people understand that rats and mice can cause infection, they may overlook problems causes by cockroaches and other insects. Such pests can transmit infection in food stores and food preparation areas as well as in the home. It is important that staff in homes are alert to infestations and report these so that they can be dealt with.

How can infection control protect patients, staff and visitors?

If micro-organisms enter the body the immune system reacts by raising body temperature and attacking infection. In healthy people the body can usually fight off infection without antibiotics or other therapy. People requiring healthcare are often unhealthy. The person may have a disease such as diabetes or heart failure. The person may have poor health. The person may be old or undernourished. The person may have been treated with antibiotics or drugs that increase the risk of infection.

Infection control aims to help us all to be aware of infection risks and to work in ways that reduce the risk of infection on a day-to-day basis. When there is an outbreak of infection then we have additional policies and procedures that help us work to get the infection under control and to reduce the risks to patients and staff.

Medical emergencies

All staff working in care homes come face to face with emergencies from time to time. It is important that you have some basic knowledge of first aid. The aims of first aid are to:

- Preserve life
- Prevent the emergency worsening
- Help recovery.

What to do if you find a resident has collapsed

- Remain calm
- Use the call bell to call for help
- Check what is happening – is the patient conscious or unconscious? How serious is the situation?
- The most important things can be remembered by 'ABC'. Ensure that the person's:
    - **airway** is open and he is able to breathe
    - **breathing** is taking place
    - **circulation** is satisfactory.

Airway obstruction

The airway enables us to breathe air in and out of our lungs. It can become obstructed for a number of reasons, but the commonest causes of airway obstruction are choking or loss of consciousness. If the person is choking this could be because food or dentures are blocking the airway. The person may have vomited and vomit has collected at the back of the

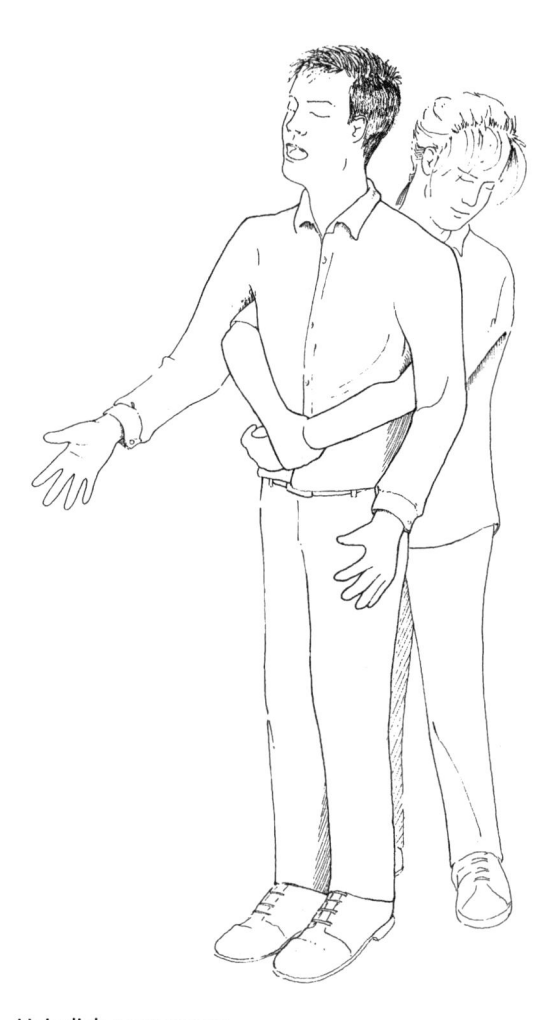

Figure 2.5 Heimlich manoeuvre.

throat. Open the person's mouth gently. Use two fingers to feel around for any food, vomit or dentures that may be causing the person to choke. Remove anything that is blocking the airway.

If the person is unable to speak and is turning blue, use the Heimlich manoeuvre (Fig. 2.5).

There are many reasons for loss of consciousness, including strokes, fits and diabetes. Staff who know as much about the older person's condition as possible can respond more effectively. People who become unconscious should be placed in the recovery position (Fig. 2.6). You may require help to place a person in this position. If possible remove the person's dentures as they may slip in the mouth and block the airway. Loosen tight clothing and call for help immediately.

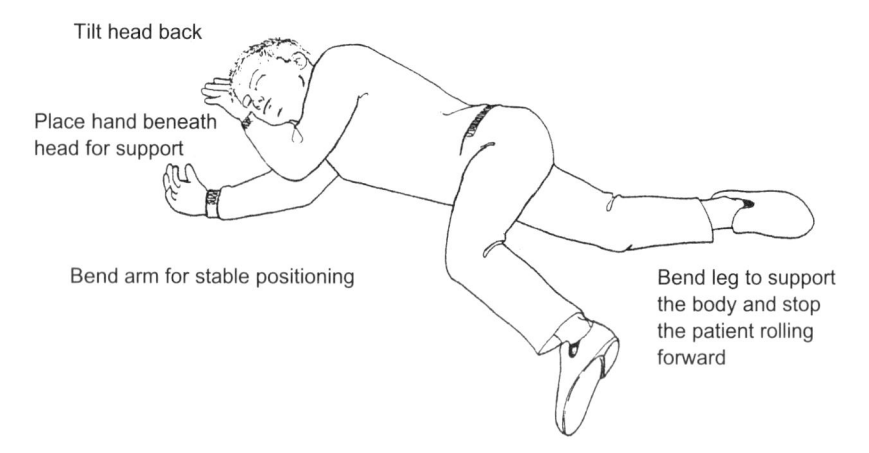

Figure 2.6 Recovery position.

Breathing

Some older people suffer from asthma and carry inhalers that help them to breathe more easily. It is important that you find out whether any of the people in the home where you work suffer from asthma. If a person in the home does suffer from asthma and may require help to use an inhaler if he or she has become breathless, find out how to do this before an emergency occurs. If the person is having difficulty breathing but is conscious, help him to sit up. Loosen any tight clothing, such as a tie, shirt collar or belt. People who have difficulty breathing feel very frightened and this fear makes breathing more difficult. Do your best to reassure the person as this will help prevent breathing problems worsening. Ask the person to take slow deep breaths, and seek assistance.

Circulation

If a person becomes unconscious, it is important to be able to decide quickly if the situation is a life-threatening emergency or simply a faint.

Check the person's colour – blue or grey skin indicates a life-threatening emergency. Check breathing – is the person breathing at all, with difficulty or normally? Check the pulse – is the pulse absent or does it appear weak? If the person's skin colour is abnormal or breathing is absent, or the person is breathing with difficulty, or the pulse is absent or weak, call for help immediately. This is a medical emergency perhaps caused by a stroke or heart attack. Check that the airway is clear and place the person in the recovery position while waiting for help.

Fainting is a brief loss of consciousness. People who have fainted may appear very pale but their skin does not become blue or grey. Breathing is normal and the pulse is always present, though it can appear weak. Fainting can occur in adults of all ages. It may be caused by hunger, shock or even getting up too quickly. The person faints because the brain is not receiving sufficient blood. A person who has fainted should not be sat up because sitting up reduces the flow of blood to the brain.

If you find a person unconscious, it is important to check their colour. Clothing should be loosened and the person should lie down until they feel well enough to sit up. Drinking from a glass of cold water may help the person to feel better.

Chest pain

Chest pain and circulation problems can be caused by angina or a heart attack.

In both cases, the heart muscle will not be getting sufficient blood and oxygen. If the person is unconscious, place them in the recovery position. If the individual is conscious, help them to breathe by helping to sit up and loosening clothing. Call for help at once.

If the person is known to have a heart condition, their GP may have prescribed tablets or a spray of the drug glycerine trinitrate. This drug acts by helping the arteries that bring blood to the heart to expand, which improves the supply of blood to the heart.

Check if any of the patients in the home where you work are known to have a heart condition. If anyone has been prescribed glycerine trinitrate by a GP find out how this is given in an emergency before the emergency occurs.

Bleeding

Bleeding can be caused by a fall. If the patient is bleeding, remain calm. A clean towel or item of clothing can be applied to the wound and pressure applied to control bleeding. A sterile dressing pack can be fetched when help arrives, and the wound can be cleaned and examined to decide what further treatment is required.

Suspected fractures

A fracture is the medical term for a broken bone. The commonest fractures in older people are fractures of the femur (thigh bone), hip or wrist. In all fractures there is acute pain around the site of the injury, there may be swelling or redness around the injury, and the joint may be in an odd position.

The clinical features of a leg fracture are outlined in Box 2.1 and illustrated in Fig. 2.7. Notice in particular that the affected limb appears shorter and twists outwards (external rotation).

Box 2.1 Clinical features of leg/hip fracture

- Inability to weight bear
- Inability to walk
- Shortening (check if knees line up using a ruler)
- External rotation (see Fig. 2.7)
- Groin pain
- Thigh pain
- Unable to raise leg straight
- Tenderness over hip joint
- Increase in size of greater trochanter on affected leg

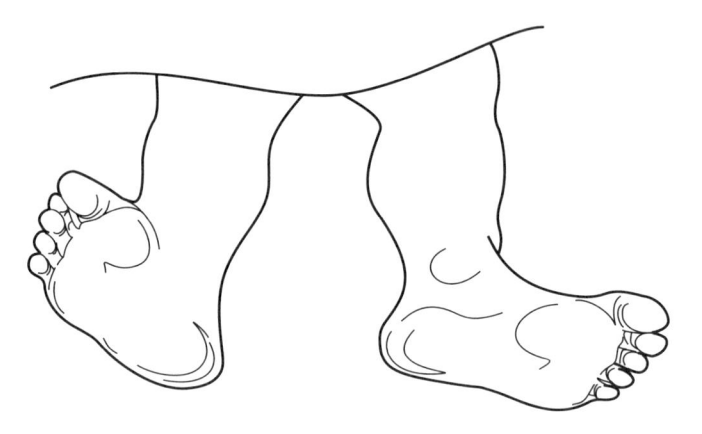

Figure 2.7 Features of leg fracture.

Action if fracture is suspected

Do not move the person if you suspect a fracture. If the person is bleeding, apply direct pressure to the wound to control bleeding. Make the person as comfortable as possible, covering them with a blanket. Do not give the person anything to eat or drink, as emergency surgery may be required. Call for an ambulance as the person needs to be diagnosed and treated in hospital.

Burns and scalds

Burns are caused by dry heat; scalds are caused by hot liquids. The treatment of burns and scalds is the same. The aims of first aid are to:

- Stop the pain
- Relieve pain and swelling
- Prevent infection.

You should:

- Assess the severity of the burn and call for professional help
- Place the burnt area under cold running water for at least ten minutes
- If the hand has been burnt remove rings and watches if possible
- Do not try to remove clothing which may be stuck to the skin
- Do not apply any creams to the burn
- Do not burst blisters
- Do not apply a dressing to the burn – this may stick and cause further damage
- If the burn is severe the skin can be wrapped in clingfilm or placed in a clean plastic bag until help arrives.

Learning more about first aid

All care assistants should have some basic knowledge of first aid. Sometimes it is possible to take a first-aid course as part of your NVQ training. If you are working in a residential home in a senior capacity, you will require training to equip you with the skills needed to cope in an emergency. Care assistants working in nursing homes may also benefit from such training. The St John Ambulance run first-aid courses locally and further details can be obtained from:

Medical Department
St John Ambulance
27 St John's Lane
London EC1M 4BU
Telephone: 08700 10 49 50
Website: http://www.sja.org.uk/

Summary

Staff working in homes should aim to provide an environment that is as safe as possible for older people. There is, however, no such thing as a 'safe' environment. Staff should work with older people and support them in living their lives as they wish. Many homes have policies that help determine the risk of people falling or having accidents. Accidents should be recorded and where possible action should be taken to prevent similar accidents occurring.

Portfolio preparation

Your assessor must have evidence that you can meet the performance criteria for this unit. Before beginning this unit, discuss assessment strategies with your assessor. Most of the evidence for this unit can be gained by direct observation of your work. You may be asked to provide the following types of evidence:

Products: This might be a copy of a hazard report you completed after identifying a hazard. It could be a note in a resident's notes giving details of how you dealt with an accident. It could be details of a first-aid dressing that you have applied to a colleague after an accident.

Witness testimony: This is a statement from a senior member of staff. It might be a statement detailing how you have met certain performance criteria.

Written work: You might be asked to prepare a piece of work about the factors that increase the risk of accidents occurring.

Your assessor may also use other methods to help you gain evidence for this unit. These may include:

- Verbal questioning
- Written questions
- **Simulations** to demonstrate that you have the skills to work effectively in emergencies.

Further information

Health and Safety at Work Act 1974. The Stationery Office, London. Your home will probably have a copy of the Act; if not, the local reference library or your college library will have one.

Health and Safety Executive (1974) *A Guide to the Health and Safety at Work Act 1974.* HSE Books, Sheffield.

Health and Safety Executive (1996) *Everyone's Guide to RIDDOR 95.* Single copies are available free from HSE Books, PO Box 1999, Sudbury, Suffolk, CO10 6FS, telephone: 01787 313 955.

The Health and Safety Executive produces a range of leaflets on health and safety. These include guidance on risk assessment and legal requirements. Copies can be downloaded from the HSE website or obtained by contacting:

HSE Information Centre
Broad Lane
Sheffield S3 7HQ
Telephone: 0541 545 5000
Website: http://www.open.gov.uk/hse/hsehome.htm

Fire safety: The local fire station will have a number of videos that you may find of interest. Fire brigade staff use these when giving talks to various groups.

Notes

1. Tullett S (1996) *Health and Safety in Care Homes: A practical guide*. Age Concern, London.
2. Health and Safety Executive (2003) Press release (www.hse.gov.uk/press/2003/e03072.htm).
3. Health and Safety Executive (1996) *Everyone's Guide to RIDDOR 95*. HSE Books, Sheffield.

Further reading

Counsel and Care (1993) *The Right to Take Risks*. Counsel and Care, London.

St Andrew's Ambulance Association and British Red Cross St John Ambulance (2002) *First Aid Manual*, 8th edition. Dorling Kindersley, London.

Tullett S (1996) *Health and Safety in Care Homes: A practical guide*. Age Concern, London.

Chapter Three

Developing Your Knowledge and Practice
HSC23
Develop your knowledge and practice

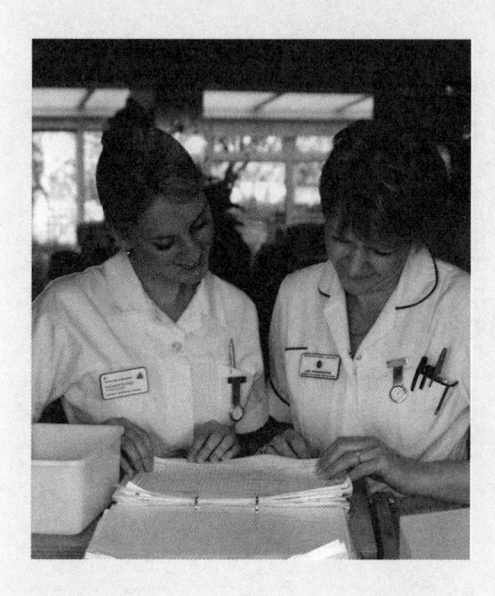

This unit consists of two elements:
HSC23a Evaluate your work
HSC23b Use new and improved skills and knowledge in your work

This chapter

- Provides information about how to assess how well you carry out activities in work
- Explains how you can encourage others to provide you with feedback on your work
- Explains how to identify your values and beliefs and understand how they may affect your work with individuals
- Provides information to help you to work with others and to identify any skills, knowledge and support required to help you develop your practice
- Explains how to develop networks and access support and information
- Provides information on how to use your new skills and knowledge in practice
- Discusses the importance of developing and reviewing how you can use your skills and knowledge in work
- Explains the legal context in which you practise and the importance of confirming that it is safe and legal for you to use certain skills
- Aims to enable you to use your new skills appropriately in work
- Provides information on the importance of working with others to evaluate how your new skills and knowledge have improved your work

How well do you carry out activities at work?

Every caring, conscientious person wants to believe that they are good at their job. Sometimes thinking about how well we do our jobs or, worse still, being evaluated, can feel very uncomfortable and threatening. It can appear threatening because if we admit that we're not very good at something then we may fear that colleagues or senior staff might think less of us. They might think that we're not very good at our jobs.

This is usually a groundless fear. Attitudes in the workplace are changing and the workplace is becoming healthier because of those changes. In the past, some organisations might have considered that staff knew everything there was to know, but such organisations are now thankfully rare. Organisations and senior people in organisations know that, if the organisation is to work well, people need to develop and grow. Most organisations now aim to be a learning organisation.

The learning organisation

In the past it was thought that the people who knew most about an organisation were the managers. People who served in restaurants or provided care were less skilled and needed to be told what to do and how to do it. J. Edward Deming, who worked with Japanese companies, did a great deal to change this sort of attitude. Deming says that the people who know about a particular service are the people who actually deliver the service. The person who serves meals in the care home knows what the problems are and usually knows how to fix them. Deming stresses the importance of empowering front-line workers to provide quality services.

They do this by working as a united team to give customers what they want. This work has been adapted by others and has led to the development of the learning organisation. In a learning organisation people acknowledge that they do not know all that there is to know. They recognise that they need to cooperate and collaborate. Learning organisations make people feel valued and enable them to give of their best. The learning organisation is built on basic principles, as outlined in Box 3.1.

The need to develop knowledge and practice

In the past, education was considered to be something we did when we were young. When we had learnt how to do our jobs we carried on doing them in the same way until we retired. This is now considered to be very poor practice because the world has changed. Our knowledge of healthcare has changed and if we are to continue to provide quality care we must continue to update our skills and knowledge throughout our careers. Expectations have also changed. In the past, shared bedrooms were

> **Box 3.1** Principles and assumptions of a learning organisation
>
> - Humans retain their childlike curiosity and drive to learn.
> - People urge themselves to ever-higher standards of quality and performance in activities that are important to them – hobbies, sports, professions – and they make much (voluntary) use of feedback data.
> - People fear, resist and deceive external evaluations by those in power.
> - All perceptions are structured by our assumptions and categories. These mental models can be surfaced, tested, revised and reframed.
> - Personal knowledge and understanding is constructed through individually processing new information – using it, discussing it, reflecting on it, etc.
> - Data is meaningless if we do not view it in context.
> - People tend to cooperate with people they see regularly, to meet their expectations, especially affirming the identity-self claimed by the other; this leads to tacit acceptance of a taboo on 'non-discussible' topics.
> - Most workers are capable of organising and planning their own work.
> - People's capabilities are vastly under-utilised in most workplaces. Their efforts to break out of those limitations are usually discouraged or punished.
> - Managers who attempt to get the most out of staff will experience resistance initially because of mistrust and barriers.

common and facilities such as en suite toilets were rare. Older people and their families did not expect the facilities and level of service that they now consider essential.

If we are to continue to provide the best possible care for older people we must become life-long learners.

Developing your knowledge and practice

The key to developing your knowledge and practice is to take a long, hard look at what you do. Think of what you do well and what you need to improve on. It's impossible to develop unless you have self-knowledge. You could try doing this at home using a table like Table 3.1.

Developing self-knowledge can be uncomfortable. Some people are all too aware of their own shortcomings and are not aware that other people also have shortcomings. Admitting that you don't know everything and developing plans to improve your skills and knowledge is a sign of strength, not of weakness.

Table 3.1 Mapping your existing knowledge.

Activity/ Skill	Can do/ Will do	Will do/ Need to learn how	Can do/ Need to develop confidence	Action

As others see us

Sometimes we are unaware of our own shortcomings although they are obvious to others. When I began a management course at university a few years ago we were asked to keep a work diary. This aimed to show our lecturer how we managed time. I'd always prided myself on being a really good time manager. Imagine my shock when my lecturer confronted me with the brutal truth. I was lousy at managing my time and had a big problem in saying 'no' to anyone. Of course it's not pleasant to be faced with the bald reality that you are not 'Miss efficient' but 'Mrs lousy time manager'. So I used the classic defence mechanism of denying the truth of her words: 'How on earth can that be true?' I said. 'Look how much I get done!' Amalia looked at me sadly – it was clear that self-awareness was some way off. 'Listen, the only reason you get so much done is because you work yourself very hard. If you were just a little bit more efficient and learnt how to say "no", life would be so much easier.' I have learnt the wisdom of her words and I do try to say 'no'; occasionally I succeed. I still work too hard but I *have* improved and I now know a little more about who I am.

All of us are a little like diamonds with many facets and sometimes we are unaware of facets of our own personality. In the 1950s two Americans, Joe Luft and Harry Ingham, were researching human personality at the University of California. They devised a way to explain these facets of personality and called it the Johari window[1] (see Fig. 3.1).

The Johari window explains these different facets of our personality.

1. The public area or 'open' quadrant contains things that are openly known and talked about – and which may be seen as strengths or weaknesses. This is the self that we choose to share with others. The knowledge that the window represents can include not only factual information, but

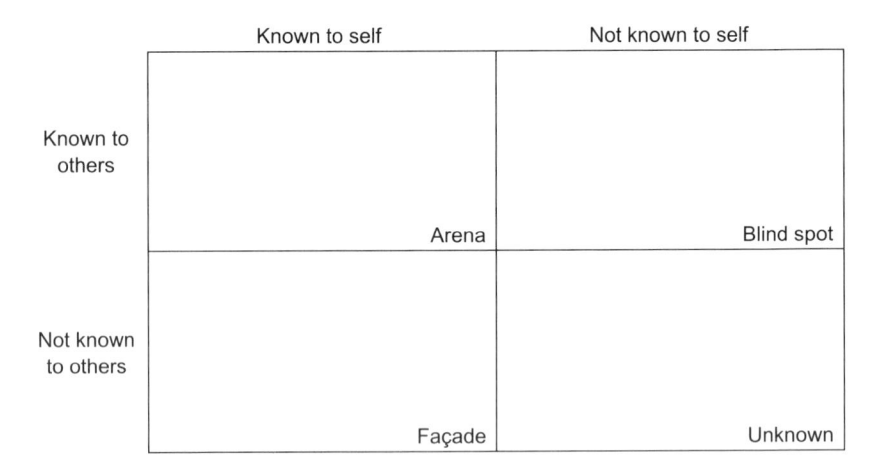

	Known to self	Not known to self
Known to others	Arena	Blind spot
Not known to others	Façade	Unknown

Figure 3.1 Johari window.[2]

also feelings, motives, behaviours, wants, needs and desires – indeed, any information describing who a person is. When we first meet a new person, the size of the opening of this first quadrant is not very large because there has been little time to exchange information. As we get to know one another, the window shades move down or to the right, placing more information into the open window, as described below.

2   The hidden or 'blind' area contains things that others observe that we don't know about. Again, they could be positive or negative behaviours, and will affect the way that others act towards us. The 'blind' quadrant represents things that you know about me, but that I am unaware of. So, I might think that I am efficient at managing time but it might be clear to you that I am not. This information is in my blind quadrant because you can see it, but I cannot. If you tell me that I'm not as efficient as I think, then the blind moves to the right, enlarging the area of the open quadrant. Now, I may also have blind spots in other things. For example, you may notice that I am wearing non-matching shoes. You may not say anything, since you may not want to embarrass me, or you may decide that I have completely lost the plot. Then the problem is, how can I get this information out in the open, since it may be affecting our relationship? How can I learn more about myself? Unfortunately, there is no readily available answer. I may notice that you keep glancing at my feet, or we may have a relationship that is open enough to enable you to tell me.

3   The unknown area contains things that nobody knows about us – including ourselves. This may be because we've never exposed those areas of our personality, or because they're buried deep in the subconscious. Being placed in new situations often reveals new information not previously known to self or others. The process of self-discovery and moving things

that we didn't know about ourselves into the open window is like Maslow's idea of self-actualisation (see page 87).

4   The private or 'hidden' area contains aspects of our self that we know about and keep hidden from others. The 'hidden' quadrant represents things that I know about myself, that you do not know. So if we become friends and learn to trust each other, I move the information in my hidden quadrant and enlarge the area of the open quadrant. This process is called 'self-disclosure', and we are only open to those whom we trust. If we do not trust people then it is best (for our own protection) to keep some things private.

Encouraging others to provide feedback on your work

It is important to examine your work and practice so that you can continue to develop. However, as you can see, it is difficult to get to know ourselves. Sometimes we delude ourselves that we're better at things than we really are. Sometimes we lack confidence in what we do and although people consider that we do something well it doesn't feel like that. Receiving feedback on our work helps us to get a full picture of our performance and to begin to build on our strengths and combat our weaknesses.

It's difficult to ask for feedback and sometimes it's even harder to hear what others have to say about us. Sometimes we don't hear what others say or distort what they say through the prism of our personality and values. Case Study 3.1 illustrates this.

Dealing with negative feedback

None of us is perfect – though sometimes we like to think we are. Our actions and inactions affect others and sometimes hurt them. When people provide critical feedback we have two main reactions: fight or flight.

Fight means that we deny that the feedback is true. We may do this pleasantly, arguing with the person: 'But how can that be true because . . .' We may do it unpleasantly by running the person down to our friends.

Flight means that we run away from what is being said. We may get upset and even cry or we may get so upset that we can't face coming into our place of work and facing the person.

Neither of these emotional reactions is helpful. It can come as quite a shock to be told something about yourself that you were unaware of. In this situation the best thing to do is say, 'This is a bit of a surprise. I was unaware of this. I'd like some time to think about it.'

You can then go away, make some notes and think things through. You can also use your informal networks to discuss these issues and obtain some support.

> **Case Study 3.1**
>
> Hannah Storey had always wanted to be a nurse. When her youngest child was 16 Hannah applied for a job at The Pines, a 30-bed care home. She worked hard, was popular with residents and staff. She was caring and her work was thorough. She worked well with others and was very enthusiastic.
>
> The home manager was very pleased with Hannah and suggested that she study for an NVQ. Hannah planned to use the NVQ qualification to enter nurse training.
>
> Then Sister Gates retired. Sister Gates had been at the home for many years and Hannah always asked for her help and advice when she was unsure. Sister O'Connor was appointed and Hannah found it difficult to ask her for advice.
>
> The home manager asked Hannah why she was having problems with Sister O'Connor when she'd got on so well with Sister Gates. Hannah replied, 'It's very difficult. Sister Gates was very experienced but Sister O'Connor is only two years older than my eldest daughter. She really can't know very much.'
>
> The home manager pointed out that Sister O'Connor was a registered nurse with several years' experience in caring for older people and asked Hannah to respect her and work with her in the way that she had done with Sister Gates.
>
> Although the home manager had been careful and gentle with Hannah and had told her that she was doing very well and that there was only one area of her behaviour that needed to be changed, Hannah was devastated. She burst into tears and felt that she'd never be good enough to be a nurse.

Informal networks

When we begin our career our informal networks are usually limited to the people we work with. As we develop we get to know others working in the same area of practice in other settings. As you are studying your NVQ your network is growing. You are probably meeting others who work in different homes and also in hospital settings. This network is valuable to you because it broadens your horizons, gives you ideas about development and provides a source of support.

Hannah Storey was at college the day after she received her upsetting feedback. She chatted about it with Janet Daley, a care assistant who had worked in a nearby home for many years. Janet and Hannah had become friends and Janet felt that she was able to tell Hannah about her 'blind side'. She explained: ' Hannah, you are really good and enthusiastic and I think that you will do well and make a great nurse but you have a problem with younger people. We have two tutors here. You get on well with

Mrs Williamson but you are a bit dismissive of Mrs Johnson. I notice that you don't pay so much attention to her and tend to argue with her.'

Hannah though about this. She was 45 years old, had brought up a family while her husband worked long hours at his business. She thought of herself as having acquired knowledge and experience as the years passed. When she thought about how she'd been in her 20s she was embarrassed by her youth and inexperience. If she was really honest then she could see how she tended to treat younger people in positions of authority more as a daughter than as an experienced fellow professional.

Hannah's values were influencing her practice.

How your values influence your practice

We are all individuals and bring our values to our practice. We have different interests, personalities and beliefs. Although we all strive to be professional, our values, personality and beliefs can influence our practice.

If, for example, you believe that people should take care of themselves and maintain good health you might deal with certain residents differently. If Mrs Jones has diabetes and needs insulin you might find yourself judging her if you discover that she is not sticking to her diabetic diet and is eating chocolate bars in her room. Although you may strive to be professional your body language might signal your disapproval of her actions. This may make it difficult for Mrs Jones to tell you about any difficulties she might have.

If you believe that people should not waste food you might find Mr Adams' complaints about the food in the home irritating. If you believe that food should be a pleasure and that it is one of the few pleasures that Mr Adams has left, you are more likely to make a special effort to ensure that he has food which tempts his jaded appetite.

All of us are entitled to have views and values. It's what makes us unique human beings. It is important to be aware of your values and to ensure that you don't impose those values on others. If, for example, you believe that people shouldn't complain and should 'suffer in silence' you may be less likely to be sympathetic to Mrs Patel when she confides that her arthritis is getting worse and that the pain makes it difficult for her to sleep at night. You might if you are unaware of your values simply reassure Mrs Patel rather than reporting her plight to a Registered Nurse who may be able to arrange for Mrs Patel to have stronger painkillers.

It's important to be self-aware. You can develop self-awareness by taking some time in a quiet place and thinking about yourself. How do you view the world? What values are important to you? Begin to think about a specific situation in your place of work. What impact did this have on you? Did it conflict with your values? If so, how did you react? Was your reaction appropriate or did you try to force your values on others? What have you learnt and how will you use what you have learnt?

Listening

Listening is a skill. You can use this exercise to show how easy it is not to hear what someone is saying.

> What did you hear 'Hannah' say?
> What did you (Janet) hear 'Hannah' say? etc. etc.
> Ask Hannah if you heard what she meant for you to hear.
> Continue to check out each message for each person.

The usual response to this exercise is: 'I know you think you heard what I said. But I'm not sure you know what I meant. Therefore, we may not be on the same page or even in the same book.'

So how can we learn to listen better? When we communicate with each other, there are two parts to the message: the content and the feelings. There are four components in listening skills:

1. Clarification
2. Paraphrasing
3. Reflecting
4. Summarising.

The first two components have to do with the content of the message. When the message you receive is unclear, vague or ambiguous, a listening response is to say: 'I'm not sure I understand. Can you clarify that for me? Do you mean that? Are you saying . . . ?' We wish to check that we're picking up the right message and also want to encourage the person we are talking with to elaborate. It sometimes takes strength and courage to ask these questions, because we may be encumbered with our own personal baggage: for example, we don't want to look stupid. When we paraphrase, we help the person focus on the key content of the message.

Reflecting has to do with the affective part of the message – the feelings. When we reflect, we restate or clarify the feelings that are being expressed. This encourages the other person to become more aware of them, to express more of them, to express them with more intensity, or more accurately.

Summarising is what ties everything together. It condenses the content and emotion of what has been said and identifies major themes of the message. It may be used to review progress in solving the problem.

Sometimes if you ask a person for advice you can learn a great deal. If, for example, a senior member of staff provides you with some critical feedback, you might ask for their advice on how to deal with the situation or improve your behaviour in certain situations. You can gain a great deal from this. You can learn what the person's expectations are. You can learn about their values and you can learn about yourself. The ability to learn from constructive criticism is valuable. You can remain true to yourself but improve how others see you and react to you.

Reflective practice

Sometimes we think about something that happened in work and think that we didn't handle a situation very well. If we could go back we'd do it differently. Reflective practice gives us the opportunity to work through situations and learn from them. There are no right or wrong ways to reflect on practice but sometimes it is helpful to use a certain approach (see Box 3.2).

> **Box 3.2** An approach to reflective practice
>
> - Be tolerant of others. There are different ways of thinking, viewing and interpreting the world.
> - Be curious. You have to be willing to ask questions and want to find out the answers.
> - Be patient. The world is not black and white. It's full of shades of grey. There are no simple solutions and 'right' answers. The solution to a problem is sometimes the 'least worst' rather than the best solution. The solution has to take into account the time, the place and the people in that time and that place. If you were to come back to those people in that place in the future the solution might be different because things change.
> - Be open and learn from this situation.
> - Be honest with yourself. Be aware and be honest about your doubts and uncertainties. Be aware of what you don't know. It's impossible to learn and to move forward if we pretend to ourselves that we know everything there is to know.

Strategies for reflection

Reflection can be difficult at first and it helps to have some formal way to reflect on practice and to record what you have learnt from this. There are two main ways to do this. You can use either a learning log or a reflective diary.

How to use a learning log

Some courses provide sheets with the main learning log headings. You can copy these and use them to keep your own log. Logs should have headings to guide your reflection. These can include the following headings:

Event/activity

Use this section to work out what happened. What was the sequence of events? What did I do? What did others do? How did I react to others? How did they react to me?

Reflection/analysis

Use this section to work out what questions this event raised for you. How did I feel? How did I act? Could I have done better? Why didn't I? What can I learn from this experience? How will I deal with such situations in the future?

Underpinning knowledge and understanding

Use this section to work out what was happening. What knowledge of theory helps me to understand this event?

Issues for future development and learning

Use this section to work out what you need to know to increase your knowledge and understanding. In this case you might have found that a resident had fallen out of bed and was injured and you did not know what to do, so you might decide that you need to learn more about first aid. Are there any unresolved issues? In this case you might feel that you panicked and did not appear competent. So you might decide to discuss this with your colleague who came to assist.

Key message

Use this section to work out what you have learnt from this and how you will change your practice as a result of it.

How to use a reflective diary

A reflective dairy is just a different way of reflecting. I prefer to use a reflective diary rather than a learning log but we are all different and as you become skilled at reflection you will work out which style of reflection best suits you.

Reflective diaries, like learning logs, should have some headings to guide you. You may find these headings helpful.

Description

Use this heading to set out what happened. Put the events in sequence.

Critical analysis

Use this section to work out what we know about the activity, what is good practice and what should happen.

Synthesis

Use this section to work out what happened in this case and why it happened in this way.

Evaluation

Use this section to talk about any issues, how they were dealt with and how you have evaluated the incident. Work out how you did, what you have learnt and what you will do in future. Identify any learning issues in this section.

Conclusion

Use this section to summarise the reflection and list any action points.

Talking things through with a colleague or learning partner

Reflection doesn't always have to be done on paper. We can learn a great deal by talking things through with a colleague whom we respect and trust or with a learning partner. In some colleges students are allocated or choose a learning partner. You can often learn a great deal and move your practice forward by discussing things with someone else who can help you to widen your perspective of the situation.

Learning from our mistakes

The only people who do not make mistakes are people who don't do anything. We all make mistakes and those mistakes are painful. What we can learn from those mistakes actually improves our practice. It also makes us better human beings because we have acknowledged that we're not perfect. We have made mistakes and we've learnt from them. Sometimes we have to make mistakes so that we can learn and go forward. One in every ten ideas is successful so that means that nine out of ten fail. Sometimes, though, we have to get it wrong before we can get it right. Some years ago I worked with my colleagues to introduce a programme in the nursing home where I worked. The aim was to increase the residents' intake of fluids and fibre and thus prevent bowel problems. I led the project and got many things wrong. It was a spectacular failure and I was quite upset at the time. I learnt so much from that failure, mostly about how not to do things, and was able to use that knowledge to successfully introduce a programme six months later. I tell everyone who's starting a project about that failure because I'm proud of it. I tried, I got it wrong, I acknowledged the failure, I learnt from it and I was able to grow in ways that would not have been possible if I'd got it right first time.

Hardly anyone gets everything in life right first time. Most of us make mistakes and if we're open to change we admit this, learn and develop. Mistakes are not a sign of failure, they are a sign of maturity and growth.

Identifying your learning needs

Care homes in England and Wales are currently regulated by the Commission for Social Care Inspection (CSCI). CSCI will merge with the Healthcare Commission in 2007. Homes in England and Wales must meet National Minimum Standards.

In Scotland homes are regulated by the Care Commission and must meet the Regulations of Care (Scotland) standards. In Northern Ireland there are similar arrangements and homes are inspected by the Social Services Inspectorate.

These standards require homes to ensure that staff have the skills and knowledge required to do their jobs. Some training, such as training in moving and handling, is statutory and the law requires that staff have regular updates.

Your learning needs will depend on what you do now and what you intend to do in the future. For example, if there are plans for the home to care for people with dementia, you may need to learn about dementia and how to care for people who have dementia. If the home plans to offer intermediate care you may need to learn about how to help people recover after illness or accident.

The best way to identify your learning needs is by using a personal development plan.

Personal development plans

Although care homes are not required to ensure that staff have personal development plans, it is considered to be good employment practice and many homes have introduced these as part of the appraisal process. If the organisation that you work for uses personal development plans then they will provide the paperwork for your personal development plan.

Figure 3.2 is an example of a personal development plan.

The personal development plan should examine different development areas. These may include practical skills, such as learning how to use a new piece of equipment, and also skills such as customer care or communication

PERSONAL DEVELOPMENT PLAN – Learning and Development Objectives

This pulls together all of your learning and development needs for the post, specific work objectives and also any career development.

Relevant dimension	What is the development need?	What will I do to develop myself in this area and how will I do this? *(Action to be taken)*	What do other people/my manager/the organisation need to do to support me? *(Action to be taken)*	What are the barriers? How can I overcome these?	How will I know that I have completed this development and that it is successful? *(Success criteria)*	Review dates

Signature of Reviewee _____ Date _____ Name of Reviewee _____
Signature(s) of Reviewer(s) _____ Date _____ Name of Reviewer(s) _____

Figure 3.2 Personal development plan.

skills. In many organisations statutory training is not included in a personal development plan because all staff will receive this training so it's not personal or individual.

Choosing suitable training

There are many ways to develop your skills. You may decide to visit another home to learn how something is done there. You may decide to read books or articles. You may ask someone in your place of work to show you how to do something, and practise until you feel confident. Sometimes certain skills are best learnt in certain ways. If you are learning a practical skill, such as taking blood, you need to learn a little theory, watch someone perform the skill and then get plenty of practice.

Sometimes there are different ways that you can gain skills and knowledge and it helps if you understand about the learning style that you prefer. We all have different learning styles.

What are learning styles?

Learning styles are simply different approaches or ways of learning. Some people are visual, auditory or tactile learners.

Visual learners

Visual learners learn through seeing. They ask to be 'shown' how to do things and say 'Yes, I see' when they understand. They need to see the teacher's body language and facial expression to fully understand the content of a lesson. They tend to prefer sitting at the front of the classroom to avoid visual obstructions (e.g. people's heads). They may think in pictures and learn best from visual displays including diagrams, illustrated textbooks, overhead transparencies, videos, flipcharts and handouts. During a lecture or classroom discussion, visual learners often prefer to take detailed notes to absorb the information. Visual learners find that they need to write things down to remember them. Visual learners tend to write themselves notes as reminders.

Auditory learners

Auditory learners learn through hearing. They say they've 'heard' about something and say 'Yes, that rings a bell' when something is familiar. They learn best through verbal lectures, discussions, talking things through and listening to what others have to say. Auditory learners interpret the underlying meanings of speech through listening to tone of voice, pitch, speed and other nuances. Written information may have little meaning until it is heard. These learners often benefit from reading text aloud and using a tape recorder. Auditory learners may repeat or paraphrase something so that they can remember it.

Tactile learners

Tactile or kinaesthetic learners learn through doing and touching. They say they 'feel comfortable' and say 'I've got it' or 'I have a handle on it' when they understand something. Tactile learners learn best by doing something. They appreciate demonstrations and practical sessions.

Your learning style may influence the way you choose to study and develop. If you are a tactile learner you might prefer to go on a study day or course that combines theory with demonstrations and practice.

Other considerations

Your circumstances also influence the way you choose to study. If you live in the country it may be difficult to travel to a study day or educational event so you might prefer to use other learning methods. If you have small children or other family responsibilities it may be difficult for you to attend study days. You might decide to use other ways to develop. You might decide that attending study days suits you best and make an extra effort to attend (see Case Study 3.2).

Case Study 3.2

Sandra Williams has four children; the youngest is aged 3. She's a farmer's wife and works part time. When Sandra found out that an interesting study day was taking place in the middle of the lambing season she didn't hesitate. She organised childcare (and extra help on the farm) and set off. She felt that this was important to her and that her husband and family could manage without her for one day.

Using your new skills and knowledge in practice

One of the hardest things about gaining new skills and knowledge is putting them into practice. Some people say that an NVQ course only proves what you already knew. I disagree. My experience of supporting NVQ students is that it opens up a whole new world to them. They benefit from an increased knowledge, and in time gain greater confidence.

A student once said to me: 'Before I did my course I did things a certain way because you'd taught me to do them that way. Now I do things a certain way because I understand the principles. Sometimes the way that you showed me doesn't always work best. I know other ways to do this now but if I use these methods how will you feel?' Annie was feeling unsure about how to act now that she knew more because when we know that there is more than one way to do things we can, for a while, feel unsure about the best way. I explained that this was an important part of her development. There was always more than one way to do a certain thing but I didn't have time to teach her every way. I had time to teach her the way that was most useful most of the time. One of the benefits of her new skills was that she could pick the right method for a particular person at a particular time. That increased knowledge and skill leads to care that is more sensitive to an individual's needs. I told her that I'd be proud as punch to see her putting her new skills into practice. Annie made me very proud and is now in her second year of student nurse education.

Staying safe and legal

The role of the care assistant is changing. In the past some care assistants performed tasks that were not considered part of their role but they did this very quietly and their work was unrecognised. Now the changing role of the care assistant is being acknowledged. Care assistants in the UK, working in hospitals, community settings and care homes, are undertaking roles that were once considered the domain of the Registered Nurse. Care assistants take blood, take ECGs, catheterise, do dressings, check blood sugars and look after people with percutaneous gastrostomy (PEG) tube feeds. There is no reason why you cannot expand your role within the home but it is important to find out what is expected of you.

The place to start is your job description. Check that it gives some indication of what you are to do. If it doesn't then arrange to meet your supervisor and ask what her expectations are. If there are plans to change your role then your job description should reflect this.

Some homes recognise the increased skills that NVQ-qualified staff have and pay a small premium for NVQ-qualified staff to reflect this. You may also require additional training to enable you to expand your role.

If your role is to change it is important to explain this to colleagues and to say that you have been asked to take responsibility for a certain task or area of work. If you are feeling nervous about this, tell them and ask them for their support and help.

Using your skills and knowledge appropriately

Care assistants are part of the nursing family and deliver nursing care on a day-to-day basis. Nursing has two components – the art and the science of nursing. There are the technical skills such as learning how to take blood and the caring, compassionate skills that enable us to make people feel that we value and care for them. It is important as we develop not to lose sight of the fact that the caring skills are just as important as the technical skills.

Evaluating how your skills and knowledge have improved your practice

It can be difficult to work out how our practice is improving because we don't stand still. We're moving and changing all the time. Healthcare doesn't stand still either: as we learn more, practice changes. One way to keep a sense of perspective is to write a list of what you want to learn and achieve. Evaluate this list every two or three months and see how you are doing. If you keep the old lists and look at them after a couple of years you'll be shocked to realise where you were then. It is always good to look back and be surprised because it shows that you are not standing still. You are moving on and developing.

Key points

- Most organisations now understand that ongoing staff development is vitally important if they are to provide a quality service.
- We need to continue our education throughout our working lives because healthcare and expectations of healthcare are changing.
- Appraisal and feedback are important aspects of self-development.
- It is important to be aware of your attitudes and beliefs and ensure that they do not affect your practice.
- Reflective practice enables you to learn from mistakes and to continue developing.
- There are many ways to continue your development. Understanding your preferred learning style helps you to choose suitable methods of continuing your professional development.

Portfolio preparation

Your assessor must have evidence that you can meet the performance criteria for this unit. Before beginning this unit, discuss assessment strategies with your assessor. Most of the evidence for this unit can be gained by direct observation of your work. This might include observing how you have developed your practice while studying for the NVQ award.

Products: This might include a reflective account of how you acted in a particular situation, what you did and why you did it, how you have learnt from this and how it has affected your practice. You might take part in a group or one-to-one discussion that reflects on practice.

Witness testimony: This is a statement from a senior member of staff. It might be a statement detailing how your practice has developed and improved.

Written work: In this unit, written work usually takes the form of a reflective diary.

Your assessor may ask questions to clarify certain aspects of your practice or to check your understanding of the reasons for working in a certain way, using:

- verbal questioning
- written questions.

Simulations are not normally permitted for any part of this unit.

Notes

1 Luft J & Ingham H (1955) The Johari window, a graphic model of interpersonal awareness. *Proceedings of the Western Training Laboratory in Group Development.* UCLA, Los Angeles, CA.
2 Luft J (1970) *Group Processes: An Introduction to Group Dynamics.* The McGraw-Hill Companies, New York.

Chapter Four

Care, Protection and Well-being of the Older Person

HSC24
Ensure your own actions support the care, protection and well-being of individuals

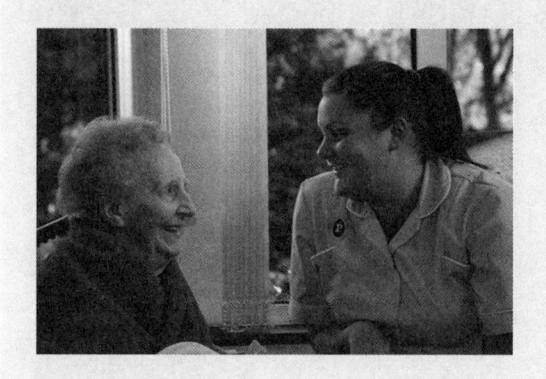

This unit consists of three elements:
HSC24a Relate to and support individuals in the way they choose
HSC24b Treat people with respect and dignity
HSC24c Assist in the protection of individuals

This chapter

- Provides information and guidance to enable you to find out an individual's needs, wishes and preferences
- Explains the importance of developing relationships with people
- Discusses how an individual's culture and background can affect choices
- Explains the importance of caring for and valuing the whole person
- Provides information on how to enable the older person to function at the highest possible level
- Explains why some older people are vulnerable to abuse
- Discusses types of abuse and how to recognise abuse
- Informs you of action to take if abuse is suspected

Importance of choosing how we live our lives

One of the best things about being an adult is that we can make choices about how to live our lives. As an adult no one tells us what to wear, what to eat, what time to go to bed or what time to get up. There are limits to our choices though. We have to be able to get up for work and to wear suitable clothing for work. Generally, however, we can make real choices about our lives most of the time. Imagine what it must be like for the older person who comes into a care home. The older person has to give up her home and move in with others. Each home has its own culture and its own routines and they may be very different from the way in which the individual wishes to live.

Everyone who provides care likes to think that the care they provide is of the highest quality, but what does it feel like for the person receiving the care? Nicholls, when writing about the NHS, stated:[1]

> 'Only when we can see through patient eyes can we be confident that we are building into organisations and systems deliverables that are meaningful for the patients at their centre.'

Reflect on practice

Make a list of the choices that you have made in the last week and think about how they have affected you. Now imagine that you live in the care home where you work. Could you have made those choices? If not, can the way the home is managed be changed so that people have more opportunities to make choices?

Human needs for well-being

Abraham Maslow, a psychologist, noticed that some needs were considered more important than others. If you are hungry or thirsty then these needs are more important than feeling well regarded by your colleagues. Maslow used these observations to create a *hierarchy of needs*. This is shown in Fig. 4.1. He outlines five layers of need: the physiological needs, the need for safety and security, the need for love and belonging, the need for esteem and the need to be fulfilled.

1   **Physiological needs:** These include the need for oxygen, water, protein, salt, sugar, calcium and other minerals and vitamins. They also include the need to maintain a pH balance (necessary for health) and body temperature, the needs to be active, to rest, to sleep, to get rid of wastes (carbon dioxide, sweat, urine and faeces), to avoid pain, and to have sex.
2   **Safety and security needs:** When the physiological needs are met, this second layer of needs takes priority. You will become increasingly

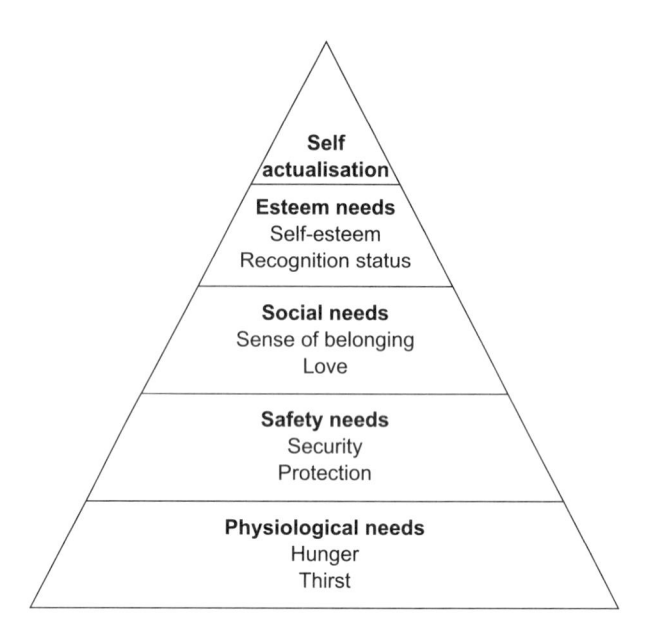

```
                    /\
                   /  \
                  / Self\
                 /actualisation\
                /──────────────\
               /  Esteem needs  \
              /   Self-esteem    \
             /  Recognition status \
            /──────────────────────\
           /     Social needs       \
          /    Sense of belonging    \
         /           Love             \
        /──────────────────────────────\
       /         Safety needs           \
      /           Security               \
     /           Protection               \
    /──────────────────────────────────────\
   /         Physiological needs            \
  /               Hunger                     \
 /                Thirst                      \
/──────────────────────────────────────────────\
```

Figure 4.1 Maslow's hierarchy.[2]

interested in finding safe circumstances, stability and protection. You might develop a need for structure, for order, some limits. The older person living in a care home who has physiological needs met may wish to have a nice room, to feel secure and know that staff will reliably meet their needs.

3 **Love and belonging needs:** When physiological needs and safety needs are met, we turn our attention to third-layer needs. You begin to feel the need for friends and people who care for you and to feel that you belong to part of a community. The older person living in a care home may wish to have visits from family and friends, may want to develop friendships within the home and to feel part of the community in the home.

4 **Esteem needs:** When lower needs have been met we turn our attention to self-esteem. Maslow noted two versions of esteem needs, a lower one and a higher one. The lower one is the need for the respect of others, the need for status, fame, glory, recognition, attention, reputation, appreciation, dignity, even dominance. The higher form involves the need for self-respect, including such feelings as confidence, competence, achievement, mastery, independence and freedom. This is the 'higher' form because, unlike the respect of others, once you have self-respect, it's a lot harder to lose. The older person living in a care home may wish to feel that staff and fellow residents respect her. She may wish to feel that she is competent in certain things and that her achievements are recognised and appreciated.

Maslow calls all of the preceding four levels **deficit needs**, or **D-needs**. If you don't have enough of something – i.e. you have a deficit – you feel the need. But if you get all you need, you feel nothing at all! In other words, they cease to be motivating. We don't seek out food if we're not hungry and we don't feel the need to be respected if we are respected. We just accept that we are respected.

Treating people as individuals

Older people are not all the same. Older people come from a variety of cultures and from different social classes. This affects their lifestyle and expectations of care. It is also important not to make assumptions about a person's lifestyle on the basis of limited information. Mrs Cohen may be an orthodox Jew who eats a strict kosher diet or she may be non-observant and fond of bacon sandwiches. Mrs Walsh may be Irish but that doesn't necessarily mean that she is a practising Catholic.

Maslow suggests that we can ask people for their *philosophy of the future* – what would their ideal life or world be like? – and obtain significant information as to what needs are unmet. Our perception of how we are meeting a person's needs may be different from that person's perception.

Staff working in care homes are in a unique position. The people they care for remain in the home for a long time and you have the opportunity to get to know the person well and to meet individual needs in a way that is not possible in settings such as hospitals where the average length of stay is measured in days.

The easiest way to find out how an individual would like to be treated is to ask them. It's important to record a person's preferences so that others can also meet the individual's needs. Important aspects of care for older people are:

- How the person is addressed
- What the person eats (or does not eat)
- What the person wishes to wear
- Respecting the person's daily routine.

Addressing older people

It is important to ask the older person how he or she wishes to be addressed. If you address Miss Smith, a retired schoolteacher, by her first name without asking if she is happy with this she may consider that you are being over-familiar or even treating her as though she were a child. Mrs David, on the other hand, may think you are being too formal if you don't call her by her first name, Maggie.

Dietary preferences

A person may eat a specific diet because of religious, cultural or medical reasons but may also have specific dietary preferences. The person may eat a traditional English diet but dislike offal or onions. If the person is able to communicate effectively then she can choose food that meets dietary preferences. If the person has communication problems it's important to note their dietary preferences so that you respect preferences and the person is able to enjoy their food.

Clothing

Clothing says a lot about us, who we are and how we want to be seen. Many people living in care homes are no longer able to get out to choose new clothes because of limited mobility. Relatives and staff may choose clothing that they consider comfortable, but how does Mr Johnson, who always wore tailored trousers, a shirt and tie, feel about wearing tracksuit bottoms and a polo shirt?

We can enable older people to choose clothing in a number of ways. Some companies will visit homes with a selection of clothes so that the older person can choose clothing. It is also possible to buy clothes by mail order or over the internet so that the older person can still make choices about what to wear.

Respecting the older person's routine

When we live at home we can decide what to do and when to do it. In care homes this might be more difficult because of staffing levels and other considerations. If we are to respect an individual's choices we have to communicate effectively and work together (Case Study 4.1).

Sometimes it's not possible to get exactly what we want in life and we have to make compromises (Case Study 4.2).

Enabling people to fulfil their potential

Older people are admitted to care homes at a low ebb. Acute illness, worsening illness or the inability of family to provide care can lead to admission. The person may have had a stroke or have made an incomplete recovery following a fall and fracture. The person may grieve for lost abilities and feel that she is totally dependent on staff. This can become a self-fulfilling prophecy if staff do not offer active support that enables the person to function to capacity.

Case Study 4.1

Mr Sterling is a retired actor. He worked in the theatre for over forty years. Normally he rises at 11 am, has breakfast and begins his day.

Mr Sterling has recently been diagnosed as diabetic and has been prescribed insulin injections twice a day. His doctor has prescribed the first injection of insulin at 7:30 am and Mr Sterling is expected to have breakfast at 8 am. Mr Sterling says that he has no intention of waking before 11 am as it is 'totally uncivilised'. Mr Sterling has every right to make decisions about when he wakes and eats – how could you balance his need to make choices about his life with the need to control his diabetes?

In Mr Sterling's case his doctor was aware that he was a retired actor but had no idea that he was a late riser. When the doctor was informed of the problem he adjusted the insulin timing to take account of Mr Sterling's lifestyle.

Case Study 4.2

When Mrs Mason entered the home she requested a bath at night. She found that a hot bath eased the pain of her arthritis and helped her to sleep.

Mrs Mason wanted to have a bath at 10 pm and then to be assisted to bed. Unfortunately this was difficult for staff at the home because Mrs Mason needed someone with her while she bathed and she liked a long soak. Staff were busy helping other residents to bed at this time. A compromise was reached and Mrs Mason agreed to bathe at 11 pm when staff were less busy.

The older person may have lost some ability but often much remains. The challenge is to enable the person to succeed at some things. The older person may feel that she is surrounded by people who are competent (the staff) and that she is incompetent and reliant on staff for all care. It is often possible to enable people to regain skills or to retain some skills and to meet self-esteem needs by retaining as much independence as possible. Assessment, goal setting and care planning help you to offer support when it is needed but not to offer care that disables.

If the person is having difficulty dressing it may be possible to help the person to dress independently by helping her to choose clothing that meets her individual style but is easier to get on and off. Blouses with square armholes, for example, are easier to put on than those with tighter armholes. It may be possible for an older woman who struggles to put on a skirt with a zip and buttoned waistband to dress independently if she wears wrapover skirts or skirts with elasticated waists.

In recognising the uniqueness of each human being we can enable people to communicate their needs and treat the person with dignity and respect.

Elder abuse

Adult abuse was first identified by Robert Butler in 1969[3] when he outlined cases of older people being abused by those who were close to them. In recent years our understanding of adult abuse and how to detect it has grown.

What is abuse?

There is no legal definition of abuse.[4] It has been defined as:

> The systematic maltreatment, physical, emotional or financial, of an elderly person. This may take the form of physical assault, threatening behaviour, neglect, abandonment or sexual assault.

> A single or repeated act or lack of appropriate action occurring in a relationship where there is an expectation of trust, which causes harm or distress to an older person.[5]

> Violation of an individual's human or civil rights by any other person or persons.[6]

It can be difficult for care assistants to work out what is and is not abuse. Registered nurses are often unsure because there is no requirement to teach student nurses about abuse.[7] Sometimes staff think that abuse is about broken bones and bruises, but this is only one aspect of abuse.[8] Many different types of abuse have been identified. These include:[9]

- physical
- sexual
- psychological/emotional
- financial/material
- neglect and acts of omission
- social
- institutional
- discriminatory.

The most common type of abuse reported is verbal abuse; physical and financial abuse are the next most common types of abuse. The least common type of abuse is sexual abuse.[10]

Physical abuse

Information from the charity Action on Elder Abuse indicates that older women are more likely to experience physical abuse than older men.[11] Box 4.1[12, 13] provides indicators of physical abuse.

Physical abuse ranges from deliberately hitting and hurting the older person through to neglect. The person abused may be hit or slapped. She may be handled roughly and may develop bruises on forearms and shins as a result. She may be pulled or pushed.

> **Box 4.1** Indicators of physical abuse
>
> - Unexplained injuries, cuts, bruises, tears
> - Signs of overmedication
> - Quiet and withdrawn
> - Nervous and eager to please
> - Poor hygiene
> - Poor diet
> - Insufficient fluids, may be very dehydrated
> - Isolation
> - Aids are forgotten or lost

Psychological abuse

Psychological abuse is shouting, swearing, laughing at, humiliating, ignoring or frightening an older person. The abused person can be bullied, isolated and denied basic rights such as the right to privacy and dignity. Psychological abuse can affect the older person to just as great an extent as physical abuse. Staff should be sensitive to the older person's feelings, as a thoughtless comment can cause great offence to an older person living in the home.

Financial abuse

Information from the charity Action on Elder Abuse indicates that older men are more likely to experience neglect and financial abuse than older women.[14] The indicators of financial abuse are outlined in Box 4.2.[15,16]

> **Box 4.2** Indicators of financial abuse
>
> - Insufficient money to pay bills etc.
> - Insufficient money for food and basics
> - A 'disappearing' pension
> - Sudden and/or large withdrawal from bank
> - Inadequate clothing
> - Reluctance of person controlling funds to pay for replacement clothes or other necessities
> - Legal documents requiring signature

Financial abuse is stealing an older person's money or belongings. The abuse may be carried out by a member of staff, a member of the family or a 'friend'. The older person may be duped into signing papers giving access to savings or property. She may be asked to give valuable jewellery to a carer, relative or 'friend' for safekeeping.

Older people who have their nursing home fees met by the local authority receive a 'personal allowance'. In some circumstances either relatives or staff members may defraud the older person of this money. Financial abuse includes theft of an older person's money, valuables or possessions. Good record keeping including keeping receipts for items bought for the older person protects staff from allegations of financial abuse and enables homes to detect theft if it occurs.

Sexual abuse

Sexual abuse is the least common form of elder abuse, however it can and does happen. It is important to be aware of such cases. Male staff in care homes have been convicted for sexually abusing residents.[17] The indicators of sexual abuse are outlined in Box 4.3.[18]

Sexual abuse is forcing an older person to take part in any sexual activity without consent. Sexual abuse occurs when an older person is involved in sexual activities to which they have not consented or, if they are in a confused state, do not truly comprehend. Sexual abuse includes inappropriate touching, fondling, kissing, oral contact, genital contact, digital penetration, rape, and being forced to watch videos or read pornographic magazines. Residents can be sexually abused by staff, other residents, relatives or visitors.

Box 4.3 Indicators of sexual abuse

- Changes in behaviour (e.g. more withdrawn, depressed, confused, fearful, agitated)
- Difficulty in walking or sitting; torn, bloody or stained underclothes
- Pain or itching in the genital area
- Bruising or bleeding in external genitalia, vaginal or anal areas
- Unexplained repeated bouts of cystitis
- Venereal disease
- Sexualised behaviour

Neglect

An older person may neglect herself because of illness or frailty.[19] However, there have been disturbing reports of neglect in hospitals[20, 21, 22]

> **Box 4.4** Indicators of neglect
>
> - Weight loss
> - Unkempt appearance, dirty clothing, poor hygiene
> - Pressure ulcers
> - Problems with continence
> - Inadequate nutrition and hygiene
> - Inadequate or inappropriate medical treatment
> - Leaving the person in a wet or soiled bed

and care homes. In these reports the older person's basic needs have not been met. A person's meal is served but no one helps her to eat. Some of the indicators of neglect are outlined in Box 4.4.[23]

Neglect is also referred to as passive abuse. The older person's needs may be unmet: the call bell may be 'dropped' on the floor out of the person's reach; the walking frame may be too far away for the person to reach it. These acts effectively cut the person off and prevent her from moving around or calling for help.

Aids that the older person depends on may be 'lost' or the person may not be able to reach them without help: without a hearing aid, the person cannot hear; without glasses, she may be unable to see; and without teeth, she will have great difficulty eating. The individual may not be helped to wash or bathe. In some cases people are left in nightclothes during the day or dressed in shabby, soiled clothing. The person who requires help to eat or drink may not receive it and may become dehydrated and ill as a result. Neglect affects a person emotionally and physically.

Sometimes neglect occurs because staff have not received sufficient training and have not developed the skills required to help care for the older person. In other cases, staff do not receive sufficient supervision and support. But even in the best of environments, where staff are well educated and supported, abuse can occur. That is why it is so important that homes have procedures to detect abuse quickly.

Abuse of medications

Abuse of medications may occur when staff are unable to meet the person's needs and ask medical staff to prescribe sedatives. The older person who is wandering around the home upsetting other residents has a reason for wandering. Educated staff who are aware of this will try to find out the reason. The older person may be hungry, cold, searching for a book or a handbag, or may simply be bored. Giving a sedative solves nothing. The person will continue to walk around because his needs remain unmet.

Now, however, because he has been sedated he is at greater risk of falling and injuring himself. Professionals are increasingly aware that prescribing sedatives in an attempt to control behaviour can lead to many problems. Sedatives are prescribed less often than before. Staff need to observe people who are prescribed sedatives carefully. Sedatives can build up in the body gradually and the person can become too drowsy to eat, drink or function normally. If you notice such symptoms, report them immediately.

Abuse from other residents

Residents can abuse other residents in the home. This abuse can take many forms. It ranges from ignoring or 'putting down' an individual, to bullying, theft and physical or sexual abuse. You need to be aware that this can occur and report any suspicions you have to your manager.

How common is abuse?

A recent report suggested that up to half a million older people may experience abuse.[24] Although there are lots of estimates on the prevalence of abuse we simply do not know how common it is. Research data is limited[25, 26] and tends to be carried out on specific groups of older people.[27] Older adults who experience abuse may not recognise it as abuse or they may be unable or unwilling to tell people about it. We do know that it is a significant and often hidden problem.[28]

Where does abuse take place?

Research based on calls to the helpline at Action on Elder Abuse indicate that most abuse takes place in an older person's own home[29] (see Fig. 4.2). However the Nursing and Midwifery Council (NMC), the body that regulates registered nurses, reports that 37% of professional conduct cases completed in October 2005 involved the maltreatment of older people. Most of these related to nursing homes. The NMC now intends to compile detailed statistical evidence on elder abuse brought together from completed fitness-to-practice hearings.[30]

Who abuses?

The older person is most likely to be abused by his or her own family (see Fig. 4.3). The next most common group of abusers are paid carers. Men are statistically more likely to abuse than women.[31]

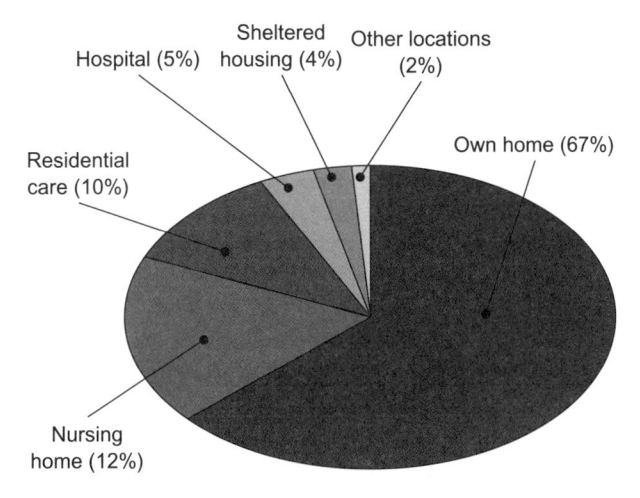

Figure 4.2 Settings of abuse of older people (based on approx. 10 000 calls reporting abuse to Action on Elder Abuse between 1997 and September 2003).

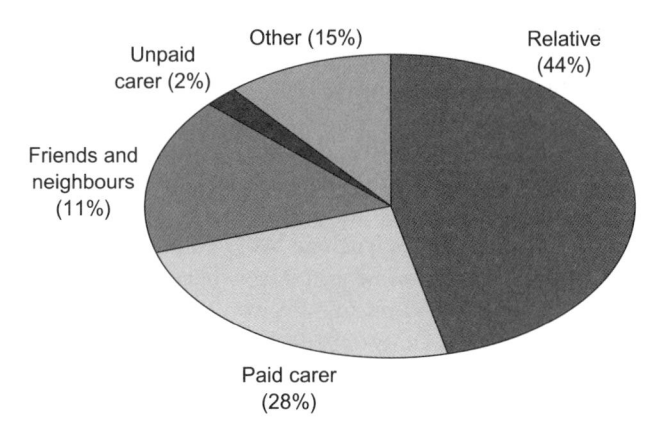

Figure 4.3 People who abuse older people.

Who is abused?

Abuse in caring situations has been recognised for some time. Abuse is rare in settings where people are alert. It occurs more frequently when staff are caring for people who are unable to protect themselves or to protest. A profile of the typical abused person is outlined in Box 4.5.

Research has shown that older people living in homes who require high levels of care are particularly at risk. Older people who are 'difficult' and whom staff find it a strain to care for are at risk. People who have communication problems are at greater risk of abuse than those who are able to communicate and build relationships with staff. People with

> **Box 4.5** Profile of the abused person
>
> - Female
> - Over 80 years old
> - Physically dependent on staff
> - Requiring high levels of care
> - May have communication problems
> - May be confused

communication problems are more vulnerable to abuse because they are usually unable to report the abuse.

Why abuse can occur in homes

Abuse within homes is completely unacceptable. It is more likely to occur in poorly managed homes; in homes where there are insufficient staff to meet older people's needs, staff are under greater pressure. In some homes, staff are expected to give care they have not been trained to give and may find themselves 'out of their depth'. In other homes, staff may feel that they cannot turn to registered nurses or their manager for help and advice. In some homes, carers do not receive sufficient supervision.

Older people now living in care homes are more acutely ill than before and require greater amounts of care. In many homes training and education programmes (such as NVQ courses) have been introduced. Abuse is more likely to occur in homes where staff feel overworked, unsupported and unable to cope and receive little training and education. It is important though to be aware that abuse can happen in even the best-run homes. The home may, despite checks, inadvertently employ someone with a history of carrying out abuse. The home may admit a resident who has been abused at home by a relative or 'friend'; if staff are not alert this abuse may continue unchecked in the home.

What systems exist to protect vulnerable adults?

At present Protection of Vulnerable Adults (POVA) legislation aims to protect vulnerable adults. Now a vetting and barring scheme has been introduced to provide fuller protection.

Protection of vulnerable adults legislation (POVA)

Government response to concerns about abuse of vulnerable adults was to set up a working group at the Department of Health. The group produced a paper, *No Secrets*, and made recommendations to protect vulnerable adults.[32] These recommendations led to Directors of Social Services being required to develop local codes of practice with health and voluntary sector partners. These arrangements were to include an emphasis on prevention and robust measures to address suspected or actual abuse.[33] In April 2004 the Protection of Vulnerable Adults (POVA) scheme was introduced.[34]

Aims of POVA

In the past vulnerable adults have been abused by people who have been supposed to protect and care for them. There have been cases of nurses removed from the register who went on to work as care assistants. The introduction of Criminal Records Bureau checks only identified people who had been *convicted* of abuse. POVA aims to add an extra layer of protection to the employment process. It aims to ban people who have harmed vulnerable adults or placed them at risk of harm from working with them.

How POVA works

Two POVA lists are held, provisional and confirmed. When a person is on the provisional list and a POVA check is made, the employer will be informed that the person cannot be employed. If the person is on the confirmed list the employer will be informed that the person cannot be employed and the police will be informed that an offence may have been committed.

If the employer receives allegations of abuse, the disciplinary policy is used to investigate. The employer notifies the Commission for Social Care Inspection (CSCI) and the local authority adult protection scheme of actions and outcome. If the outcome of employer's investigation and/or the adult protection scheme is that abuse is proven, the employer must notify the Secretary of State for Health. Referral does not mean automatic inclusion on the POVA list. The Secretary of State writes to the employer and to the individual. The individual has 28 days to reply. If no reply, the Secretary of State makes a decision. A person confirmed on the list has the right to appeal to the Care Standards Tribunal. If the Care Standards Tribunal upholds the decision, then further appeals are only possible on points of law.

The manager's responsibilities

Employers are required to check with the Criminal Records Bureau (CRB) before employing staff. CRB Disclosures are made under the Police Act

1997. A disclosure is a document containing information held by the police and government departments. Disclosures are provided by the CRB, an executive agency of the Home Office. There are currently two types of disclosure – standard and enhanced. A standard disclosure gives details of criminal convictions, cautions, reprimands and warnings held on the police national computer. An enhanced disclosure may also include relevant information held by local police forces. A POVA check is available with either type of disclosure.

POVA was introduced on 26 July 2004 and is not retrospective. This means that organisations are required to check people who join the organisation after this date or people who move from a non-care to a care position within an organisation.

POVA legislation applies to people working in care homes and domiciliary care. It does not cover NHS organisations or private hospitals. A new system of vetting and barring is being introduced. This will cover all people working in a care capacity with vulnerable adults.

Employers must also refer a care worker to the Secretary of State in the following circumstances:

- The employer has dismissed the worker on the grounds of misconduct that harmed or placed at risk of harm a vulnerable adult. This dismissal might not be related to employment.
- The worker has resigned, retired or been made redundant in circumstances such that the provider would have dismissed him, or would have considered dismissing him, on such grounds if he had not resigned, retired or been made redundant.
- The provider has, on such grounds, transferred the worker to a position which is not a care position.
- The provider has, on such grounds, suspended the worker or provisionally transferred him to a position which is not a care position but has not yet decided whether to dismiss him or to confirm the transfer.

The role of CSCI

The Commission for Social Care Inspection and the Care Standards Inspectorate for Wales have the statutory power to refer individuals to the Secretary of State for inclusion on the POVA list.

CSCI may make referrals to the POVA list when they come across evidence of misconduct that has not been referred to the Secretary of State by the employer. This might apply where registered persons themselves warrant referral for inclusion on the POVA list (for example, because the provider is directly concerned in care provision).

Providers of care (and employment agencies and businesses) have the primary duty under the Act for referring care workers to the POVA list as and when required, rather than CSCI. Failure to fulfil this statutory duty may be evidence of a lack of fitness and could potentially lead to cancellation of the registration of providers of care. When abuse is reported, CSCI informs the local authority social services department.

The role of social services

Social services departments are the main agency responsible for coordinating the response to cases of alleged or suspected abuse and working with the police when they need to investigate. The guidelines emphasise a multidisciplinary approach to a complex task requiring the professional knowledge, experience and skills of a range of staff.

Adult Protection Committee

Each local authority has an Adult Protection Committee that monitors the implementation of these guidelines and develops policy and practice. The committee aims to provide guidance to local agencies and to act when a vulnerable adult is believed to be suffering abuse or neglect. The aim is to set up robust procedures to prevent abuse from taking place and to change these to prevent further incidents of abuse.

Vetting and Barring Scheme

The objective of the Vetting and Barring Scheme (VBS) is to reduce the incidence of harm to children and vulnerable adults by helping to ensure that:

- Employers get a better vetting service when recruiting people who come into contact with children and/or vulnerable adults through their work
- Those who are known to be unsuitable are barred from working with children and/or vulnerable adults at the earliest opportunity.

The Vetting and Barring Scheme will introduce online checks of people who are barred from children and vulnerable adults. It will cover all staff who work with children and vulnerable adults in all care settings. It will also cover people working in the vulnerable adult's home.

Barring

The bar will only apply to jobs that involve substantial access to children or vulnerable adults.

The bar will not cover administrative and (non-clinical) support work in health, housing and other settings. Where the bar does not apply, employers will have the discretion to employ individuals on the barred list with safeguards in place. It may be possible for some barred people to be employed safely in posts that do not involve close involvement with children or vulnerable adults.

Vetting and barring information will allow employers to think carefully about whether to employ the individual with appropriate safeguards in place.

Adult protection meetings

The key tasks of adult protection meetings are to:

- Decide what further action is necessary, if any, to investigate/assess the alleged abuse.
- Establish how the abused person can best be protected and cared for in the future. Factors leading to the abuse should be identified and a plan made to address these. The full range of support and services should be considered to meet assessed needs.
- When police proceedings are ongoing, to ensure that there is a plan to support the abused person (and her/his carer where appropriate) through them.
- To plan how the abused person can be helped to overcome the feelings aroused by the abuse.
- To assist the abused person and the person responsible for the abuse to re-establish their relationship, where this is appropriate.
- To identify a key worker (most usually a care manager) whose role it is to ensure that the decisions and plans made at the meeting are coordinated and implemented.
- To fix a date for a review meeting within three months.

How effective is legislation?

Legislation improves the protection of vulnerable adults. But it is not foolproof.[35]

It is dependent on staff and employers reporting abuse. That means that staff and employers need to be well informed about what is and what is not abuse.

POVA only covers vulnerable adults receiving care in care homes or those using domiciliary care agencies. The district nurses, care manager or podiatrist coming to the home will not have been checked under POVA. The new vetting and barring system will cover all staff.

Analysis of the first 100 referrals shows that 58% were placed on the POVA list, 8% on the provisional list and the remainder were not listed. There were fewer referrals from social services home care than might have been expected. The type of abuse was mainly physical (33%), financial (29%) and verbal/psychological (33%). Financial abuse was more common in domiciliary care. Women were more likely to be involved in financial abuse and men in physical abuse. Most of the abuse involved people caring for older people with challenging behaviour.[36]

What to do if abuse occurs

In some situations, the inexperienced care assistant may be unsure whether an older person is being abused. You may witness a colleague appearing to argue with an older person but it may be that the colleague and the older person are teasing each other. In another situation, you may feel that a colleague is refusing to help an older person, for example:

'Mary, get a wheelchair and wheel me downstairs please . . .'
'Why don't you get your walking stick and I'll walk down with you, Mr Blackburn?'

In this case the care assistant may be encouraging Mr Blackburn to maintain his independence and to continue walking. If you feel unsure in such situations, you could ask the person who is with you. Many care assistants who are new to the home do not wish to risk upsetting staff. Find someone in the home you can trust, perhaps the matron or manager, and ask, 'Does Mr Blackburn normally walk to the lounge?' You may discover that Mr Blackburn has come to the home for a period of convalescence, has lost confidence in his ability to walk, and needs support and encouragement.

In other cases, sadly, there can be no doubt that a colleague's behaviour is unacceptable and the older person is being abused. You may be on a placement or may be a new member of staff. You may fear that you will be seen as a trouble-maker and that you will suffer as a result of reporting the abuse. You cannot ignore it; you must tell someone. The older person may be unable to tell staff what is happening; they may be too frightened to speak out. If you turn a blind eye the abuse will continue and may get worse. Care homes take the issue of abuse very seriously and will have a policy on action to take if abuse is suspected. This should be in the home's procedure book. This will give you information and advice about what to do if you suspect abuse.

Normally you should ask to speak to the manager and discuss the situation. Action can then be taken. If you do not feel able to approach the manager perhaps you could send a letter or leave a note giving information about the situation. Even if you are not able to sign the note, at least you will have informed the manager. Many homes have a 'whistle blowing' policy to enable you to do this. If no action is taken you can contact CSCI.

You can inform CSCI of your concerns; your call will be in complete confidence and the inspection unit will investigate. Even if you do not wish to leave your name, the call will still be treated seriously. You can, if you prefer, inform the person's care manager of the situation. You may wish to call a helpline for advice and support. Details of these are given at the end of the chapter.

Preventing abuse

The way a home is managed can make abuse more or less likely to occur. In homes where older people are respected and treated with dignity and respect, the possibility of abuse is reduced. In this atmosphere older people and their families will have developed a good relationship with the manager and staff and will be able to raise concerns. Listening to and communicating with older people individually and at regular patient meetings will help prevent abuse or detect it quickly.

A home where staff are supported and supervised will prevent staff from feeling 'useless', 'out of their depth' and reaching the end of their tether because they are unable to cope with certain situations. A programme of staff education and training helps all staff to develop a greater understanding of the needs of older people. An educational programme helps staff to feel valued, and increased knowledge leads to improved care. In many homes where older people have been neglected the main problem has been that the staff did not know how to meet the needs of older people. In homes where abuse has occurred unchecked, staff morale is poor, many staff have had no training for many years and management has been ineffective.

The home should have a series of procedures in place that help to detect signs of abuse quickly.

Caring for older people who are confused

It can be more difficult to treat people who are confused in the way that they wish because it is difficult to find out the person's wishes. Older people who are confused may be more at risk of abuse than other residents.

Staff may find caring for confused residents less rewarding and more exhausting. This section deals with the causes of confusion and aims to enable you to provide sensitive care to people who are confused. This reduces behavioural problems and the risk of abuse developing.

It is easy to label older people as confused. Some years ago, a nurse who was studying for a qualification in care of older people conducted a survey on how older people are treated. She went shopping and got on buses. When she lost her way and asked for help people were helpful. When she misheard, people repeated what they had said. Then, wearing make-up and a wig so that she looked old, she did exactly the same things. People were less helpful and treated her as a confused old lady, not because of her behaviour but because of her age.

As adults we are allowed to mishear, misunderstand or be absent-minded, but older people who behave in the same way can quickly be labelled as confused. People who have difficulty in communicating can easily be wrongly labelled as confused. The deaf person who understands only part of the conversation may be thought confused. The person who has suffered a stroke and who uses the wrong word may be thought of as confused. It is important that staff listen to the older person and make sure that the person is not having difficulty in communicating, before deciding that they are confused. Chapter 1 gives details of how to communicate with people who have communication difficulties.

Causes of confusion

Confusion is not a disease, it is a symptom. The first sign of illness in many older people is that they become confused. If this happens, you should ask a registered nurse or doctor to see the person and to find out the cause of the confusion. There is often a physical cause for sudden confusion. Many people who become confused will recover if the cause of the confusion is treated; however, there is no cure for dementia at present. Some of the causes of confusion are listed in Table 4.1.

Table 4.1 Some causes of confusion.

Type of cause	Cause
Physical	Infection, e.g. chest infection
	Metabolic causes, e.g. thyroid disease
	Electrolyte imbalance, e.g. dehydration or low sodium levels
	Oxygen lack
	Physical trauma
Medication	Sleeping tablets
	Some painkillers
	Drugs used to treat incontinence
	Tranquillisers
	Antidepressants
	Diuretics (water tablets)
	Digoxin
	Drugs to treat Parkinson's disease
Sensory	Poor eyesight
	Poor hearing
Environmental	Moving to new environment
	Poorly designed environments

Treatment of physical causes of confusion

Infection can cause confusion. If the infection is caused by a virus (such as the flu virus), antibiotics will not help. Antibiotics are only effective in treating bacteria. There are two main types of bacteria, known as gram negative and gram positive because of their appearance under the microscope. Certain antibiotics are only effective in treating gram-negative or gram-positive bacteria. Other antibiotics are effective in treating diseases caused by both gram-negative and gram-positive bacteria; these are known as broad-spectrum antibiotics.

In recent years more of the bacteria that cause infections in older people living in homes have become resistant to the more commonly used antibiotics. If the bacteria are resistant to the antibiotic, the antibiotic will not cure the infection. Many homes now have policies to prevent the spread of infection. These often include the taking of specimens to ensure that the correct antibiotic is used. The person with a suspected urine infection would have a specimen of urine sent to the microbiology laboratory, where the staff would check for the presence of infection and advise the doctor on the most effective antibiotic to use.

If diabetes is suspected, investigations will be carried out and treatment given. This may include insulin injections or tablets or, if the diabetes is mild, a diabetic diet.

If thyroid disease is present a blood sample will be sent to check the level of thyroid hormone, and tablets containing the hormone thyroxine will be given if required.

If the person is thought to be suffering from Parkinson's disease the doctor will examine them and prescribe medication to treat the disease. This is usually very effective in the early stages of the disease. If anaemia has caused confusion this will be investigated. Any disease which has caused the anaemia will be treated. Iron tablets will normally be prescribed, and the older person will be encouraged to eat a diet rich in iron. An imbalance in the chemicals in the blood (known as electrolytes) can cause confusion. This imbalance may be caused by medication such as diuretic tablets, diarrhoea, overuse of laxatives or prolonged vomiting. Any imbalance will be treated.

If medication has caused the confusion, the person's doctor will alter the medication. If head injury has caused confusion, urgent hospital treatment will be required. If depression has caused the person to become confused, the doctor may prescribe antidepressant tablets.

Dementia may also cause confusion. There is no cure for dementia at present. Dementia is the name used for a group of diseases affecting brain function. There are two main types: multi-infarct dementia and Alzheimer's disease.

Multi-infarct dementia

Multi-infarct dementia is thought to be responsible for 20% of all cases of dementia. A small clot interrupts the blood supply to an area of the brain, and this leads to the death of an area of brain tissue and is known as an infarction. Many of these small infarctions cause brain tissue to die and the person loses the ability to remember and reason.

Multi-infarct dementia is more common in men, because it is a disease of the arteries supplying the brain. Men are more at risk of arterial disease than women, who are protected from the effects of arterial disease by female hormones that are produced until the menopause. Women of the older generation are less likely to have smoked than men and smoking increases the risk of arterial disease. People with multi-infarct dementia often have other arterial problems such high blood pressure (hypertension) or heart disease and problems such as angina. People can deteriorate suddenly and then stay at that level until another brain infarction occurs.

Medical treatment aims to prevent or reduce the number of infarcts that will cause brain damage. If the person's blood pressure is high, this will be treated. If the person is overweight, he should be encouraged to lose weight. If he smokes, he should be encouraged to give up. If the person has arterial disease, this will be treated by the doctor. Many people who suffer from multi-infarct dementia are prescribed a junior aspirin each day. Research has shown that this small dose of aspirin helps prevent blood clots forming and greatly reduces the risk of further brain infarction.

Alzheimer's disease

Alzheimer's disease is named after a German neurologist who first described the disease at the beginning of the last century. The cause of Alzheimer's disease is not known. There have been many theories over the years but none has been proved. It is known that the number of people suffering from Alzheimer's disease increases with age. Research has shown that 25% of all people over the age of 85 suffer from dementia, and that 80% of those people suffer from Alzheimer's disease.

Alzheimer's disease is a gradual slow deterioration of mental function; memory loss is the first sign. The person has difficulty in learning new things but old memories are retained: the person remembers family but may forget about the new grandchild who was born recently; old skills and habits are retained but the person can easily become lost in new places.

Caring for people with dementia

Dementia is a progressive disease. People with dementia have a vast range of abilities. In the early stages of dementia, the individual may be forgetful, have difficulty handling money or remembering what is for lunch. In the advanced stages, the individual may be unable to recognise her daughter or her own face in the mirror. She may be unable to wash, dress, use the toilet, eat independently, or walk without a great deal of help from staff. Obviously, the type of care required is very different, but the aims of care remain the same.

Some people who have dementia cope well because they have a routine. This gives the day structure and the person depends on this routine to cope. It is important, if a routine is established, that everyone maintains it. If the person normally has breakfast and then bathes, dresses and has coffee in her room, a change in the routine can cause the person to become confused and disorientated.

The older person should be treated with dignity and respect. Their preferred title should be used. A retired doctor may wish to be referred to as Dr Lawson and a retired headmistress may wish to be known as Miss Anderson. Staff who use first names to address people who have been referred to all their lives by their titles deprive the older person of dignity and respect and may increase confusion.

It is easy for staff to see all confused older people as lacking in personality and to treat all people with dementia in the same way. Staff should aim to care for the individual. If the person is unable to express preferences, relatives and friends can often tell staff about the person's preferences. The woman who liked to have her hair permed and set should be encouraged and helped to maintain her usual hairstyle. The woman who preferred to wear trousers and blouses should not be discouraged from wearing these clothes just because dresses are seen as 'easier'. The person who detests fish and who is unable to request an alternative should have this noted so that she does not refuse lunch and go hungry or spend the afternoon trying to get into the kitchen to find some food. People suffering from dementia are often able to continue to perform activities that they have been doing for decades, such as washing or dressing, although they may forget the way to the dining room. You should aim to provide support and help without taking over and without encouraging the person to depend on staff for care before this is required.

If the person enters the home suffering from mild confusion and the early stages of dementia, staff can get to know the person. When the person deteriorates and is unable to communicate needs to staff, this is seldom a problem because staff know the person very well. If a person is admitted to the home with advanced dementia, it can be difficult to provide the type of care the person would prefer because staff do not know the person. Relatives and friends can be a great help in these circumstances. They can tell staff what food the person prefers, what her interests are and how she likes to dress and style her hair. Good record keeping and care planning enable all staff to treat the person as she would wish to be treated and promote well-being.

Wandering

Some older people wander around the home. This wandering can upset other residents and can make staff feel on edge. Although the older person appears to be wandering around aimlessly, they have a reason for wandering. People with dementia wander for the same reasons. Research has shown that people who wander have great difficulty in communicating their needs. It has been suggested that the person's wandering is an attempt to meet those needs.

Shouting and screaming

You may meet residents who shout, scream, or sing continually. Staff and other residents can find this behaviour difficult to cope with. A great deal can be done to help people who behave like this. You should seek professional advice. Often the person's GP will ask a nurse specialising in psychiatric nursing to see the person. The aim of treatment is first to discover the reasons for the person behaving in this way, and then to plan care to eliminate or reduce such behaviour.

Aggression

Some older people lash out and shout, hit, kick and bite. In many cases the person is confused and may be unaware of your intentions. You should do everything possible to ensure that the older person is aware of what is about to happen, for example: 'Mrs Greendale, I'd like to help you to have a bath now.' If the person understands what your intentions are and what is happening, aggression is less likely to occur. If the person refuses to bathe, dress or get up, you must not try to force the person. This is unlawful and can lead to aggression. Try leaving the person and returning a little later. The way you approach people is very important. If you have a good relationship with the person and have the right approach, problems are rarer. If a resident becomes aggressive, inform your manager.

If a person is aggressive the reasons for the aggression should be determined and care planned to avoid such incidents. Sometimes the older person is extremely aggressive and could injure staff or other residents when lashing out. Residents and staff should not be placed in this situation. If the person is very disturbed, he or she will require care from registered nurses specially trained in caring for people with mental health problems. These nurses are known as registered mental nurses (RMN). This specialist care may be given either in hospital or more usually in a specialist nursing home known as an elderly mentally infirm (EMI) home.

Conclusion

Older people are just like us. They are individuals with a range of abilities, hopes, needs and aspirations. They need, as we do, to feel safe and secure and to be treated decently and respected. Caring for older people who are confused, who appear to wander aimlessly, who scream, shout or sing, can be difficult and frustrating. The way that staff handle residents who suffer from dementia influences that person's behaviour. Staff attitudes and care can reduce or increase problems.

You may see staff treat people with dementia as if they are children. You may even be told: 'They're just babies really.' Older people with dementia are not babies and are not 'in their second childhood', but are older people suffering from an incurable disease that affects brain function. Treating such people as babies not only denies them the dignity and respect that they deserve, but also worsens problem behaviour and increases the likelihood of abuse. The likelihood of abuse is increased because staff can come to view residents as less than human. People with dementia can be seen not as people suffering from a dreadful incurable disease, but as objects. If you provide thoughtful, sensitive care and ensure that the older person is treated with dignity and respect you will find the older person responds to such care and that problem behaviour is rare.

Abuse in homes is rare. I hope that you never see it. Most staff do a wonderful job of caring for residents. I hope that throughout your career you see people treated with dignity and respect. If you do see abuse occur, you must do something to stop it.

Key points

- All human beings have a range of needs.
- Individuals have different perspectives, hopes, needs and aspirations.
- Older people are as individual as we are.
- If we are to meet the needs of the older person we must treat the person as an individual.
- Abuse of older people is a real problem.
- Abuse can take many forms.
- Abuse is less likely in homes where staff are supported and enabled to give of their best.

Portfolio preparation

Your assessor must have evidence that you can meet the performance criteria for this unit. Before beginning this unit, discuss assessment strategies with your assessor. Most of the evidence for this unit can be gained by direct observation of your work. You may be asked to provide the following types of evidence:

Products: This might be a copy of a care plan you completed showing how you met an individual's needs. It could be a note in a resident's notes giving details of how you provided individualised care. It could be details of a person's life history or food preferences.

Witness testimony: This is a statement from a senior member of staff. It might be a statement detailing how you have met certain performance criteria.

Written work: You might be asked to prepare a piece of work about the factors that increase the risk of abuse occurring.

Your assessor may also use other methods to help you gain evidence for this unit. These may include:

- Verbal questioning
- Written questions
- Simulations to demonstrate that you have the skills to work effectively in situations where a resident's behaviour is challenging.

Further information

These are national organisations that provide advice and information.

Action on Elder Abuse
Astral House
1268 London Road
London SW16 4ER
Telephone: 020 8679 2468
Website: http://www.elderabuse.org.uk

This charity provides information and leaflets including *Elder Abuse in Care Homes* and *Abuse of Elderly People: Guidelines for action*. These are available free of charge and can be downloaded or obtained by post (send a stamped, self-addressed envelope).

Age Concern (England)
Astral House
1268 London Road
London SW16 4ER
Telephone: 020 8765 7200
Website: http://www.ageconcern.org.uk/

Age Concern offers information and advice on all aspects of ageing including nursing and residential home care. You'll find a range of information, and downloadable fact sheets on their website.

Alzheimer's Society
Gordon House
10 Greencoat Place
London SW1P 1PH
Telephone: 020 7306 0606
E-mail: enquiries@alzheimers.org.uk
Website: http://www.alzheimers.org.uk

The Alzheimer's Society provides information about Alzheimer's disease for people with dementia, carers and professionals. Their website contains information on dementia including many downloadable booklets.

Counsel and Care
Twyman House
16 Bonny Street
London NW1 9PG
Telephone: 020 7241 8555 (administration and general enquiries)
Advice line: 0845 300 7585
Website: http://www.counselandcare.org.uk/

Counsel and Care offer information and advice for older people and carers. This includes advice on care homes. Their website contains information on dementia including many downloadable booklets.

Public Concern at Work
Suite 306
16 Baldwin Gardens
London EC1N 7RJ
Telephone: 020 7404 6609
Website: http://www.pcaw.co.uk/

Public Concern at Work is a legal advice centre. They offer information and support.

Notes

1. Nicholls S, Cullen R, O'Neill S & Halligan A (2000) Clinical governance: its origins and its foundations. *Clinical Performance and Quality Health Care* 8:3: 172–178. MCB University Press. (http://www.cgsupport.nhs.uk/PDFs/articles/Clinical_Governance_Origins_Foundations.pdf)
2. This figure is reproduced in numerous publications. Copyright resides with the American Psychological Association.
3. Butler RN (1969) *Testimony, Subcommittee on Retirement and the Individual*. The US Senate Special Committee on Aging. 15 July 1969. US Senate, Washington DC.
4. Neno R & Neno M (2005) Identifying abuse in older people. *Nursing Standard* 20:3: 43–47.

5 Action on Elder Abuse (1995) *What is Elder Abuse?* Action on Elder Abuse, London.
6 Department of Health (2000) *No Secrets: Guidance on Developing Multi-agency Policies and Procedures to Protect Vulnerable Adults from Abuse.* Department of Health, London.
7 House of Commons Health Committee (2004) *Elder Abuse Second Report of Session 2003–2004 Volume 1.* The Stationery Office, London.
8 Gray-Vickrey P (2001) Protecting the older adult. *Nursing Management* **32**:10: 36–40.
9 World Health Organization (2002) *Missing Voices: Views of Older Persons on Elder Abuse.* WHO, Geneva.
10 Action on Elder Abuse (2004) *Hidden Voices.* Age Concern, London.
11 Action on Elder Abuse (2004) *Hidden Voices.* Age Concern, London.
12 Decalmer P & Glendenning F (eds) (1997) *The Mistreatment of Elderly People*, 2nd edition. Sage, London.
13 Action on Elder Abuse (2005) *Indicators of Abuse.* www.elderabuse.org.uk (accessed 12 November 2005).
14 Action on Elder Abuse (2004) *Hidden Voices.* Age Concern, London.
15 Kleinschmidt KC (1997) Elder abuse: a review. *Annals of Emergency Medicine* **30**:4: 463–472.
16 Neno R & Neno M (2005) Identifying abuse in older people. *Nursing Standard* **20**:3: 43–47.
17 Hill A (2001) *Hidden plague of sexual abuse grips care homes.* http://society.guardian.co.uk/longtermcare/story/0,8150,443114,00.html
18 Garner J & Evans S (2000) *Institutional abuse of older adults.* Report CR84. Royal College of Psychiatrists, London.
19 Cooney C & Hamid W (1995) Review: Diogenes Syndrome. *Age and Ageing* **24**: 451–453.
20 Health Advisory Service 2000 (1998) *Not because they are old.* An independent inquiry into the care of older people on acute wards in general hospitals. Health Advisory Service 2000, London.
21 Help the Aged (2002) *Hospital Care: Problems in hospital care.* Help the Aged Policy Statement June 2002, Help the Aged, London.
22 Covinsky KE, Palmer RM, Fortinsky RH et al. (2003) Loss of independence in activities of daily living in older adults hospitalised with medical illness increased vulnerability with age. *Journal of American Geriatrics Society* **51**:4: 451–458.
23 Counsel and Care (2005) *Older People at Risk of Abuse.* Counsel and Care, London.
24 House of Commons Health Committee (2004) *Elder Abuse Second Report of Session 2003–2004 Volume 1.* The Stationery Office, London.
25 Penhale B (1999) Researching elder abuse: lessons for practice. In: Slater P & Eastman M (eds) *Elder Abuse Critical Issues for Policy and Practice.* Age Concern, London, pp. 1–23.
26 Community and District Nursing Association (2003) *Responding to Elder Abuse.* CDNA, London.
27 Compton SA, Flanagan P & Gregg W (1997) Elder abuse in people with dementia in Northern Ireland: prevalence and predictors in cases referred to a psychiatry of old age service. *International Journal of Geriatric Psychiatry* **12**:6: 632–635.

28   Lachs MS & Pillemer K (2004) Elder abuse. *Lancet* **364**: 1263–1272.
29   Action on Elder Abuse (2003) *Hidden Voices: Older People's Experience of Abuse*. Action on Elder Abuse, London (http://www.elderabuse.org.uk/).
30   Nursing and Midwifery Council (2005) *NMC to tackle elder abuse*. Press release, 8 November 2005. NMC, London.
31   Action on Elder Abuse (2004) *Hidden Voices*. Age Concern, London.
32   Department of Health (2000) *No Secrets: Guidance on Developing Multi-agency Policies and Procedures to Protect Vulnerable Adults from Abuse*. Department of Health, London.
33   Centre for Policy on Ageing (2002) *No secrets, the protection of vulnerable adults from abuse: local codes of practice*: 1–12 (http://www.cpa.org).
34   Department of Health (2004) *Protection of Vulnerable Adults (POVA) Scheme in England and Wales for Care Homes and Domiciliary Care Agencies. A Practical Guide*. The Stationery Office, London (http://www.dh.gov.uk/assetRoot/04/09/03/20/04090320.doc).
35   Belfield P (2005) *Abuse of Older People: British Geriatrics Society Compendium of Guidelines, Policy Statements and Statements of Good Practice*. British Geriatrics Society, London.
36   Steven M & Manthorpe J (2005) *POVA referrals: the first 100. Summary report*. Kings College London and Social Care Workforce Research Unit, London.

Further reading

Action on Elder Abuse (2004) *Hidden Voices*. Age Concern, London.
Action on Elder Abuse (2005) *Indicators of Abuse* (www.elderabuse.org.uk).
Eastman M (ed.) (1995) *Old Age Abuse: A New Perspective*. Age Concern and Chapman Hall, London.
Pritchard J (1996) *Working with Elder Abuse: A training manual for home care, residential and day care staff*. Jessica Kingsley, London.
Stokes G (1988) *Wandering*. Winslow Press, Bicester, UK.
Stokes G (2000) *Challenging Behaviour in Dementia: A person-centred approach*. Speechmark Publishing, Bicester, UK.

Chapter Five

Care Planning
HSC25
Carry out and provide feedback on specific plan of care activities

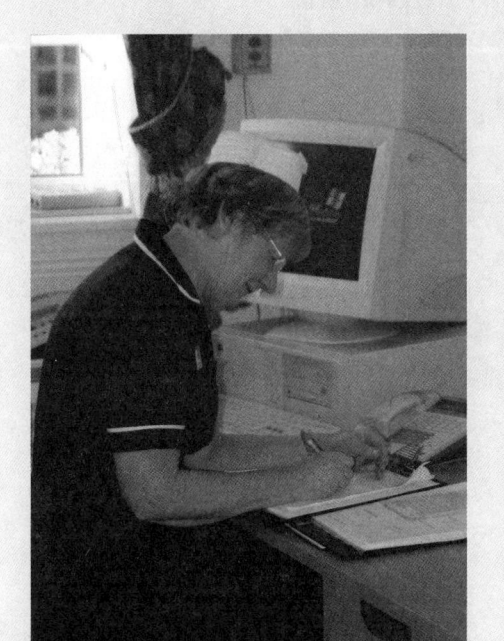

This unit consists of three elements:
HSC25a Carry out specific plan of care activities
HSC25b Provide feedback on specific plan of care activities
HSC25c Contribute to revisions of specific plan of care activities

The aim of this chapter is to outline how you can carry out a plan of care specified on a care plan, provide feedback on the effectiveness of that care and contribute to updating the care plan.

This chapter

- Provides information and guidance on nursing models and how they are used to develop care plans
- Explains the principles of care planning
- Provides information on the care planning process
- Explains the common pitfalls in care planning
- Explains legal requirements on care planning
- Provides information on how to deliver planned care
- Provides information and guidance on how to review and amend care plans

Why use care plans?

In the past, care was planned based on 'task allocation'. Each member of the team was allocated tasks that took account of the abilities of that member of staff. One member of staff might have been asked to check everyone's temperatures, pulses and blood pressures. Another staff member might have been asked to make all the beds. This system of care had several drawbacks. The first was that residents were cared for by many different staff and few residents got to know staff. Also, staff felt as if they were working on a production line and that they had little opportunity to get to know residents. Using a task allocation system meant that most residents with the same condition were treated in exactly the same way.

The system now used is that of individualised patient care. This aims to treat the person as an individual. Two people who have arthritis in the knees may have entirely different priorities and needs. Mrs Cain, for example, may have difficulty in walking because of her arthritis and this may be preventing her from attending church on Sundays. Mr Edwards may find that the pain in his knees is preventing him from getting a good night's sleep. The basis of individualised care is the care plan. This plan is drawn up in consultation with the person requiring care.

Nursing models

In the past nursing and medical staff were considered experts, and they informed patients in all settings about the care they would receive.[1] This began to change in the 1970s with the introduction of care planning, and over the last 30 years we have moved to a more collaborative model of care. People receiving care are consulted, or at least that's the theory. The reality is that many people in all care settings are still unsure of what care they are receiving and why.[2] Although care planning is now well established there are ongoing problems with identifying problems and needs, consulting the person, and planning and managing care.

The idea of a nursing model can appear complex and offputting but nursing models are really very simple. They are simply tools that provide a framework. This framework is used to enable us to assess need, set goals, implement and evaluate care.

The Roper model is the most widely used in the UK (see Box 5.1). It was introduced by Roper, Logan and Tierney in the late 1970s and has been evolving ever since.[3] It identifies activities of daily living that the authors consider should be used to plan care. It is the most widely used nursing model in the UK.[4] Critics of this model state that it places too much emphasis on physical aspects and not enough on the psychological.

There are many nursing models but they all have a common core. They assess the person, the environment, the person's health and nursing needs.

Box 5.1 Roper, Logan and Tierney activities of daily living

1. Maintaining a safe environment
2. Breathing
3. Communication
4. Mobilising
5. Eating and drinking
6. Eliminating
7. Personal cleansing and dressing
8. Maintaining body temperature
9. Working and playing
10. Sleeping
11. Expressing sexuality
12. Dying

The principles of planning care

Care planning consists of four key areas, illustrated in Fig. 5.1.

Assessing needs

Nursing models provide structured assessment and enable staff to identify problems that could otherwise be overlooked. You can only begin to set

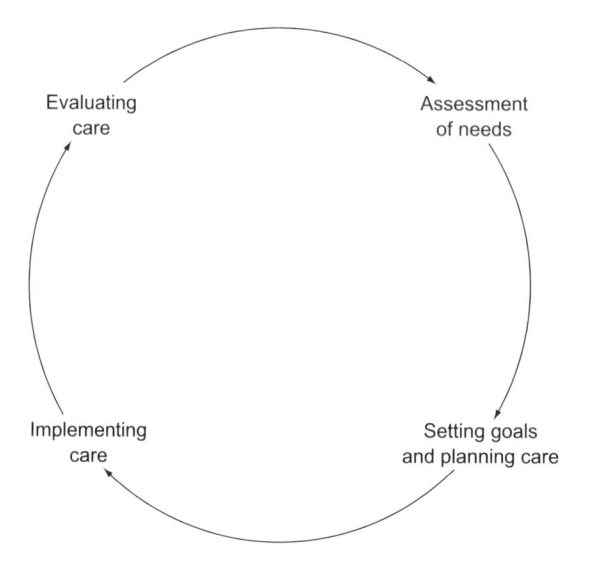

Figure 5.1 The care planning cycle.

goals and plan care when you have accurately identified needs. Assessment is crucial to the whole care planning process. Yet often staff rush assessment in their haste to set goals and plan care. One of the problems of assessment is that if you assess everyone for everything then you don't have time to actually provide care. You can avoid this trap by using a general assessment with trigger questions.

General assessments

General assessments are also called core assessments. They aim to obtain general information about a person such as their GP and next of kin and also ask a series of trigger questions which trigger a specialist assessment. You might use trigger questions in your general or core assessment to find out whether a person is at risk of developing a pressure sore. Trigger questions might include questions about mobility, conditions that increase the risk of pressure sores such as stroke, or confusion. If you identify risk factors on the core assessment then you carry out a specialist assessment. This approach is now being used by social services and in the NHS where it is called the single assessment process. It aims to avoid asking people the same questions over and over again and to cut down on unnecessary paperwork. Table 5.1 gives details of trigger questions related to falls.

Specialist assessments

If core assessments indicate the need for specialist assessments you then either carry out these specialist assessments or refer to a specialist. If you examine one area, such as continence care, there are differing levels of assessment which are carried out by people with different skill levels. A level 1 continence assessment is a series of trigger questions that can be asked by anyone working in health or social care. A level 2 continence assessment is usually carried out by a registered nurse. This assessment will have triggers for further referral. A level 3 continence assessment is carried out by a nurse specialist or a doctor. A level 4 assessment is carried out either by a medical specialist or occasionally by a nurse consultant.

The assessment will enable you to work out what the aim of care is. In continence, for example, you need to be clear about whether you aim to promote continence or to manage incontinence. You then move on to setting goals and planning care.

Table 5.1 The STRATIFY falls assessment tool.[5]

Question	Score
Admitted because of a fall or has fallen since admission? Yes = 1. No = 0	
Do you think the person is agitated? Yes = 1. No = 0	
Visually impaired to the extent that everyday function is affected? Yes = 1. No = 0	
Needs to use the toilet especially frequently? Yes = 1. No = 0	
Walks independently and safely with or without aid? Yes = 0	
Walks independently but is unsteady? Yes = 1	
Is unable to walk/stand without help or prompting? Yes = 2	
Total score	

Setting goals and planning care

The older person must be actively involved in planning and reviewing their care whenever possible.[6, 7] The planning process must set specific, realistic, measurable and achievable goals. Objectives are concrete statements describing what you are trying to achieve. Objectives should be written in a way that enables you to find out if you have achieved these at the end of a specific time. A well-written objective will be Specific, Measurable, Attainable/Achievable, Realistic and Time-bound ('SMART').[8]

Specific: An objective should address a specific target or accomplishment. Goals must be realistic and attainable.

Measurable: Establish a standard that indicates that an objective has been met. If your aim is to improve mobility your standard might be that within two weeks Mrs Smith can transfer from bed to chair with one person assisting.

Attainable: If an objective cannot be achieved, then it is probably a goal. Goals that are set too high or too low become meaningless, and staff may ignore them.

Realistic: Limit objectives to what can realistically be done with available resources. If you set unrealistic objectives everyone will become demotivated. If it is not possible to set a goal because of lack of resources, senior staff may be able to reorganise work to free up time.

Time-bound: Objectives must have starting points, ending points and fixed durations. Commitment to deadlines helps everyone to focus their efforts on completion of the objective on or before the due date. Objectives without deadlines or schedules for completion tend to be overtaken by the day-to-day crises that invariably arise in an organisation.

Table 5.2 gives a SMART checklist to help plan care.

Actions should be clear and concise. Everyone in the team should be able to understand them. It's important to break down a large goal such as 'Enable Mrs Mary Evans to regain mobility' into a number of smaller, easily measured goals. Breaking down the process into smaller, more easily measured goals means that the task does not appear overwhelming

Table 5.2 SMART checklist.

Do the Objectives describe concrete achievements and outcomes that support the stated goal?	
Are your Objectives	Tick here
Specific – Does your Objective specify an achievement? **M**easurable – Does your Objective have a measurable outcome? **A**ttainable – Is it actually possible to obtain your specified Objective? **R**ealistic – Is the proposed Objective attainable within the constraints of available resources? **T**ime-bound – Is there a definitive date by which the Objective will be reached?	

and unachievable. A goal should not plan to take Mrs Jones from inability to weight bear to walking independently with a frame. Set interim goals such as standing with a standing frame, transferring from bed to chair with help, rising unaided from a chair. People are more motivated by a series of small wins rather than one big win.

When planning care, consider:

- What is the problem?
- What does the individual want to achieve?
- What can we do about the problem?
- What are the benefits of treatment or care?
- What are the costs or pitfalls of treatment or care?
- What resources (e.g. equipment and staff) are required?
- Who is the best person to deliver this care?
- How will this care be delivered?
- What do we want to achieve?
- How will we know when this has been achieved?
- When will we review treatment or care?

Delivering care

When implementing a plan of care, consider the person's safety but do not lose sight of the person's needs, hopes and fears. It is important to work with other professionals and with the person's family.[9]

Evaluating care

The evaluation process is concerned with the outcome of the plan of care. Evaluation, like all other stages of care planning, should be ongoing but often it isn't. If you look at care plans many of them are never evaluated. Staff often shrink from evaluating care because evaluation may reveal that they have 'failed' to achieve their goals. The real problem usually isn't failure, but evaluation may show up the fact that we've not set the right goals. When evaluating, you need to ask:

- Were the goals realistic and achievable?
- Was the time scale in which the goals were to be met realistic?
- Did we really have the person's consent and active participation?
- Did we set the right priorities?
- Did we have sufficient staff to realise these goals?
- Did staff have the skills to achieve these goals?
- Was the care plan flexible and adapted to the person's changing needs?

Evaluation is a learning process. Be forgiving of yourself and others. If staff are condemned for 'getting it wrong' you'll develop a culture where no one is prepared to take risks. Then all innovation will be stifled and morale will suffer.

Common care planning problems

The most common care planning problems are:

- Incomplete initial assessments
- Unrealistic care plans that lack clear objectives
- Incomplete or absent evaluation

The main reasons for these problems are because some staff do not contribute to care planning. This might be because the policy in the home is that only certain people are allowed to carry out assessments and to update care plans. When this is the case it's usually the responsibility of senior staff to plan and manage care. Senior staff have many responsibilities and priorities and may find the task of completing large numbers of assessments and care plans overwhelming. Senior staff are also less likely to know the individual so well as the person providing day-to-day care.

Sometimes staff who deliver day-to-day care and who know most about the individual are worried that they have little to contribute to care planning. This is a mistaken view. If care plans are to be real and to accurately reflect care given, then the people delivering care must contribute to the care plan.

National minimum standards on care planning

Standard 3 of the national minimum standards requires all older people to be comprehensively assessed prior to admission. Box 5.2 gives details.

> **Box 5.2** National minimum standards on assessment and care planning
>
> 3.1 New service users are admitted only on the basis of a full assessment undertaken by people trained to do so, and to which the prospective service user, his/her representatives (if any) and relevant professionals have been party.
> 3.2 For individuals referred through Care Management arrangements, the registered person obtains a summary of the Care Management (health and social services) assessment and a copy of the Care Plan produced for care management purposes.
> 3.3 For individuals who are self-funding and without a Care Management Assessment/Care Plan, the registered person carries out a needs assessment covering
>
> - personal care and physical well-being
> - diet and weight, including dietary preferences
> - sight, hearing and communication
> - oral health
> - foot care
> - mobility and dexterity
> - history of falls
> - continence
> - medication usage
> - mental state and cognition
> - social interests, hobbies, religious and cultural needs
> - personal safety and risk
> - carer and family involvement and other social contacts/relationships.

Standard 7 relates to social and health needs. This requires homes to:

- Draw up a plan of care
- Set out in detail actions to be taken to meet needs
- Meet relevant clinical guidelines
- Include a risk assessment and a falls risk assessment
- Review care plan at least monthly
- Involve the older person in the care plan
- Record it in a style accessible to the person
- Have it signed by the person (when possible) and/or their representative.

Information recorded on a care plan

The care plan contains information about the person's day-to-day care. It should give details of any assistance required to wash or bathe; this may include using a bath hoist. It will also include the person's preferences, for example if the person prefers to bathe or shower. It should give details of the person's mobility. If the person uses a frame to walk, this should be recorded. If the person requires a walking aid and the help of one or two members of staff to walk, this will be recorded. If the person has a continence problem, this should be recorded. A separate continence assessment will also have been undertaken and this will be kept separately. Treatment to promote continence such as a toileting programme or bladder retraining will be noted on the care plan. If the older person requires a special diet, has difficulty in eating independently, or requires aids to enable him or her to eat independently, this will be noted on the care plan.

The care plan should identify the person's needs and the aims of care, and give details of how that care is to be given. After a time, the effectiveness of the care given will be evaluated.

Care assistants should read the older person's care plan so that they are aware of the care required and the reasons that this particular care is given. A care assistant might think that it is cruel to expect a person to begin walking again who has recently had surgery to repair a fractured femur. The care plan should explain the reasons why the older person should be encouraged to walk again. Care assistants can often help registered nurses and senior staff give better care by informing them of how the person is feeling. The individual may tell you that pain is making it difficult for her to walk but she does not want to 'bother' the nurse. If you find out and inform the nurse, arrangements can be made to ensure that the patient receives satisfactory pain relief. In this way nurses and care assistants can work together to ensure that the older person receives care of the highest quality.

Sometimes Registered Nurses use technical terms that you may not understand. In this book, all technical terms used are explained. Nursing staff sometimes use abbreviations and initials and these can appear confusing to care assistants. You can look these up in the glossary. The Nursing and Midwifery Council (NMC), the body responsible for regulating nurses, recommends that nurses do not use abbreviations and initials in nursing records. Abbreviations are confusing and can lead to error. If you do not understand terms or see abbreviations used in a person's records, ask the nursing staff to explain. They will usually be pleased to do so and will be delighted that you are keen to learn.

Following a care plan

The care plan shown in Fig. 5.2 gives details of Mrs Cooper's diet. Mrs Cooper has had a stroke and has difficulty chewing and swallowing. The care plan states that Mrs Cooper is to have a soft diet. This means that you do not offer Mrs Cooper foods that are hard to chew and swallow. Mrs Cooper has fish pie or minced meat rather than a roast meal. She does not have dry food.

Your role in following the care plan is to ensure that Mrs Cooper has food that meets her needs and her preferences. Your role also includes checking how effective this plan of care is and whether any changes are required. This should be documented in the daily record or progress notes.

People change, and care plans should be real and up to date and should accurately reflect the person's care needs.

Providing feedback on care plans

Your role and your observations are very important and enable the team to provide care that is appropriate for the individual at any given time. Case Study 5.1 illustrates this.

Reflect on practice

Think about the care plans in your workplace. Do they accurately reflect the care required? Are they up to date? Would a new member of staff be able to pick up the care plan and work out what care a person requires? If not, why do you think this is? Is it clear who is responsible for individual care plans? Do staff consider care plans to be important? What can you do to ensure that care plans are accurate and up to date?

Case Study 5.1

When you bring Mrs Cooper her fish pie you notice that she's just finishing fish and chips. She tells you: 'I don't want lunch. My friend Dorothy brought me in some lovely fish and chips. It was such a change from this dreary food I get here.'

Mrs Cooper has managed her lunch and she's enjoyed it. Obviously something has changed and her ability to swallow has improved.

You need to report this to a senior member of staff so that Mrs Cooper's ability to swallow is reassessed. Sometimes people improve after stroke but you need to be sure.

Your role in informing senior staff can lead to a reassessment and Mrs Cooper may be able to enjoy a much better quality of life.

NUTRITION

Risk factor identified	How to assess	Results of assessment	How are we treating	Who leading	Outcome/evaluation
Malnutrition	Use the nutritional assessment questions in the admission pack to check if the person is malnourished or at risk of malnourishment. ■ Have you unintentionally lost weight recently? ■ Have you been eating less than normal? ■ What is your normal weight? ■ How tall are you?	Has lost 15 kg in last six months following stroke. Difficulty chewing due to stroke. Difficulty swallowing due to stroke.	Identify factors leading to weight loss and address. Note action to address below. Difficulty chewing and swallowing. Provide soft diet, offer food such as fish pie and minced meats. Do not give dry food or food that is difficult to chew such as roasts.	Nurse but may require expertise and advice of dietician.	
Difficulty eating	■ Identify any problems that prevent the person eating independently. ■ Does the person normally use any aids to enable independent eating? ■ Would the person benefit from an OT assessment to enable independent eating?	1. Difficulty cutting up food. Assist by cutting up food. 2. Use non-slip placemat to prevent plate slipping. 3. Use plate with a deep rim to prevent food slipping off plate.	Identify factors leading to weight loss and address. Note action to address below.	Nurse to identify initial problems then refer to OT who will provide appropriate aids. Nurse continues to lead on this.	

Difficulty swallowing	• Check if the person is taking any medicines that can cause swallowing difficulties. • Check if the person is taking medication as prescribed. • Check for dehydration. • Request swallowing assessment from Speech and Language therapist if the following symptoms present: dysphasia, coughing after eating/drinking/feeling of food stuck halfway down or if you have other concerns re swallowing.	1. Unable to swallow paracetamol tablets – give soluble paracetamol if Mrs Cooper has pain. 2. Can swallow digoxin tablets. 3. Not dehydrated, hates water, loves tea.	Prescriber to review any medication that could cause swallowing difficulties. Inform prescriber if person is not taking medicines as prescribed. If dehydrated, increase fluid intake if possible. If not possible, inform responsible clinician so that fluid balance can be addressed.	Nurse Nurse Nurse

Figure 5.2 Care plan (nutrition) for Mrs Cooper.

Contributing to care planning

The policy on who writes care plans will vary from organisation to organisation. Sometimes the same care home will have different policies in different parts of the home. In a care home with nursing, Registered Nurses may complete the care plans. In care homes where Registered Nurses are not employed, care plans may be completed by senior staff. In other homes, care assistants may write the care plan and have this countersigned by a Registered Nurse or senior member of staff. In all cases it is important that the person delivering day-to-day care and the person receiving care are involved.

Sometimes the person receives care from people who visit the care home.

If a person living in a residential home is being visited by a district nurse, perhaps to treat a leg ulcer, the district nurse may write a care plan. If the person is receiving therapy from another professional, such as speech therapy, the speech therapist may wish to write in the care plan. The speech therapist may write instructions and advice that help you to enable the person to make progress with their speech between treatments.

Check it out

Find out what the policy is in the home where you work. How is the older person involved in planning care? What is your level of involvement? Can you think of any changes to improve the way care is planned and delivered?

Beyond care planning: patient care pathways

Care plans originated in the US in the 1970s. The world has moved on and in the future care plans may be replaced in some care settings by care pathways. Integrated care pathways are defined as: '*structured multidisciplinary care plans, which detail essential steps in the care of patients with a specific clinical problem*'.[10] Care pathways are research based, reduce paperwork and enable staff to demonstrate that care has been delivered. They can also be used to check quality of care and change practice. If the care given should deviate from the pathway, a variance is recorded. This allows a record of what was done differently, why it was done differently and what action was taken.[11] Integrated care pathways are particularly suited to some areas of work. People who are receiving healthcare move through different healthcare systems and receive care from people in different organisations. An integrated care pathway can help ensure that the person receives continuity of care and that different staff communicate effectively.

If you are providing intermediate care you may be asked to use a care pathway. The care pathway aims to take the person from home, to hospital, to intermediate care and back home again.

Conclusion

Care planning is very simple and straightforward but it is an area that many staff have difficulty with. Staff fear that there is a 'right' and a 'wrong' way to write a care plan. The most important aspects of care planning are that you produce a simple, comprehensive and up-to-date plan that is relevant to the person and is easily understood.

Key points

- All older people admitted to care homes should have a comprehensive assessment of their needs.
- Staff are legally required to assess need and plan care.
- Care plans should be drawn up with the older person whenever possible.
- Care plans should be comprehensive and easy to understand.
- Care plans should be updated at least monthly.
- The older person should whenever possible sign the care plan.
- If the older person is not able to sign the care plan the person's representative should do this.
- You should follow the care plan. If the person's care needs changing, you should inform senior staff.
- You should contribute to updating care plans so that they accurately reflect care needs.

Portfolio preparation

Your assessor must have evidence that you can meet the performance criteria for this unit. Before beginning this unit discuss assessment strategies with your assessor. Most of the evidence for this unit can be gained by direct observation of your work. You may be asked to provide the following types of evidence:

Products: This might be a copy of an assessment you completed. It could be a note in a resident's notes giving details of how you delivered care detailed on a care plan. It could be a care plan that you have drawn up to meet the assessed need of an individual.

Witness testimony: This is a statement from a senior member of staff. It might be a statement detailing how you have met certain performance criteria.

Written work: You might be asked to prepare a piece of work on how you assessed needs, drew up a plan of care and evaluated the care you delivered.

Your assessor may also use other methods to help you gain evidence for this unit. These may include:

- Verbal questioning
- Written questions
- Simulations to demonstrate that you have the skills to assess care needs, plan care and provide feedback on a plan of care.

Notes

1. Aggleton P & Chalmers H (2000) *Nursing Models and Nursing Practice*, 2nd edition. Macmillan, London.
2. Butterworth C (2005) Ongoing consent to care for older people in care homes. *Nursing Standard* **19**:20: 40–45.
3. Roper N, Logan W & Tierney J (2001) *The Roper–Logan–Tierney Model of Nursing*. Churchill Livingstone, London.
4. Holland K, Jenkins J, Solomon J & Whittam S (eds) (2003) *Applying the Roper–Logan–Tierney Model in Practice: Elements of Nursing*. Churchill Livingstone, London.
5. Oliver D, Britton M, Seed P *et al* (1997) Development and evaluation of evidence based risk assessment tool (STRATIFY) to predict which elderly inpatients will fall: case-control and cohort studies. *British Medical Journal* **315**: 1049–1053.
6. Department of Health (2001) *The Care Homes Regulations*. The Stationery Office, London.
7. Department of Health (2002) *Care Homes for Older People: National Minimum Standards*. The Stationery Office, London.
8. Nazarko L (2004) *Managing a Quality Service*. Heinemann, Oxford.
9. Coleman V, Regan D & Smith J (1999) *Who Cares Plans: A Guide to Care Planning in Homes for Older People*. Counsel and Care, London.
10. Campbell H, Hotchkiss R, Bradshaw N & Porteous M (1998) Integrated care pathways. *British Medical Journal* **316**:7125: 133–137.
11. Johnson S, Smith J (2000) Factors influencing the success of ICP projects. *Professional Nurse* **15**:12: 776–779.

Further reading

Holland K, Jenkins J, Solomon J & Whittam S (eds) (2003) *Applying the Roper–Logan–Tierney Model in Practice: Elements of Nursing*. Churchill Livingstone, London.

Chapter Six

Recreational Activities
HSC210
Support individuals to access and participate in recreational activities

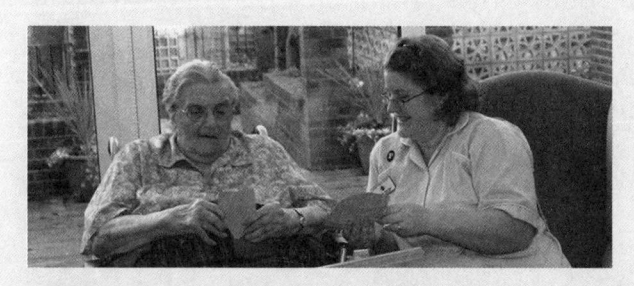

This unit consists of three elements:
HSC210a Support individuals to identify their recreational interests and preferences
HSC210b Encourage and support individuals to participate in recreational activities
HSC210c Encourage and support individuals to review the value of the recreational activities

This chapter

- Explains why it is important to identify the older person's recreational interests
- Provides information on the value of activities and interests
- Provides information on a range of activities available in homes
- Explains how to enable older people to enjoy activities
- Provides information about why some people may decline to participate in activities
- Provides practical advice on how to encourage and support older people in participating in activities
- Provides information to enable you to recognise problems

Enabling older people to identify activities and interests

Many older people who enter homes have lived alone for some time. The person may be widowed. People who enter homes have mental or physical impairments. The person may have difficulty with mobility or an impaired memory. Research suggests that 78% of people who enter homes have mobility problems and 40–60% have some level of cognitive impairment.

People who enter homes have physical care needs. The person may have been housebound for some time and their world may have shrunk. Some people may have benefited from attending a day centre and have been able to maintain activities, interests and contact with others. Before entering the home many people will have received care at home. Homecare is delivered according to a package of care worked out by social services unless the person has a private carer. In most cases care at home involves meeting physical care needs but not activities and interests. Often the person receiving home care only sees people who provide care. The person may not have been able to pursue leisure activities for some time.

Care homes have a negative image and older people are not immune from such perceptions. The older person may have resisted entering the home because she thought that moving to a care home was a sign that she was becoming more disabled and more dependent. The person may enter the home because of increasing disability or because a carer is no longer able to cope. In such circumstances leisure activities are the last thing on a person's mind.

Older people may think that they have come to a home to die but many find that entering a home is a positive experience. Older people can blossom in a home and enjoy the freedom from worry, knowing that care needs will be met when they occur and not when home care is scheduled. Many older people benefit from company. Living alone can be lonely when the only people you meet are the home care team. It is good to have company and conversation available at all times. Life is for living and recreational activities are an important part of life. They add richness to what would otherwise be a dull and boring existence.

It is important to enable the older person to identify her individual activities and interests. Bingo, for example, is heaven for some and hell for others. The easiest way to enable individuals to access and participate in recreational activities is to ask the person about his or her interests (see Case Study 6.1). You can then identify opportunities for the person to engage in these activities.

People come from many different backgrounds and they have different skills, interests, experiences and personalities. Older people who live in homes differ in their interests just as much as any other group of people. The activities offered in the home should take account of the different interests and personalities of the people living there. Staff in homes have to work hard to identify individual needs and to develop a range of activity programmes that provide something for everyone.

> **Case Study 6.1**
>
> When Dr Patrick Lister, a retired GP, was admitted to The Pines residential care home his key worker, Alice Burgess, asked Dr Lister about his interests.
>
> Dr Lister was a keen cricket fan. Alice worked out a number of ways to enable Dr Lister to continue to enjoy cricket. She checked newspapers to find out when a test match or a one-day match would be televised and told Dr Lister about these. She organised any care activities so that Dr Lister was free to watch cricket. She also checked the times of radio commentary on cricket matches.
>
> Dr Lister had a poster of cricket fixtures from the local cricket club in his room. Alice discovered that he'd been an active member of the cricket club for many years. As the doctor's Parkinson's disease had worsened he'd become more isolated and lost touch with his friends in the cricket club. Alice encouraged Dr Lister to make contact with the club again. The club secretary put an item about Dr Lister moving to The Pines in their newsletter and friends came to call. Dr Lister enjoyed their visits and said how he missed watching live matches. The club secretary was able to organise transport and Dr Lister began to attend matches in a wheelchair.
>
> In finding out about Dr Lister's interests and supporting him in following them, Alice was able to make Dr Lister feel that he could live a full life even though he needed assistance with care because of having Parkinson's disease.

Benefit of activities and interests

Homes are for living in and activities and interests make life worthwhile and interesting for many people. Activities have been shown to improve concentration and reduce boredom. Taking part in activities helps people to live full lives and this improves physical and mental well-being.

In the early 1980s, many older people requiring long-term care were cared for in NHS units. These units were usually in geriatric hospitals built many years earlier. Older people were nursed in wards. There was little privacy and they were dressed in clothes supplied by the hospital laundry rather than in their own clothes. In many hospitals, older people were not treated as individuals and there were few opportunities for them to pursue their interests. It was thought that older people would enjoy a better quality of life if they were cared for in nursing homes. Four experimental nursing homes were set up and people were asked if they wished to move from the hospital to the nursing home. The homes aimed to provide care in an environment that was more like the older person's home than a hospital. Individuals had their own rooms, wore their own clothes and were encouraged to take part in activities and pursue their own interests.

The results were dramatic; people who had lived in hospital for years began to take an interest in life again and their physical and mental health improved. Activities encourage older people to move around, to sit up, to concentrate and to take an interest in life. People who are more alert and involved are less likely to spend half the day dozing in a chair and will normally sleep well at night without sleeping tablets.

What happens when people stop engaging in activities?

Tessa Perrin of NAPA has worked with people in care homes for many years. Most of her work is with people who have dementia. Tessa believes passionately that, although most of us would consider it unthinkable not to meet physical care needs, we sometimes consider that psychological needs are less important. She points out that physical and psychological well-being are linked. She states that people who stop engaging in activities experience physical and psychological changes. The physical changes are outlined in Box 6.1.

Box 6.1 Physical changes caused by inactivity

- Muscles atrophy and joints develop contractures
- Bone loses calcium leading to osteoporosis and fracture
- Heart atrophies and blood pressure increases
- Risk of thrombosis and embolism increases
- Appetite diminishes
- Gastrointestinal movement decreases and constipation increases
- Potential for urinary infection and incontinence increases
- Potential for respiratory infection increases
- Potential for pressure sores increases
- Sleep pattern is disrupted

Human beings are designed to be active and when people become inactive the body changes. Joints stiffen if we are inactive for eight hours or more. If we are inactive for a few days our muscles become weaker, our bones start to lose calcium and become weaker and our heart muscles become less able to pump blood efficiently. People living in care homes are old and often have long-term conditions that limit the ability to exercise and to move around and be active. However, activities that are tailored to the person's ability lead to improvements in health and well-being. The older person who has enjoyed activities during the day is more likely to sleep well than one who has sat alone, unstimulated and anxious.

Inactivity also affects people psychologically. These changes affect both young and old, people in good health and in poor health. They start to

> **Box 6.2** Psychological changes caused by inactivity
>
> - Decreased alertness
> - Diminished concentration
> - Increased irritability, impatience and hostility
> - Increased tension and anxiety
> - Listlessness and restlessness
> - Depression and lethargy
> - Feelings of oppression
> - Problem-solving difficulties
> - Confusion and disorientation

take place within 48 hours of a person becoming inactive. These changes are outlined in Box 6.2.

The older person who enters a care home may have had weeks, months or even years of inactivity and may be unused to company and to taking part in activities and interests. At first it may be difficult for you to get the person to open up and tell you about their activities and interests. It is important to persist in a sensitive way because the person will benefit enormously from engaging in activities. Engaging in activities improves both physical and mental well-being. Box 6.3 outlines the physical benefits of activity.

> **Box 6.3** Physical benefits of activity
>
> - Muscle strength and joint mobility increases
> - Bone loss diminishes and healing time of fractures reduces
> - Blood pressure and potential for thrombosis/embolism diminish
> - Appetite increases
> - Gastrointestinal movement increases and defecation normalises
> - Continence improves
> - Potential for respiratory disorders decreases
> - Potential for skin disorders decreases
> - Sleep pattern normalises

If you look at Dr Lister's case history (Case Study 6.1) you can see that he became more active in pursuing his love of cricket. He began to have visitors so he greeted them at the door of the home and walked them back to the entrance after their visits. He walked to the car when going out, got into the car and got out at the other end. He got some fresh air and his appetite improved. This activity and his eating a better diet helped to improve his bowel and bladder function. Before he became involved in cricket Dr Lister would sit and worry. He is by nature a bit of a worrier.

At night it took him ages to fall asleep. When he began to watch cricket, his sleep pattern improved and he felt and looked better.

Taking part in activities has psychological benefits. Activities can provide a sense of continuity and enable the person to feel that life continues when she enters the home. Although the person may be old and may require assistance with the activities of daily living she can still enjoy lifelong interests. Box 6.4 outlines the psychological benefits of activity.

Box 6.4 Psychological benefits of activity

- Smiling, laughing and talking increase
- Initiation of, and engagement in, social interaction increases
- Alertness to environmental stimuli increases
- Concentration and memory improve
- Emotions are more readily expressed
- Agitation diminishes and relaxation increases

Encouraging individual activities and interests

Some people are naturally chatty and outgoing and love company. Some patients rush to get ready and get to the lounge for coffee and a chat. Others are quieter and prefer to spend their days quietly away from the bustle and activity of others. Sometimes well-meaning staff encourage residents to join in activities that have been organised. It is important to realise that organised activities aren't for everyone.

If a person does not wish to take part in an activity you should ask why; some people long to join in but lack confidence. You can help, support and encourage people who lack confidence to take part in activities. Some older people are embarrassed by their disabilities or worry that because of illness it will be difficult to participate. You can help by encouraging and offering practical help in such situations. Activities in the home should be organised to take account of disabilities and to enable individuals to participate.

Some older people prefer their own company or that of their family and friends who visit. If the individual prefers not to take part in activities, you should respect their wishes.

Sometimes the older person is worried or upset and needs assistance to sort out problems before it's possible to engage in the life of the home. Case Study 6.2, which appears on the following page, illustrates this.

When Mr Mann felt assured that Charlie would be cared for even if Elsie was unwell, he relaxed and was able to take part in some of the activities in the home.

> **Case Study 6.2**
>
> Mr Frederick Mann appeared happy although he took little part in the activities in the home. The highlight of his day was when his friend Elsie visited with Charlie, his dog. Elsie had taken Charlie in when Mr Mann had a stroke and she looked after the dog.
>
> When Elsie received news that she could have her hip operation she worried about who would care for Charlie and exercise him until she got back on her feet. Mr Mann confided in Judith Evans, his key worker, that Elsie was considering turning down the operation because of worries about Charlie. Judith discussed the problem with her manager, who suggested they contact the Cinnamon Trust (contact details at end of chapter). The Cinnamon Trust provides a fostering service and its volunteers care for animals while their owners are unable to provide care.
>
> The Trust arranged for Charlie to be cared for by a volunteer while Elsie was in hospital. After Elsie returned home the volunteer exercised Charlie until Elsie was well enough to do this herself. The volunteer also took Charlie to visit Mr Mann each day.

Providing activities for residents

Many larger homes employ an activities organiser. This person works with staff and residents to organise and coordinate activities within the home. Many people, when they think of activities, imagine a large group of people all doing the same thing. Well-organised activity programmes involve working with small groups of people and with individuals as well as large groups.

At some homes a number of people come to the home for a few sessions each week. Activity sessions from different people offer a variety of activities. In smaller homes, staff are required to work with residents to organise activities. In this situation staff have to ensure that activities are not squeezed out by the other work in the home. Homes are busy places and there is always something to do. Activities are important and helping patients to pursue their interests and activities is a very important part of working in homes. Ask any older person who mattered most to them: the person who tidied the lockers, or the one who found time to help residents begin a game of Scrabble.

Types of activities

If you are involved in activity programmes, aim to offer as wide a range of activities as possible. This enables you to cater for as wide a range of interests as possible and also to prevent boredom that can set in if only a limited range of activities is offered.

Games

Many older people enjoy games. Some older people have poor eyesight even with spectacles. Playing cards that are twice the normal size can be seen by people with poor eyesight. A large-print version of Scrabble is available. People with poor eyesight can see this more easily and people suffering from diseases such as motor neurone disease, multiple sclerosis and arthritis will find them easier to handle.

Large, easy-to-handle dominoes (Fig. 6.1) are also available. Bingo is popular in many homes and large-print bingo cards are available. Many homes have radios or music centres, which have microphones. The microphone can be used to call out numbers so that people who do not have perfect hearing can join in.

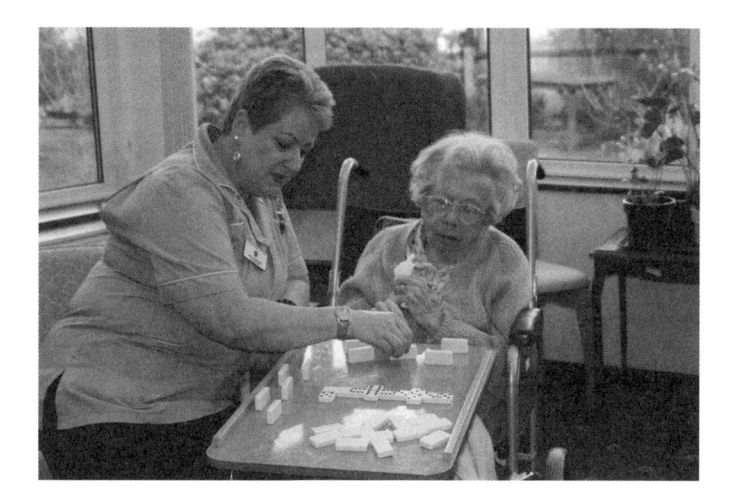

Figure 6.1 Enjoying a game of dominoes.

Music

Many people enjoy music. It is easy to build up a record collection for the home. A notice on the home's notice board and a letter to the local newspaper asking for records usually works well. If you ask what type of music people prefer you will normally find this varies from classical to popular music of the 1920s, 1930s and 1940s. In some homes, popular music is played during the morning and classical in the evening.

It is important to get the music right, as Case Study 6.3 illustrates.

Most local hospitals have hospital radio stations, and many of these also offer a tape service. A member of the radio team visits the home and speaks to a group of residents asking what type of music they prefer. The music is then taped and sent to the home. Tapes are usually exchanged

> **Case Study 6.3**
>
> Mrs Ethel Donnelly had been struggling at home for some time. Her rheumatoid arthritis made it impossible for her to get up, wash and dress independently. When Mrs Donnelly fell and fractured her femur she didn't recover her previous level of mobility. She discussed her situation with her family and felt it would be best if she went into a care home. Then she wouldn't have to worry about the upkeep of her large house and garden, her needs would be met and she'd have company.
>
> Mrs Donnelly's son Paul agreed to look at local homes and find one that his mother would like. Mrs Donnelly agreed to visit the home for a day. When she returned to she told Paul to find another home. 'I couldn't possibly go there. When I got there they were having a singsong with songs from the Edwardian music hall. I was born in 1930 and when I was a teenager we didn't sing "Daisy", we sang "I get a kick out of you". It's clear that the people running the home don't have any idea about the needs of today's older people.'

twice weekly. Individuals can also have a personal selection of music taped and sent to them regularly. This can be listened to in private or enjoyed with others.

Sometimes we think that older people won't embrace technology but many do. The growing popularity of digital music players such as the iPod mean that it is possible for the older person to have every song they ever liked recorded on their iPod and can enjoy music whenever they wish. Some digital music players such as the iPod mini are the size of a matchbox and can fit into a pocket.

Singsongs can also be popular. CDs, tapes or records of favourite songs from musicals such as *South Pacific* can be bought. It is seldom necessary to buy large-print song books because the lyrics of popular songs can often be downloaded from the internet into a word-processing program and printed off using an increased font size. You can help by encouraging residents to join in and by joining in yourself.

Many homes have pianos that are seldom used because no one can play. Often a notice saying 'Volunteer wanted to play the piano for one hour a week' will bring offers flooding in. An advertisement in a newsagent's window costs very little. Many local supermarkets offer a free notice board service, so it may be worth advertising. The local secondary school may have pupils who would enjoy playing.

Concerts

Concerts can be formal and involve the use of professional entertainers, but this can be expensive and your home may not be able to afford many such concerts. Local choirs, operatic societies and other groups may be willing to perform in the home. Details of local groups can be obtained from your local library or Citizens Advice Bureau.

Arts and crafts

Painting and drawing are relaxing activities. Many people who are no longer able to take part in more active pursuits enjoy creating drawings, pictures, prints and collages. Some older people are talented artists and create impressive paintings, while others enjoy making birthday cards, Christmas cards and prints. Paper, pencils, pens, felt-tip pens and poster paints are inexpensive and give hours of pleasure. When people have worked hard to produce work it can be admired and displayed in the person's room or in the lounge, dining room and hall.

Knitting

Many women enjoy knitting. Some, though able to knit beautifully, find that it is difficult to read a pattern because the print is too small. Now free knitting patterns are available online (details at the end of the chapter). These can be downloaded and the text can be changed to as large a print as necessary before they are printed. The older person can also use a magnifying glass if she wishes to use a favourite pattern. The latest magnifying glasses come with built-in light to make reading even easier. Large-print knitting patterns are available by post (see end of chapter).

People who have poor eyesight but are still able to knit may have difficulty sewing up garments. Often another resident who enjoys sewing may be able to help finish off garments. Both may enjoy working together.

Sport

Recently researchers asked older men living in nursing and residential homes what would improve their quality of life most within the home. A huge majority said they would like satellite television so that they could watch sport. Many older people enjoy watching sport. Football, boxing, tennis, horse racing and cricket are often shown on television, although increasingly satellite television has more coverage of major sporting events. If an individual enjoys watching, staff can help by checking the times of particular events and helping the person to enjoy them uninterrupted. The person who enjoys tennis should have treatment planned so that it will not coincide with matches at Wimbledon.

Many people enjoy watching sports events out of doors. If Mr Walters played rugby as a younger man, he may enjoy watching a local rugby team. The team can be contacted and arrangements made for him to watch local matches. Many sports teams are extremely helpful and will help transport sports enthusiasts to their games and involve them in the social activities of the team. Sitting under a tree watching a cricket match or sitting in a pub watching the darts team play is a world away from how most people view homes. You can, with a little imagination and planning, help older people live life to the full within homes.

Exercise sessions

Exercise is not only for the young and fit. People of all ages can benefit from exercise; even frail and disabled people can take part. EXTEND (Exercise Training for the Elderly) is a charity which specialises in working with older people. Using music and a series of exercises that exercise different parts of the body, EXTEND aims to make people living in homes feel as well as possible.

Reading

Homes are able to obtain books from the mobile library service, which is run by the local council. Councils deliver a selection of books to homes and hospitals, and these are exchanged every few months. A member of the library staff asks the home which types of books are required. Most older people find it easier to read large print and there is now a large selection of large-print books available. If an older person is an avid reader, the library service can deliver a book (or two) to the individual. The library asks the person to fill in a form (usually large print) asking them their reading preferences and delivers and collects books on request. Some older people may prefer to go to the library and select their own books. You can escort and help individuals who wish to do this. You can also suggest that family and friends take the individual to the local library to select books.

Books for people who are blind and partially sighted

People who have very poor vision can be registered blind. The person's doctor fills in a form and the person is registered with the local council. People who are registered blind or partially sighted are issued with special library tickets that enable them to take out tapes or books free of charge. There are two sizes of book tape. The Talking Book cassette recorders take larger cassettes. Talking Book cassettes are posted to registered blind people from a central library run by the council. The book cassettes available in local libraries fit into normal cassette players. Older people with poor vision may find it difficult to use standard cassette players. Some older people with poor vision find that cassette players designed for toddlers are easy to use. These are inexpensive and easy to obtain, with four large, bright, differently coloured buttons each with a separate function.

Television and films

Many older people enjoy watching television. It is important though that television is not seen as the only activity. In some homes, the television is on all day and no one is listening. Try to find out which television programmes individual residents like and let them know when these are on. Many people like watching films, especially old films. Many classic films are inexpensive and can be obtained easily. Videos are now often available in bargain bins in shops. If the home has a video recorder, films can be taped and film shows organised in the evening. DVDs of classic films are often given away free with newspapers. DVD recorders are becoming more widely available and films can be recorded on DVD to show in the evenings. This can be made into an event, with drinks and popcorn available.

Gardening

Gardening is a popular pastime for people of all ages (Fig. 6.2). People living in homes will have differing abilities. Some suggestions to enable people who enjoy gardening to continue their interest are:

- Caring for a raised bed or a tub of plants in the garden. Bulbs can be planted all year round.
- Planting indoor bulbs. Bulbs can be planted in bowls and containers to brighten up the person's bedroom or other parts of the home.
- Planting seeds. Usually large seeds such as nasturtium are easier to handle. Choose plants that germinate easily. There's nothing worse

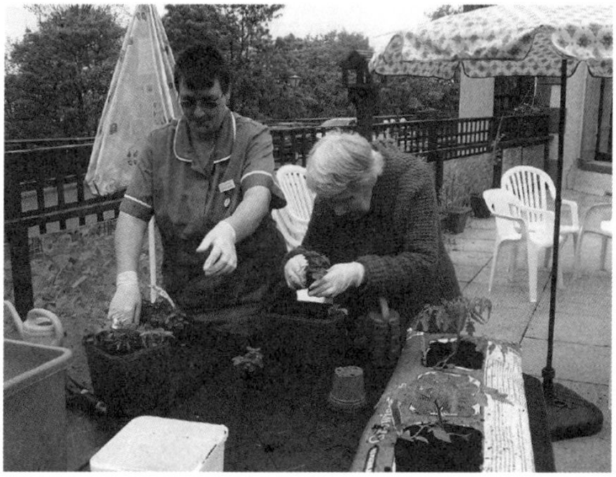

Figure 6.2 Gardening at a convenient height.

than watching and waiting for plants that fail to sprout. Plants can be transferred into pots, bowls, tubs or the garden.
- Taking cuttings from plants. Residents can give the new plants to family and friends as gifts.

Outings

Many people enjoy going out and often people in homes enjoy outings. Some homes successfully organise regular outings, while others are less successful.

If you are involved in planning an outing, do not think that the aim is to take every resident. It is better to organise several smaller outings as older people, like all of us, have differing interests. Find out what residents require. Plan the outing. Visit the place beforehand to make sure it is suitable. Involve families and friends. Ask for help and support. Remember that things rarely go exactly to plan, so be flexible.

Individual activities

Some people who come to live in homes have managed their own leisure activities for years. In such circumstances, your role should be to support the person and offer help if required. If the person is a member of the local bridge club then your role may be to welcome visitors and offer them refreshments.

Pets

Most people who enter homes lived alone before entering the home. This may be because they never married or because they have been widowed. Many people who live alone enjoy the companionship of pets. People who live alone and who have pets enjoy better health than those without pets. Stroking a cat or patting a dog has been shown to reduce blood pressure and help people to relax (Fig. 6.3 and Case Study 6.4).

Some homes have a policy of allowing the older person with a pet to bring the pet to live at the home wherever possible. This is not always possible, however, as some breeds of dog require a lot of exercise and the older person who enters a home will rarely be able to take a dog for long walks. Many older people recognise these difficulties and ask a friend or relative to care for their dog when they enter a home. Most homes now encourage family and friends to bring the older person's dog to visit. Many other residents also enjoy such visits. Cats require less looking after and in some homes the older person may bring her cat to stay.

Some people have budgies as pets and most homes allow people to bring these with them when they enter the home.

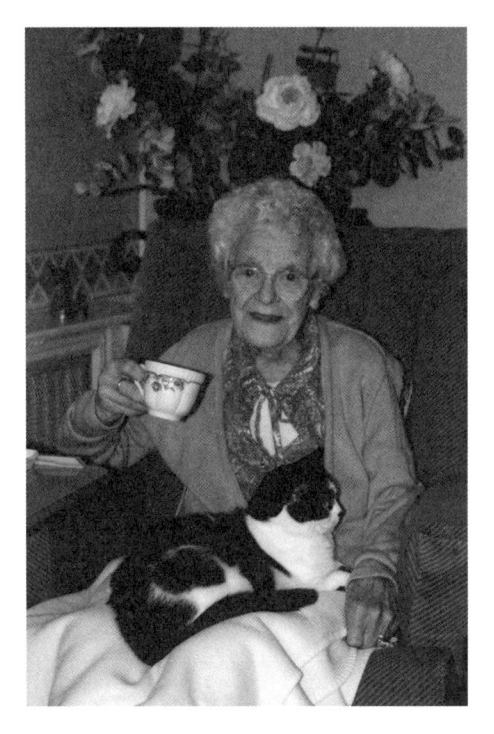

Figure 6.3 A pet provides companionship.

Case Study 6.4

Grace Andrews was admitted to a nursing home after suffering from a severe stroke. She recovered well from the stroke and regained speech and mobility but remained quiet and withdrawn. Staff at the home discovered that when Mrs Andrews was in hospital her cat had been run over and killed. Mrs Andrews missed the companionship dreadfully. The local Cats Protection League visited and Mrs Andrews 'adopted' a cat. Having the companionship of a cat made Mrs Andrews feel that life was worth living again (Fig. 6.3).

Pets as Therapy

Pets as Therapy (PAT) is a national charity. It provides therapeutic visits to hospitals, hospices, care homes and nursing homes. Volunteers visit homes with their friendly dogs and cats.

There are currently around 3500 active PAT dogs and 90 cats at work in the UK. Every week these calm, friendly dogs and cats visit more than

10 000 people, both young and old, giving pleasure and the chance to cuddle and talk to them. PAT animals visit half a million people a year. Some people who no longer have dogs of their own enjoy these visits and look forward to seeing and petting the PAT dogs.

Key points

- Older people living at home can become isolated.
- Sometimes older people entering a home have not had the opportunity to enjoy activities and interests for some time.
- The best way to find out about a person's activities and interests is to ask.
- Enabling the person to engage in activities and interests has real health benefits.
- Homes should offer a range of activities so that they can meet the differing needs and aspirations of residents.
- Skilled, knowledgeable care assistants can make a real difference to the older person's ability to enjoy activities and interests.

Portfolio preparation

Your assessor must have evidence that you can meet the performance criteria for this unit. Before beginning this unit, discuss assessment strategies with your assessor. Most of the evidence for this unit can be gained by direct observation of your work. You may be asked to provide the following types of evidence:

Products: This might be a copy of a care plan that you wrote or contributed to, outlining the person's activities and interests and how you aim to help the person engage in activities. It could be a note in a resident's notes giving details of how a resident is participating in activities and any support needed. It might say what activities the person particularly enjoyed. This might include details of an activity you have organised. One NVQ level 2 student organised a Christmas pantomime and submitted a video recording of the pantomime in her evidence. Another organised a trip to the seaside and submitted photographs of residents enjoying the trip.

Witness testimony: This is a statement from a senior member of staff. It might be a statement detailing how you have met certain performance criteria.

Written work: You might be asked to prepare a piece of work on how to identify suitable activities for an individual and how to compensate for any problems that the person might have (such as poor eyesight or stiff hands).

Your assessor may also use other methods to help you gain evidence for this unit. These may include:

- Verbal questioning
- Written questions.

Simulations may be used to help gain evidence if it cannot be gained by direct observation.

Further information

NAPA (National Association for Providers of Activities for Older People)
Bondway Commercial Centre
5th Floor, Unit 5.12
71 Bondway
London SW8 1SQ
Telephone: 0207 078 9375
Website: http://www.napa-activities.net/home.php

NAPA provides information, advice and training about activities in homes. Their website has downloadable articles, leaflets and recommended reading lists.

Pets as Therapy
Rocky Bank
6 New Road
Ditton
Kent ME20 6AD
Telephone: 01732 87222
Website: http://www.petsastherapy.org

PAT has over 8500 registered PAT dogs and owners who visit hospitals, hospices and nursing and residential homes. Their website has details of their work and how to request their services. If you write to PAT please enclose a 9-inch by 6-inch stamped self-addressed envelope.

The Cinnamon Trust
10 Market Square
Hayle
Cornwall TR27 4HE
Telephone: 01736 757900
Fax: 01736 757010
Website: http://www.cinnamon.org.uk

The Cinnamon Trust aims to enable owners to continue to care for their pets. It provides a national fostering service so that pets can be cared for when their owners are in hospital or are unwell. If a person is unable to care for a pet because of infirmity or acute illness, the trust volunteers can help with all aspects of pet care including walking the dog. The trust provides sanctuary to pets while their owner is in long- or short-term care. The owner receives visits and regular photos and letters informing them how their pet is. There are no charges for services though donations are welcome. Their website provides details of their work. If writing send a large stamped, self-addressed envelope.

Age Exchange Reminiscence Centre
11 Blackheath Village
London SE3 9LA
Telephone: 020 8318 3504
Website: http://www.age-exchange.org.uk

The Age Exchange Reminiscence Centre has a museum and shop, produces books and offers training in reminiscence therapy.

Winslow Press
Telford Road
Bicester
Oxford OX6 0TS
Telephone: 0800 243 755
E-mail: info@winslow-press.co.uk
Website: http://www.winslow-press.co.uk

Winslow Press has a free catalogue full of books, puzzles, games and music.

Knitting Pattern Central
Website: http://www.knittingpatterncentral.com

This website offers free knitting patterns. There are hundreds of patterns on the site and they can be printed in large type.

Carter & Parker Ltd
Gordon Mills
Guiseley
Leeds LS20 9PD

Send a large, stamped self-addressed envelope to obtain a catalogue of free, large-print knitting patterns.

Further reading

Perrin T (ed.) (2005) *The Good Practice Guide to Therapeutic Activities with Older People in Care Settings.* NAPA/Speechmark, Bicester, UK. It is full of practical suggestions and imaginative ideas for activities.

Ruddlesden M (1997) *You Can Do It.* Hawker Publications, London (telephone: 020 7720 2108). This is a guide to exercise for older people and is illustrated with lots of photographs of older people exercising. Highly recommended.

Chapter Seven

Food and Drink
HSC213
Provide food and drink for individuals
HSC214
Help individuals to eat and drink

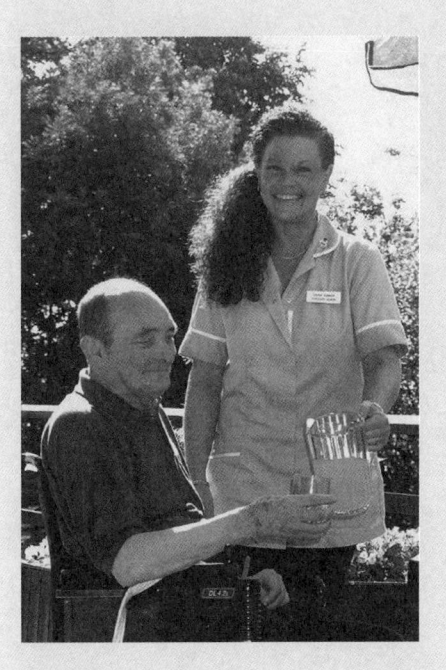

The Unit HSC213 consists of three elements:
HSC213a Support individuals to communicate what they want to eat and drink
HSC213b Prepare and serve food and drink
HSC213c Clear away when individuals have finished eating and drinking

HSC214 consists of three elements:
HSC214a Make preparations to support individuals to eat and drink
HSC214b Support individuals to get ready to eat and drink
HSC214c Help individuals consume food and drink

Please note these units cannot be used in combination.

The early part of this chapter will deal with dietary requirements and enabling older people to choose healthy food that is appropriate to their wishes, preferences and culture and that takes into account any eating difficulties the person may have. The later part will explain the difficulties that older people may face in eating and drinking and how you can help and support the person in such circumstances.

This chapter

- Explains why older people are at risk of dehydration and how fluid is required
- Provides information on how to help and encourage the person to drink
- Provides information on the importance of a healthy diet and calorie requirements
- Explains about special diets
- Provides information about meeting the dietary needs of people from different cultures
- Explains why dietary supplements may be required and how to use these

Importance of fluids

Healthy people will die within three days if they do not have fluids. Fluid is essential to life. The human body is mostly water in healthy young adults. Women's bodies contain less fluid than men's because women carry more fat on their bodies and fat contains little fluid. The amount of fluid in the body lessens with age. The average older man's body is 55% fluid and the average older woman's body is 45% fluid.

Each day we lose fluid and if the fluid lost is not replaced the amount of fluid in the body is reduced. This process is known as dehydration. Each day the average person loses fluid in:

- Urine – normally 1500 ml is produced
- Breath – normally 400 ml of fluid is lost in the breath
- Faeces – normally 100 ml of fluid is lost in faeces
- Sweat – the amount of fluid lost in sweat will vary according to the temperature and how much the individual perspires.

It is important that the individual drinks enough fluid to replace fluids lost by the body.

The dangers of dehydration

If the person does not drink sufficient fluids, the balance of chemicals (known as electrolytes) within the body is disturbed and this can lead to illness. People who do not drink enough are at risk of developing urine infections. They are more likely to become constipated, have less resistance to infection, and are at risk of developing infections, such as a chest infection, which can lead to serious ill health or even death.

Individuals who become dehydrated may become confused. Dehydration causes the blood to thicken and become more sticky (viscous). The blood is more likely to clot and blood clots can lead to strokes, heart attacks and blood clots in the legs (deep vein thrombosis). All of these can cause serious illness that can lead to the older person becoming more disabled. In some cases, the older person may die because of the complications of dehydration.

Why older people become dehydrated

Older people living in homes are more at risk of dehydration because of age-related changes and the effects of illness. These risks are outlined in Table 7.1.

Normally when it is hot or we are in danger of becoming dehydrated we become thirsty. Drinking restores the body's normal fluid balance. This is known as the thirst mechanism. As people age the thirst mechanism

Table 7.1 Risks of dehydration.

Risk	Reason
Decreased thirst mechanism	Ageing
Less able to concentrate urine	Ageing
Problems recognising thirst	Illness
Problems informing staff of thirst	Illness
Difficulty holding glass	Illness
Difficulty swallowing	Illness
Increased fluid requirements	Illness

becomes less efficient and even when older people are becoming dehydrated they do not feel as thirsty as younger people do. In hot weather or when we are in danger of becoming dehydrated, our kidneys respond by trying to conserve water. Less urine is produced. As people age the kidneys become less efficient at concentrating urine and conserving water.

Some people who live in nursing homes have problems communicating. Even if they are thirsty, they may have difficulty in asking staff for a drink. Some older people living in homes suffer from confusion and, although they are thirsty, they may have difficulty in understanding that this is the problem. Confusion gets worse if the individual does not have enough fluid. These individuals depend on staff to leave a drink where they can reach it, perhaps on the patient's locker or table.

Some people are unable to manage to drink without help even if the drink is placed in front of them. People suffering from arthritis may be unable to hold or lift the cup. People with a tremor may drop the cup or glass. The person who has had a stroke or who has poor eyesight may be unable to see the glass. Some people are reluctant to drink because they suffer from urinary incontinence and are afraid that they will have an accident if they drink. Some people have difficulty in swallowing because illness makes it difficult. People who have had strokes or have Parkinson's disease or motor neurone disease may have difficulty in swallowing. The older person may not like the drink she has been given.

Some individuals may need more fluid than others. A person who has diabetes may pass much more urine than normal. The reasons for this are given later in the chapter. The person may have a leg ulcer or pressure sore that can weep fluid and increase their fluid requirements. The older person may be vomiting, may have diarrhoea, or may feel sick, perhaps because of the medication they are taking, or perhaps because of constipation.

How much fluid do older people normally require?

Older people normally require two litres of fluids each day. Check how much fluid is held by a teacup in your home. The average teacup holds approximately 250 ml, but the cups in your home may be slightly larger or smaller than average. Remember, when measuring how much a cup holds, that cups are not normally filled to the brim and most people do not drain their cups. Usually a little tea or coffee is left in the bottom of the cup. Check how much fluid is held by the drinking glasses used in your home. The capacity of drinking glasses varies more than that of teacups. Drinking glasses hold between 200 and 330 ml on average.

When do older people require extra fluids?

While most people require two litres of fluid each day, there are times when individuals require more fluid. In hot weather individuals will sweat more and will require extra fluid to prevent dehydration. Research carried out in a Swedish nursing home found that residents liked to spend most of their day in the sunny conservatory. The sun raised the temperature and people who spent most of the day in the conservatory required an extra 500 ml of fluid a day because of increased fluid loss.

When people have an infection, the body fights it by raising the body temperature, because bacteria and viruses are usually killed by higher than normal body temperatures. When the body temperature rises the individual will sweat more and increased fluids are required to replace fluid lost in this way. Normally approximately 100 ml of fluid is lost in faeces each day. If the older person has diarrhoea, the amount of fluid lost from the bowel increases. Extra fluid is needed to replace this lost fluid.

Some older people have had surgery and a piece of small or large bowel is brought to the surface of the abdomen. This opening is known as a stoma. Faeces are collected in a bag that is attached to the abdominal wall. One of the functions of the large bowel (which is known as the colon) is to reabsorb water from faeces. People who have stomas may have either ileostomies (where the small bowel – known as the ileum – is brought to the surface of the abdomen) or colostomies (where a piece of the large bowel is brought to the surface of the abdomen). People who have stomas lose more fluid in their faeces than normal. People who have ileostomies tend to lose much more fluid than those who have colostomies. Individuals who are losing more fluid than average in their faeces must drink extra fluids to make up for the loss.

Older people, especially women, are more likely to develop cystitis and urine infections. These are normally treated with antibiotics but an important part of treating urine infections is encouraging the individual to drink plenty of fluid. This helps flush the infection out of the system.

Normally healthy people breathe in and out through the nose. The breathing rate (known as the respiration rate) varies from 12 to 20 times per minute in healthy adults. If the older person develops a heavy cold or a chest infection, the nose can become blocked and the individual breathes through the mouth. The mouth then becomes dry and the amount of fluid lost in breathing is increased. The respiration rate increases when an individual develops a chest infection and the amount of fluid lost in breathing increases. A high temperature will normally develop and this will lead to increased sweating and more fluid will be required.

Helping and encouraging older people to drink

Before you can encourage the older person to drink you need to find out what fluids the individual prefers. There is no point in offering the individual tea four times each day if she detests tea and relishes coffee. Does the person like tea? Does she like it black, with lemon, strong or weak? If the older person prefers sweet tea and cannot have sugar because she has diabetes, it is worth checking which sweetener is preferred. Some sweeteners can leave a bitter aftertaste. If the individual likes sugar in her tea, don't forget to stir the tea or provide a teaspoon, otherwise all the sugar stays in the bottom of the cup, the tea tastes bitter, and the person may not drink it.

If the individual likes coffee find out how she likes it. She may not appreciate mellow powdered coffee and may long for a rich, darkly roasted coffee. On the other hand, she may detest the pungent, almost black coffee offered and prefer coffee made with milk and two sugars.

What cold drinks does the person prefer? Not everyone likes orange squash. Some people may prefer orange barley water, fresh orange juice, lime juice, blackcurrant squash, apple juice or fruits of the forest. Some people may prefer fizzy drinks and may like lemonade, ginger beer, cola or even fizzy water. Low-calorie still and fizzy drinks are available for people who are diabetic or who are trying to lose a little weight.

The individual may like to have a can of beer in the evening. You should check with professional staff before suggesting that the older person can have alcohol as some medicines react with alcohol and increase the risk of unpleasant side effects.

Drinks should be served at the right temperature. Orange squash made with cold water is much more appealing than squash made with lukewarm water. Squashes should not be overdiluted as they then look unappealing and have no taste at all. Tea and coffee should be served hot, not lukewarm. You should make sure that tea or coffee is not so hot that it could burn the mouth of a confused person or scald someone who accidentally spills the drink onto his or her lap.

If the older person has difficulty in communicating or is confused, family and friends can often advise staff on the individual's preferences. These preferences should be recorded so that all staff can offer preferred fluids.

Some older people may not drink because staff have left a jug of orange but not brought a glass. Sometimes staff are aware that the person does not have a drinking glass and mean to bring it later but forget. Many older people worry about being thought of as 'a nuisance' and do not wish to 'trouble the staff when they are busy'. If the older person does not have a glass, she may remain thirsty for hours. Sometimes the drink is left just out of the older person's reach.

Some older people can become forgetful and may forget to have the drink that has been poured and left; popping back to remind the older person only takes a moment and can prevent dehydration. Some older people cannot manage to lift heavy pottery cups full of tea. Providing lightweight cups such as those used on picnics can mean that the individual can drink independently. These cups look and feel just like normal cups. The person or her family could choose lightweight cups if the home does not provide them.

It is almost impossible to drink if you are slumped in a chair or lying in bed. It is important to help the older person sit up comfortably so that she is able to drink. Some residents may have problems swallowing, especially those who have suffered from strokes or who have Parkinson's disease or motor neurone disease. Many of these individuals will require help to sit up and drink. If a person appears to be choking on a drink you should stop giving the drink immediately and seek professional advice. Details of how to cope in an emergency are given in Chapter 2.

Helping frail people to drink

Some older people are unable to drink fluids and rely on staff to give fluids. In many homes, it is assumed that if the person requires help a feeding cup should be used. Feeding cups are usually made of opaque white plastic and have a top with a spout on them.

Many older people can manage to drink from a normal cup if you hold it to the person's lips. It is important not to fill the cup too full and to take time helping the person to drink. Some older people manage to drink cold fluids more easily using a flexible straw that bends over. If this is not possible, you may have no choice but to use a feeding cup, but these should not be used if there is an alternative. Feeding cups give people very little control over how fast they drink. It can be easy to give the person mouthfuls that are too large to swallow comfortably.

You must always remember to offer frail older people the fluids they prefer. Some people do not like to drink a great deal of fluid at once. You should respect the older person's wishes and offer 'little and often' in such a situation.

Reflect on practice

Ask one of your colleagues to give you some tea from a teacup. Now ask to be given tea in a feeding cup. Did you feel more in control when drinking from the cup? Which drink was more enjoyable? Think about how many of the residents in your home have tea in feeding cups. Do you think that some of them would be able to use a teacup instead?

Recording fluid intake and output

Sometimes senior staff may decide that an individual's fluid intake and output should be recorded. There are a number of reasons for this. Staff may be unsure how much the individual is drinking. Recording the amount allows staff to check whether the person is drinking enough. Sometimes an individual is not drinking enough and all staff are asked to encourage and help the person to have sufficient fluids. The chart allows staff to check how successful they are in giving the person fluids. In other cases staff may be interested in how often the person is passing urine and how much is passed. This information is used to help people who have problems with continence. Further details on this are given in Chapter 11. Fluid charts are also called fluid balance charts; an example is given in Fig. 7.1.

Fluid charts are normally commenced at midnight. Some have continuous or running totals while others are added up at midnight.

All fluid taken into the body is recorded on the left-hand side of the chart. This includes fluid given by an intravenous or subcutaneous infusion (drip) or directly into the stomach using either a tube that goes from the patient's nose (nasogastric tube) or one that is stitched into the patient's stomach (gastrostomy tube). Registered nurses in nursing homes will record fluids given intravenously, subcutaneously or via gastrostomy or nasogastric tubes. Residential homes do not care for older people who require fluids given by these methods.

The right-hand side of the chart is used to record fluids that leave the body. Urine is measured and recorded. If the person vomits, the amount of vomit is usually estimated and recorded on this side of the chart. It is important to record fluids as accurately as possible. You may be asked to record fluids which patients have drunk on the fluid balance chart. Senior staff will show you how to do this.

Fluid Balance Chart

Name _____ Date _____

Time	Fluid type/amount	R/T	Output type/amount	R/T
	Total intake =		Total output =	

Figure 7.1 Fluid balance chart.

Importance of a healthy diet

Older people require the same amount of vitamins and nutrients as younger people, according to Department of Health guidance. On average, though, older people require fewer calories than younger, more active people. Food provided to older people living in homes needs to be carefully selected. It should be as full of vitamins and nutrients as possible but should normally have fewer calories than our normal diet. A healthy diet makes the person feel well and protects against infection and illness.

How many calories does an older person require?

The amount of calories required varies from person to person. The active, older person living in a home will normally require more calories than the person who is not active. The less active person may, however, sometimes require more calories than the average older person. If the person is recovering from a major operation, such as repair of a fractured femur, a diet high in calories, protein and vitamins will be required. If the person has a wound (for example, a pressure sore), extra calories, vitamins and protein are required to enable the wound to heal.

Some people living in homes will require large portions of food to meet their requirements, while others must avoid eating too much if they are to avoid gaining a great deal of weight. Weighing individuals will warn staff if the person is not having enough food or is gaining weight rapidly. In many hospitals, all elderly people are weighed each week. If the older person is not seriously undernourished, monthly weighings are adequate.

What is a healthy diet?

Over the years, experts have given different and contradictory advice about a healthy diet. No doubt this advice will change again as experts learn more about nutrition. The Department of Health issues dietary guidelines for healthy eating, but these do not apply to older people. The guidelines, for example, recommend that adults should drink skimmed milk instead of whole milk, should reduce the amount of fat in their diet, should eat only two or three eggs per week, and should eat cheeses low in fat instead of high-fat cheeses such as cheddar.

But these recommendations are not suitable for older people, who require a diet full of vitamins and nutrients and containing a balance of protein, fat and carbohydrate. One recommendation that does apply to older people though is eating more fruit (Fig. 7.2) and vegetables. The Department of Health now recommend that we eat five potions of fruit and vegetables a day.

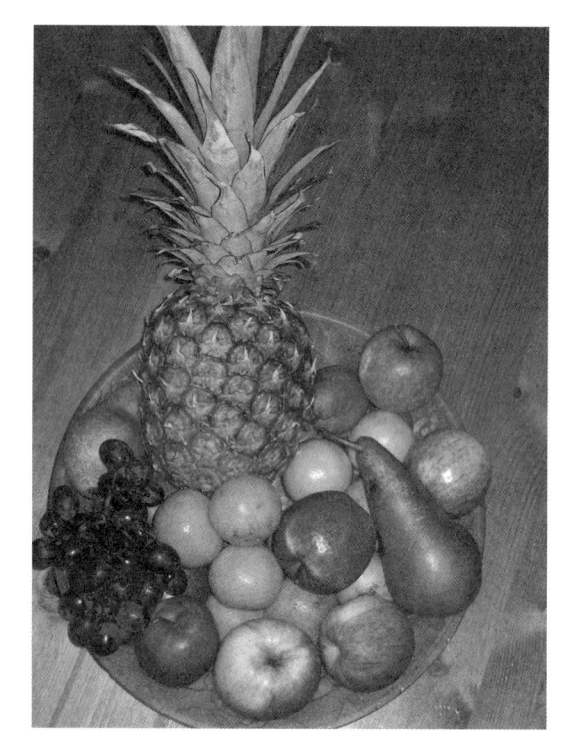

Figure 7.2 Fruit is important in a balanced diet.

Protein

Protein is found in meat, fish, nuts, lentils and beans. Protein is required to repair and replace tissues. People who have wounds, who have had recent surgery or who are recovering from a major illness require higher than normal amounts of protein.

Carbohydrate

Carbohydrate is found in vegetables and cereals. Carbohydrate is required to provide energy. It is converted by the body into glucose. Glucose is the body's main source of energy and is required by every living cell.

Fat

Fat is found in meat, fish, nuts, butter, margarine, cheese, eggs and cream. Fat is required to provide energy.

Vitamins and minerals

All food contains vitamins and minerals. Each vitamin and mineral has a function, and a shortage of vitamins or minerals can lead to illness. Some minerals and vitamins are found in most food, and shortage is rare. Others are only contained in a limited range of foods and, if the individual does not eat these foods, she may lack these vitamins or minerals. The minerals and salts required by the body are given below.

Calcium

Calcium is found in milk, butter, cheese and other foods. Calcium is required to maintain healthy teeth and bones. It also affects blood clotting and enables nerve cells to pass messages to each other. Older people can become short of calcium because they do not eat enough dairy produce. Vitamin D is required to enable the body to absorb calcium. Some older people who have osteoporosis (see Chapter 8 for details) are prescribed additional calcium and vitamin D (and often other medication) to strengthen their bones.

Copper and cobalt

Shortage of these minerals is very rare.

Iodine

Iodine is normally contained in the soil and vegetables grown in such soil absorb it. Sea fish and shellfish are a rich source of iodine. Most people living in homes eat sea fish at least once a week and are not at risk of iodine deficiency. Even those who do not eat fish get enough iodine from fruit and vegetables.

Iron

Iron is found in red meat, beef, spinach, broccoli, baked beans, apricots and chocolate. Many older people suffer from iron deficiency. This may be because they find it difficult to chew red meat, because they do not eat enough foods containing iron or because they have lost blood following an operation.

Some tablets, especially those given to people who suffer from arthritis – the anti-inflammatory drugs – can irritate the lining of the stomach and bowel. This irritation can cause the stomach and bowel to bleed a little, and this slow bleeding can cause the older person to develop anaemia. Iron tablets are usually given to treat anaemia.

Only one tenth of iron in the diet or given in tablet form is normally absorbed by the body. If the person is anaemic, the body absorbs more of the iron given. It has been found that the body can absorb more iron if vitamin C is given at the same time. Giving the older person an orange to eat or a glass of orange juice after iron tablets helps the body to absorb the iron.

Magnesium

Lack of magnesium is rare.

Sodium

This is found in normal salt. Fruit and vegetables contain salt. Processed foods usually have salt added. Most people add salt to their food and a shortage of salt is rare in this country. In tropical countries individuals may need to take extra salt on their food if they are working very hard and losing salt in their sweat.

Phosphorus

Phosphorus is found in milk, eggs and butter. It is needed to help muscles work properly, to form bones, and to balance the chemicals in the body known as electrolytes. Shortage is very rare.

Zinc

This mineral is required to allow wounds and bones to heal. It is found in liver, eggs, meat and bran. Zinc supplements are sometimes given to people who have wounds that fail to heal.

Vitamin A

Vitamin A is found in milk, butter, cream, eggs, liver, carrots and spinach. It is added to margarine. It is required to keep the skin and eyes healthy. Recent research suggests that vitamin A helps to protect the body against developing cancer.

Vitamin B

Vitamin B complex is really a series of vitamins.
   Folic acid is found in green leafy vegetables, liver, yeast, Marmite (which is made from yeast) and beer. Shortage of folic acid causes anaemia. Some people who are suffering from anaemia are treated with a mixture of iron (ferrous sulphate) and folic acid.
   Niacin is found in cereals, wheat, liver, yeast and fish. Deficiency is usually only found in countries where wheat flour is not eaten, but it

can occur in alcoholics. Deficiency causes a disease known as pellagra and the person affected suffers from confusion, dementia, diarrhoea and dermatitis. Pellagra is very rare in the UK.

Thiamine is found in eggs, peas, beans, nuts, yeast, liver, kidneys and the outer husk of rice. Deficiency leads to a disease known as beriberi. It is very rare in the UK as thiamine is found in such a variety of foods.

Riboflavin is found in green vegetables, milk, cheese, eggs, yeast and liver. It is needed to maintain a healthy skin. Deficiency is rare and normally only occurs in people who for medical reasons have been taking antibiotics for a long period.

Vitamin B_{12} is found in meat, especially liver and kidneys. Deficiency causes a special type of anaemia known as pernicious anaemia. Some people are unable to absorb vitamin B_{12} because their stomach lacks a substance necessary to absorb it. People who suffer from vitamin B_{12} deficiency have injections of this vitamin, given monthly or less frequently. Vegetarians can suffer from a shortage of vitamin B_{12} but eating foods containing yeast, such as Marmite, or drinking beer (in moderation) can prevent this.

Vitamin C

Vitamin C is required to maintain a healthy skin and to enable wounds to heal. It is thought that vitamin C protects the body against infection. Fresh fruit and vegetables contain vitamin C. Citrus fruits are high in vitamin C, while apples, pears and plums contain only small amounts. Vitamin C is easily destroyed by cooking, and keeping vegetables warm (for example in a hot trolley) destroys the vitamin C content. Liquidising or pureeing food reduces the vitamin C content. People who have extensive wounds or wounds that are slow to heal are sometimes prescribed vitamin C supplements.

Vitamin D

Vitamin D is required to produce and maintain strong bones. Oily fish such as herrings, salmon and tuna, butter, margarine, cheese, eggs and liver contain vitamin D. The body can also make vitamin D. Spending half an hour, even in winter, outside with the hands and face exposed to sunlight enables the body to make enough vitamin D for its needs.

Older people who are housebound and who have a poor diet may develop vitamin D deficiency. Some people who live in homes seldom go out and do not receive half an hour's sun on their skin daily. Some doctors now prescribed calcium and vitamin D supplements for such individuals. People with dark skins are more at risk of developing vitamin D deficiency in the UK. Women who cover their hands and face, such as Muslim women, are at risk of developing vitamin D deficiency.

Vitamin K

Vitamin K is required to enable blood to clot normally. Vitamin K is found in meat and green vegetables. It is also produced by the body in the small intestine. Deficiency is rare.

Special diets

Some older people living in homes require special diets because of long-term conditions.

Diabetic diet

Older people who suffer from diabetes require a special diet. Normally when we eat, the pancreas produces insulin. Insulin enables us to use the glucose that is produced when food is digested. People who suffer from diabetes do not produce any insulin, or do not produce enough insulin or cannot use the insulin that they make effectively. There are two different types of diabetes.

- Type 1 diabetes (formerly known as insulin-dependent diabetes) usually begins when the person is young. It is treated with insulin injections and a diabetic diet.
- Type 2 diabetes (formerly known as non-insulin-dependent diabetes) may also be called mature-onset diabetes. The pancreas fails to produce enough insulin for the person's needs. This form of diabetes can sometimes be treated with diet alone. Many people who suffer from type 2 diabetes are overweight, and losing weight helps to control the disease. Some older people are given tablets. These tablets make the pancreas work harder to produce insulin and enable the person's body to use insulin more effectively. Sometimes a combination of tablets and a diabetic diet is used to control diabetes. People with type 2 diabetes may require insulin if they are ill or if their diabetes worsens.

Diabetes becomes more common as people age. Research has shown that by the age of 85 one-tenth of all older people suffer from diabetes. Some people are more at risk of diabetes than others. Research shows that Asian people are more likely to become diabetic than other races. The reasons for this are not known.

The aim of a diabetic diet is to provide a diet high in fibre and low in fat and sugar. Fresh vegetables and fruit are recommended. The diabetic person can eat starchy foods such as potatoes, but baked potatoes are preferable to chips as they contain more fibre and less fat. The diabetic person should avoid sugar and sweet foods. Diabetics can eat sugar-free puddings. Many desserts are now available that use artificial sweeteners instead of sugar and these are suitable for diabetics. Special biscuits, sweets, chocolates, marmalade and jam can be bought for diabetics. However, diabetes specialists advise against the use of these special foods and recommend that the person with diabetes be allowed a small amount of a non-diabetic treat occasionally.

Overweight diabetics should avoid eating too many 'diabetic' foods. These are sweetened using a substance called sorbitol, which is just as fattening as sugar. Too much sorbitol can cause diarrhoea; a diabetic person who eats a whole packet of sugar-free mints or a packet of diabetic custard creams may suffer from acute diarrhoea. Tea and coffee can be sweetened with artificial sweeteners. An artificial sweetener that looks like sugar can be sprinkled over cereals, used to sweeten custard, and used instead of sugar in cakes.

Reducing diets

These are intended to help overweight people lose weight. Being overweight can make an older person unwell, and losing weight can make them feel better. People who have high blood pressure and are overweight may find that their blood pressure improves if they lose weight.

People who suffer from arthritis, especially arthritis of the hips and knees, place an extra strain on their joints if they are overweight. Losing weight can help reduce pain and increase movement. Researchers found that 40% of people who had such pain from their arthritic knees that knee replacement was being considered, no longer needed surgery when they lost weight.

The aim of a reducing diet is to produce a small, steady loss in weight. It is important that the older person has a diet with sufficient vitamins and nutrients. Usually the amount of sugar in the diet is reduced. Sweeteners can be used in tea and coffee and on cereals. Fat can be reduced: the older person can have grilled bacon instead of fried, a poached egg instead of a fried egg. Occasional treats such as cake or a small bar of chocolate should be allowed, otherwise the person who is on a reducing diet may decide to give up. If the older person is overweight and does not wish to lose weight, staff working in the home must respect the person's wishes.

Vegetarians

Vegetarians do not eat meat. Some vegetarians eat fish, eggs and dairy products while others do not eat any animal products. People who do not eat any animal products are known as vegans. It is important to ensure that people who are vegetarian are offered a healthy vegetarian diet. The Vegetarian Society provides a wealth of information including recipes on its website (see further information at the end of the chapter).

High-fibre diets

The diet we eat in the UK can be low in fibre and this can cause many problems. Eating a diet rich in fibre increases health and reduces the risk of problems such as constipation. Further details on the reasons why older people are at risk of developing constipation are given in Chapter 8. A diet rich in fibre can enable older people to have normal bowel actions and avoid relying on laxatives.

There are two different types of fibre: soluble and non-soluble. It is recommended that a high-fibre diet should contain a mixture of both types. This means that the diet should contain fruit and vegetables and fibre found in cereals such as porridge, Weetabix, All-bran, wholemeal bread, digestive biscuits and wholemeal flour.

A high-fibre diet can be tasty and varied but should be introduced gradually so that the person's body can become used to it. All people are different and the amount of fibre people require varies. One person may find that the diet provides too much fibre and causes diarrhoea, while another might require extra fibre perhaps, by having an extra portion of fruit, a dish of prunes or a slice of date loaf.

High-calorie diet

Many frail older people are at risk of malnourishment; around 40% of older people in care homes need to gain weight. High-calorie diets are required when the older person is thin and undernourished or has increased dietary needs, perhaps because he is more active than other patients, is recovering from a recent operation or has a pressure sore or leg ulcer. The aim is to provide enough calories to meet the patient's needs. Putting too much food on the plate can be offputting so offer snacks, encourage family and friends to bring in foods that the person is especially fond of, and give dietary supplements if they have been supplied by the doctor.

Puréed diets

Some older people who are very frail or who have difficulty in chewing, perhaps because of a stroke, may require a puréed diet. The aim is to give, as far as possible, a normal diet that has been puréed. Meat and vegetables should not be mixed together and puréed as this is unappetising and the person cannot choose which part of the meal to eat.

Food should be puréed separately. It may be served in a dish with partitions so that the different foods do not blend into each other. Thickening agents are available and the puréed food can be thickened. Moulds can be used to shape puréed food. Puréed thickened lamb can be moulded into a lamb chop mould. Using thickening agents and moulds helps make a puréed diet look more attractive. Sometimes the person receiving a puréed diet may also require dietary supplements.

Meeting the dietary needs of people from different cultures

Some older people come from different backgrounds to those of the majority of people living in homes. People who come from different cultures or who practise different religions may require a different diet. The aim of care in homes is to provide a similar type of life to that which the person would lead living at home. Research shows that although there are a significant number of people from different cultures living in the UK, few people from ethnic minorities enter homes. The reasons for this are not known but there are several theories. Many people come to the UK from other countries when they are young. In the 1950s, many people came to the UK from the West Indies. They were recruited by London Transport to work on the railways, tubes and buses. Since then, many younger people have entered the UK from other countries. People who came to the UK in the 1950s are only just becoming old and may require care in homes. Another theory is that already many people from other cultures require care in homes but because homes do not provide special services to meet their needs, they are reluctant to enter homes. It is important that all older people living in homes have their needs met and their cultures respected. People from different cultures have different dietary needs.

Jews

Jewish people may eat a special diet that is called a kosher diet. Those who follow this diet strictly have separate areas within the kitchen for preparing meat and milk dishes. Milk and meat are not eaten together and separate crockery is used for meat and milk dishes. Even people of the Jewish faith who do not have a strict kosher diet normally avoid having meat and milk at the same meal. The person may have cereal with milk for breakfast but would not eat a beef sausage at this meal. Jewish people do not normally eat pork or shellfish. If a care assistant is caring for a person of the Jewish faith, she should find out what the person prefers to eat and drink.

There are a number of care homes throughout the UK that care for Jewish people and provide kosher food and culturally sensitive care. Sometimes people of the Jewish faith who follow a strict kosher diet are admitted to care homes that do not have the ability to provide kosher food. This might be because the person has come in as an emergency placement or for intermediate care. In such circumstances kosher food can be delivered to the home.

Muslims

Muslims do not eat pork and normally avoid alcohol. Strict Muslims eat meat that has been killed in a special way, known as halal meat. This can be obtained from halal butchers and is cooked normally. If halal meat is not available, strict Muslims may prefer to avoid eating meat.

Hindus

Hindus do not eat beef. Some people of the Hindu faith are vegetarian and do not eat any animal products.

Dietary supplements

Older people who are unable to eat enough food to meet their requirements are often offered dietary supplements. There is an enormous range of dietary supplements available. These include drinks that look and taste like squash but are high in calories, vitamins and minerals. Other drinks are like milk shakes and come in a range of flavours; these too are full of vitamins, minerals and calories. Special puddings are available, and special high-protein snacks such as biscuits may be given.

If the older person is underweight, losing weight or not eating very much, professional advice should be sought. Dieticians can advise on action to be taken. The dietician will normally bring a range of dietary supplements. The older person can taste these supplements and the dietician will normally contact the person's doctor and ask for them to be prescribed. Dietary supplements are available on prescription to individuals who have difficulty in swallowing or who suffer from certain conditions.

Why some older people have difficulty eating

Chewing

Chewing can be difficult for some older people. Those who have lost their dentures or who have poorly fitting dentures will have difficulty. People who have suffered from strokes sometimes have difficulty in chewing because one side of the face is paralysed.

Swallowing

Swallowing can be difficult. People who suffer from motor neurone disease, multiple sclerosis, Parkinson's disease or who have suffered a stroke may have difficulty in swallowing. You should encourage people with swallowing difficulties to take small mouthfuls, chew thoroughly and wash food down well with water. The person should be provided with a suitable diet. The person who has difficulty in swallowing should sit up straight in the chair, as slouching makes the problem worse.

Cutlery

Cutlery can be difficult for some older people to use. The person who has lost the use of one hand may find it very difficult to cut up food and eat one-handed. Special cutlery is available to help people who can only use one hand. People who have severe arthritis in the hands can find it difficult to grip ordinary cutlery, and special cutlery is available for them. Some people find that the plate slips. Non-slip mats placed under the plate prevent this. If a person is eating one-handed, the food can easily slip off the plate. Using a plate guard that clips onto the plate prevents this.

Aids to help older people to eat can be purchased from medical supplies companies or they can be supplied by the occupational therapist for the individual's use. The person's doctor can ask the occupational therapist to visit. Occupational therapy services available to homes vary. In some areas it is difficult to obtain occupational therapy advice and senior staff have to be firm in obtaining such services. In some areas occupational therapy staff will advise on aids needed but are not able to supply them. The home must purchase such aids. Aids can enable even the most disabled person to eat independently.

Poor eyesight

Poor eyesight can prevent people from seeing the food on the plate. Using dark-coloured plates (see Fig. 7.3) to provide a contrast enables the older person to see the food more easily.

Confusion

Many residents who are confused have dementia. People who have dementia have great difficulty processing information. Too much bustle and too many things happening at once cause great distress. Some confused people can find it difficult to settle down to eat a meal. Creating a relaxed, calm atmosphere helps confused people to settle and enjoy their meal. Turning off the television, playing music and avoiding bustling about help to create a relaxing mealtime.

Research carried out in American nursing homes found that when lighting was subdued and gentle music was played, residents ate more.

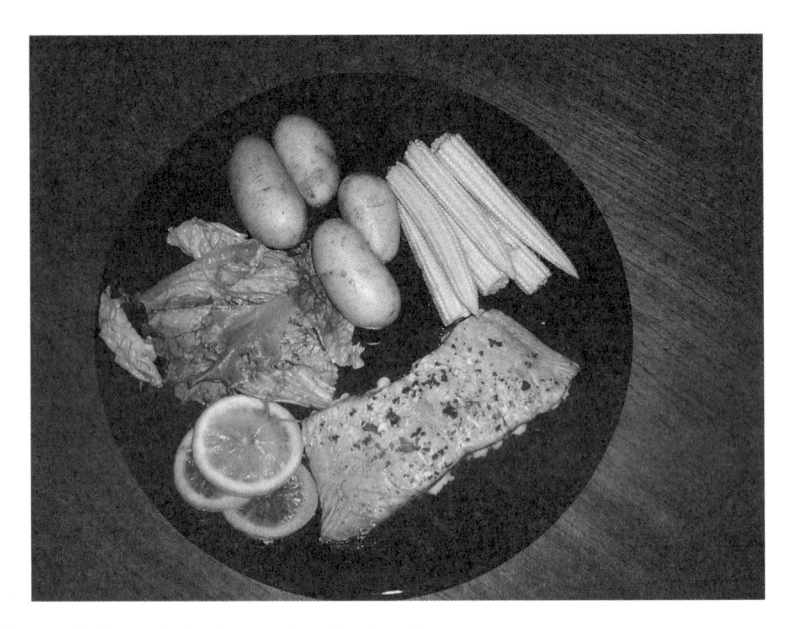

Figure 7.3 A dark plate makes food easier to see.

Residents became unsettled when country and western music was played but relaxed and ate well when classical music or nature sounds were played. In some cases confused residents benefit from eating in a small dining room where bustle can be reduced to a minimum.

Serving food and making mealtimes a pleasure

Mealtimes should be pleasant occasions and should give the older person the opportunity not only to enjoy a meal but also to chat with others and to relax over the meal. It is important that staff make an effort to make eating a pleasant experience. In some homes, breakfast is served in the person's room. The older person should be made comfortable for breakfast and helped to sit up in bed or to sit out in a chair if she requires help. Food should be presented attractively and served hot; people are not tempted by lukewarm tea and cold porridge.

Many homes encourage older people to eat lunch in the dining room (Fig. 7.4) so that they can chat with others. Tables should be set out with tablecloths, flowers, napkins, cutlery, drinks, salt, pepper and sauces. Older people who are able to help lay tables should be encouraged to do so. Playing music quietly in the background helps create a relaxing atmosphere and encourages people to relax and enjoy their meal. People who require help with eating must be helped. You should sit down with the individual who requires help, as this makes the person feel more relaxed and less hurried.

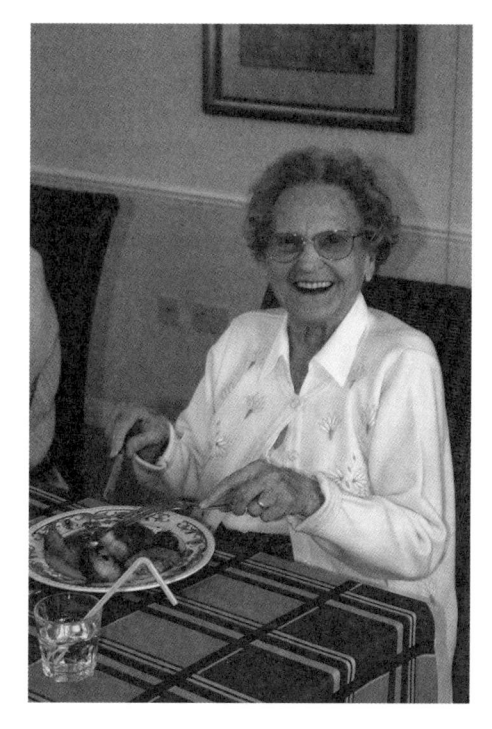

Figure 7.4 Mealtimes are enjoyable.

Preparing food and drink

Care assistants in most homes are rarely required to cook main meals. Many care assistants may prepare snacks to tempt people with poor appetites to eat. Occasionally you may be required to help in the kitchen. Most homes now employ a cook or chef who is responsible for meals.

When preparing food and drink it is important to remember that we eat with our eyes. Presentation is very important. However, all the presentation in the world is wasted if the food provided is not what the person wants so it is important to find out what the person wishes to eat.

Enabling people to choose

Information about enabling people to choose drinks is given earlier in the chapter. Choosing what to eat is something we take for granted. Yet many people living in homes have difficulty choosing food. There are many reasons for this. Poor vision can make it difficult for people to read the menu. People who have had strokes may no longer be able to read. People who do not read English will be unable to choose from a menu written in English. Some older people are expected to tick boxes on a menu to indicate their choices. People who are no longer able to write cannot complete such menus. Some older people have poor memories. The person may choose a dish for the next day but forget by morning. There are many ways you can enable people to choose what they would like to eat. Some suggestions include:

- Produce the menu in large print; many older people with visual problems can read 20-point bold with ease.
- Use pictures to illustrate the menu. Computer Clipart has made it so much easier to produce this type of menu. You can use a picture of fish and chips and large-size type to illustrate the menu. If you do not have access to a computer you can cut pictures out of magazines. People who are unable to read can see the pictures of the dishes and point to their choice.
- Allow people to choose their next meal as late as possible; in the home where I worked residents were able to choose lunch up to 11 am that morning.
- Read the menu to people with visual problems.
- Note people's likes and dislikes in the care plan.

Good practice

Eating and drinking are essential if the individual is to remain in good health. Some older people living in homes require help to eat and drink; others, especially those with special dietary needs, may require advice on what foods they should eat. Care assistants should be aware of the older person's fluid and food preferences. You should aim to provide, wherever possible, food and drink that the older person prefers. The food available should be similar to that which the older person would choose to eat at home. You should offer to assist older people who require help and should be careful to ensure that the older person maintains dignity at all times.

Key points

- Ageing and illness increase the risk of an older person becoming dehydrated.
- Older people may need assistance and encouragement to eat and drink.
- Dietary needs vary and it's important to meet individual dietary needs.
- A range of aids is available to enable the individual to eat independently.
- Some people may need assistance to eat.
- It is important to enable people to choose food.
- Making mealtimes a pleasure reduces the risk of poor nutrition.
- You role in encouraging people to eat and reporting any problems is of vital importance.

📖 Portfolio preparation

Your assessor must have evidence that you can meet the performance criteria for this unit. Before beginning this unit, discuss assessment strategies with your assessor. Most of the evidence for this unit can be gained by direct observation of your work.

Products: This might be a copy of a fluid balance chart that you completed. It could be a note in a resident's notes giving details of the person's dietary preferences or details of assistance that the person requires detailed on a care plan. It could be a care plan that you have drawn up or contributed to on meeting the assessed need of an individual.

Witness testimony: This is a statement from a senior member of staff. It might be a statement detailing how you have met certain performance criteria.

Written work: You might be asked to prepare a piece of work about how you encourage a resident to eat a balanced diet, or you might be asked to write a case history about a resident with special dietary needs and how those are met.

Your assessor may also use other methods to help you gain evidence for this unit. These may include:

- Verbal questioning
- Written questions.

Simulations can be used to increase your awareness of how it feels to be fed. Some assessors ask students to feed each other and then discuss their feelings. Often students report that they are fed too quickly, or the spoon is overloaded, or they are not told what they are having. This type of simulation improves care. Simulations can also be used to assess your ability to meet performance criteria. They may also be used to help gain evidence if it cannot be gained by direct observation.

Further information

Diabetes

Diabetes UK
Macleod House
10 Parkway
London NW1 7AA
Telephone: 020 7424 1000
Helpline: 0845 120 2960 (Monday to Friday, 9 am to 5 pm)
E-mail: careline@diabetes.org.uk
Website: http://www.diabetes.org.uk

A translation service is available for non-English speakers.

Information on all aspects of diabetes and diabetic diets is available. A range of leaflets, books and videos are available on the website and can also be obtained by post.

Vegetarian diets

Vegetarian Society
Park Dale
Durham Road
Altrincham
Cheshire WA14 4QG
Telephone: 0161 925 2000
Fax: 0161 926 9182
E-mail: support@vegsoc.org
Website: http://www.vegsoc.org

Information on vegetarian diets is available. A useful leaflet, *Healthy Nutrition in Later Life*, which contains guidance and recipes, is available free if a stamped self-addressed envelope is sent. The website has several useful sections. There are professional pages giving information on all aspects of vegetarian diet, pages for people who are vegetarian and information and recipes for caterers.

High-fibre diets

Kellogg's Consumer Services
PO Box 356
Freepost
Warrington WA4 6XY
Telephone: 0800 626066 (Monday to Friday, 8 am to 6 pm)
Website: http://www.kelloggs.co.uk/health/

Kellogg's (the cereal manufacturer) provide information on high-fibre diets, a patient education pack, and a selection of recipes.

Further reading

Nursing Times (1998) *Nutrition in Practice*. This binder contains ten articles on nutrition including one on nutrition and the elderly. You may find it in your college library.

Sandy D (1997) *Food in Care*. Macmillan Caring series. This book provides detailed advice on nutrition. You may find it in your college library.

Chapter Eight
Mobility
HSC215
Help individuals to keep mobile

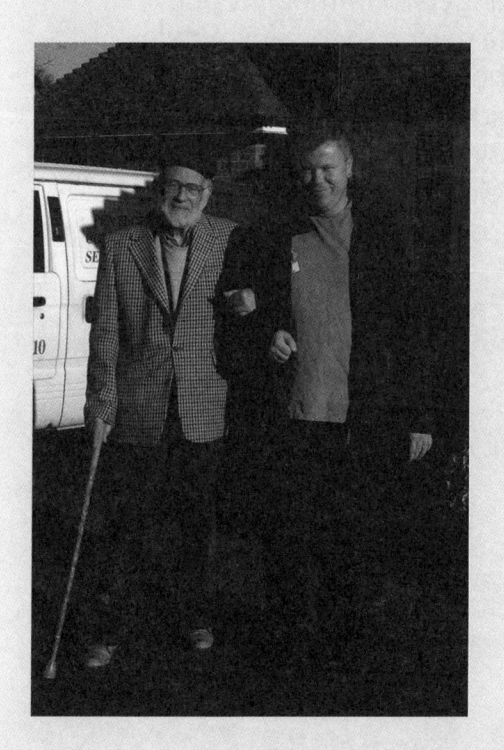

This unit consists of two elements:
HSC215a Support individuals to keep mobile
HSC215b Observe any changes in the individual's mobility and provide feedback to the appropriate people

This chapter

- Explains why older people benefit from remaining mobile and how illness affects mobility
- Provides information on the dangers of immobility and how to help and encourage the person to remain mobile
- Provides information on aids, how to encourage and assist the older person to use aids
- Provides information about maintaining safety and enabling people who use wheelchairs to remain mobile
- Provides information and advice on exercise and passive movement
- Provides information and advice on how to support people making journeys

Benefits of remaining mobile

The ability to move around freely is one of the most basic of human rights. It is an ability that we often take for granted. Many older people who enter homes have problems moving around. Some are unable to move unaided from bed to chair and some are bed-bound. Some develop deformities that mean that they can no longer straighten arms or legs, and hands may become permanently closed in fists.

Some professional staff in some homes may tell you that such changes are the inevitable effects of ageing and that older people become immobile because of ageing. While older people may become immobile in the last few months or weeks of life, many older people living in nursing and residential homes become immobile because of poorly managed care. It does not have to be this way. The way staff work within homes may not only prevent some older people from regaining mobility after illness, it can also cause older people to become less mobile and more dependent. An important goal of care in homes should be to enable older people to retain and regain mobility. This in turn enables them to retain the ability to care for themselves and enjoy a superior quality of life within the home. It also reduces staff workload.

This chapter will outline how illness affects the older person's ability to move around, the dangers of immobility, and how carers can help older people to retain independence after illness. Some older people, normally those who are extremely ill or disabled, will require greater levels of assistance and may need to be moved. This is dealt with in Chapter 12.

How illness affects ability to move around

Many older people are admitted to care homes from hospital, although some are admitted from home. Most are admitted because the effects of an accident or illness mean that the individual can no longer manage to care for him or herself at home. Some older people are admitted because a long-standing illness has worsened and it is impossible to provide the levels of support and care required at home. Others are admitted because of a sudden illness or an accident.

It is possible for many older people who are unable to care for themselves at home to enjoy life in a home where the support they require is given. There is a danger that staff who are not aware of the older person's abilities may discourage the older person from moving around the home. In other cases, older people may require encouragement, help, support and aids to help them walk. It is important that you understand how illness affects an individual's ability to walk, so that you can offer appropriate support and help.

Arthritis

Arthritis is a disease that affects all people as they age. Adults start to develop arthritic changes from the age of 40 onwards. Although all older people have arthritis, not all suffer the symptoms. Approximately 12% of men and 25% of women over the age of 70 suffer pain, stiffness and difficulties in moving because of arthritis. There are two types of arthritis: osteo-arthritis and rheumatoid arthritis.

Osteo-arthritis

'Osteo' means bone, and 'arthritis' means damage or inflammation at a joint (Greek: *arthron*). Osteo-arthritis is damage and inflammation of the bone. The ends of bone at joints are covered with a thin layer of smooth material called cartilage. The ends of the bone and the cartilage are surrounded by a thick fluid called synovial fluid. This is contained in a thin membrane known as the synovial membrane. Cartilage and synovial fluid cushion the end of the bone from the effects of movement and act as shock absorbers. The cartilage becomes thinned and roughened when osteo-arthritis is present. The bone is not so well protected from the shock of movement and thickens, the amount of fluid increases and the joint appears swollen. In severe osteo-arthritis, the cartilage can wear away completely and bone can rub on bone. The joints affected usually become visibly deformed.

Figure 8.1 shows a healthy knee joint and Fig. 8.2 shows a knee joint affected by osteo-arthritis.

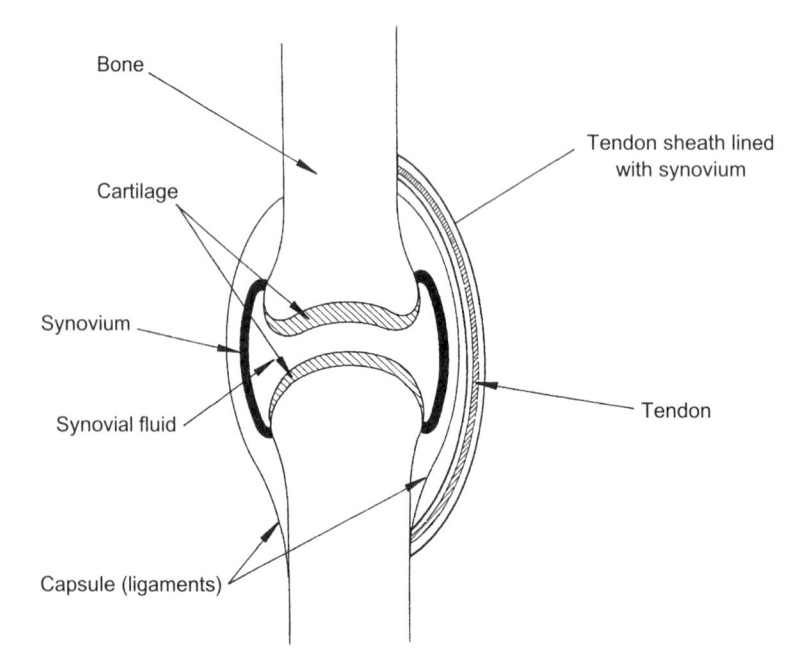

Figure 8.1 A healthy knee joint.

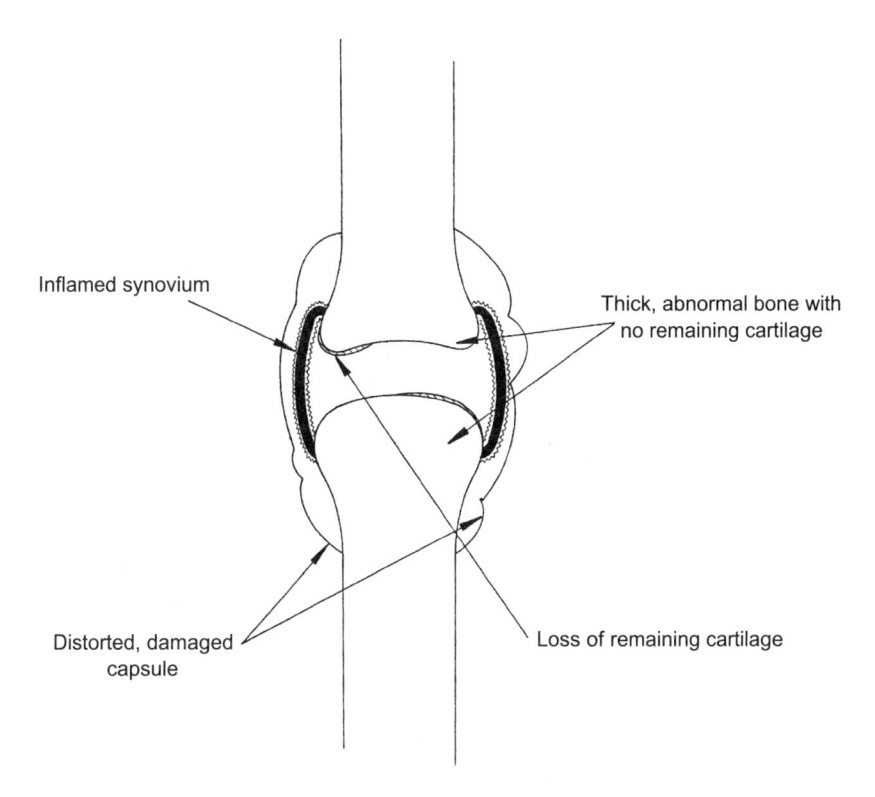

Figure 8.2 An arthritic knee joint.

The causes of osteo-arthritis are not yet known. People are more likely to develop osteo-arthritis as they become older and people who have injured a joint or had an operation on a joint are more likely to develop osteo-arthritis. It often develops in people who have taken part in active sports. The joints affected are usually the hand, hips, knees and big toes. Osteo-arthritis of the hip usually affects one hip more severely than the other. It can lead to one leg becoming slightly shorter. This can cause walking difficulties and back pain. Osteo-arthritis of the hip is more common in men than in women. Osteo-arthritis of the knee is more common in women. Osteo-arthritis normally affects only one or two joints. Although many people who suffer from osteo-arthritis find that pain and stiffness is worse in damp weather, dampness does not cause the problem. People all over the world suffer from this condition.

Osteo-arthritis causes pain, stiffness and swelling. The stiffness is made worse by remaining in one position for a long time, and will improve after a few minutes of exercise.

Pain is normally treated with pain-killing tablets, known as analgesics. Paracetamol is commonly prescribed. It is important that analgesics are given regularly. Weaker analgesics given regularly are more effective that strong analgesics given occasionally. If these are not effective the prescriber may prescribe analgesics with codeine in them. These can cause constipation and nausea in some people so it is important to observe and report any such problems.

Anti-inflammatory drugs are often prescribed. These drugs act not only by treating pain but also by reducing the inflammation in the joint. Such drugs are known as non-steroidal anti-inflammatory drugs. Nurofen, a popular painkiller that can be bought over the counter, is a non-steroidal anti-inflammatory drug. Anti-inflammatory drugs, like all drugs, have side effects. They can cause stomach ulcers and the person may bleed from the stomach. Prescribers often prescribe a drug to protect the person's stomach in such cases. People who have had ulcers in the past may not be able to take these drugs. Anti-inflammatory drugs can cause some people (especially those with heart failure) to develop swollen legs. If you notice any side effects, report them to a senior member of staff.

Overweight people who suffer from osteo-arthritis will feel much better if they lose weight, because extra weight increases the strain on joints.

Rheumatoid arthritis

Rheumatoid arthritis is an inflammatory disease of the joints. The synovial tissue that covers the joints becomes inflamed. This causes the affected joints to become hot, swollen and painful. Figure 8.3 shows how rheumatoid arthritis affects a joint.

Rheumatoid arthritis normally affects many joints. A person with rheumatoid arthritis may suffer from pain and inflammation in the shoulders, arms, wrists, fingers and toes. Although this is a chronic disease, there are often periods when it settles down and causes few problems. At other times the individual suffers an acute attack and joints become very painful. During an acute attack, people are advised to rest the joints

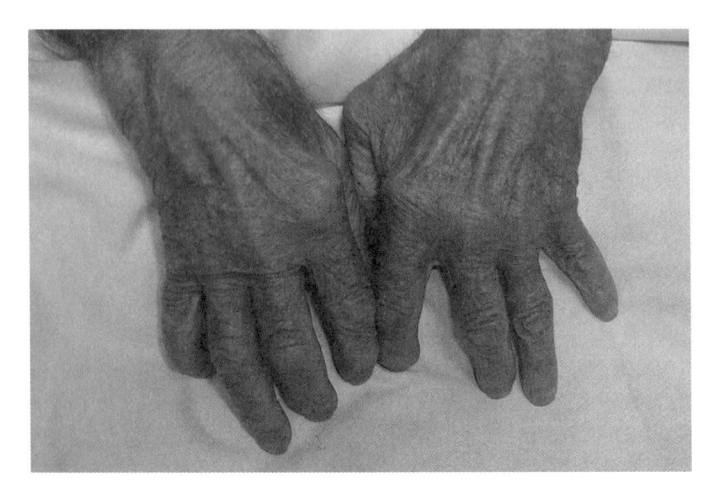

Figure 8.3 Joints affected by rheumatoid arthritis.

as much as possible. In mild cases, paracetamol is prescribed. In more severe cases, non-steroidal anti-inflammatory drugs are prescribed. Doctors may prescribe steroids in severe cases. The cause of rheumatoid arthritis is not yet known.

Benefits of exercise

It is important that people suffering from all types of arthritis keep as active as possible. Many years ago it was thought that the best treatment for all types was rest. Many people with arthritis of all types were admitted to hospital and kept on strict bedrest. Arthritic joints were often put in plaster of Paris casts to prevent any movement. It was thought then that joints became worn out by too much movement. Now people who are suffering from acute rheumatoid arthritis are advised to rest their swollen joints but to take gentle exercise to aid recovery. People suffering from chronic rheumatoid arthritis and osteo-arthritis are advised to carry on with gentle exercise and remain as mobile as possible. Some older people worry that exercise will cause further damage to joints and need reassurance that this will not happen. Gentle exercise will reduce stiffness and help them to remain as fit as possible.

Stroke

Many older people are admitted to homes after suffering from strokes. The medical term for a stroke is a cerebrovascular accident. Nursing and medical staff often refer to this as a CVA. Normally blood flows around the brain, feeding it with oxygen and sugar (Fig. 8.4). A stroke causes the blood supply to the brain to be interrupted and part of the brain is starved of oxygen.

There are two main causes of strokes. Some occur because the blood becomes too thick; blood cells stick together and form a clot, which prevents blood reaching an area of the brain (Fig. 8.5a). In other cases the blood vessels supplying the brain leak and bleed into the brain (Fig. 8.5b). In both cases, the blood supply to the brain is interrupted and the brain becomes damaged. The amount of damage a stroke causes varies enormously. The longer the person is unconscious after a stroke, the greater the damage. Once an area of the brain has been damaged, it cannot recover (Fig. 8.6). It is estimated that we use only about a tenth of our brain and often other parts of the brain learn to do the job of the damaged area.

People who have suffered from strokes often develop weakness or paralysis down one side of their body. A weakness is known as hemiparesis and paralysis as hemiplegia. Many older people who have a stroke can regain movement and continue to recover for up to two years after a stroke. Some older people remain paralysed down one side but can learn to walk with special aids. Others can learn to move around freely in

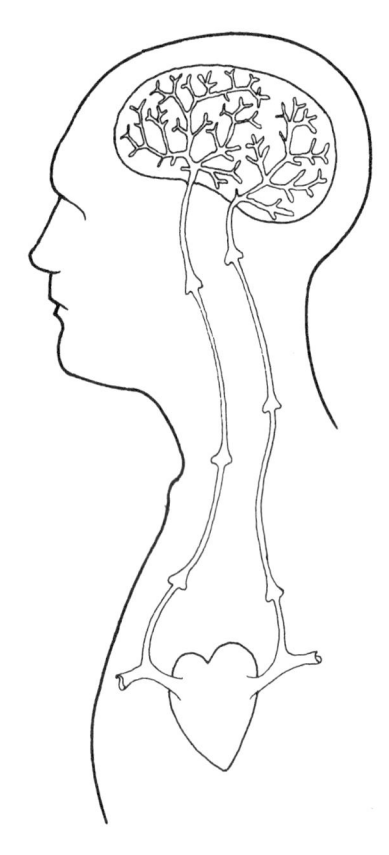

Figure 8.4 Blood flows from the heart to the brain via the arterial circulation.

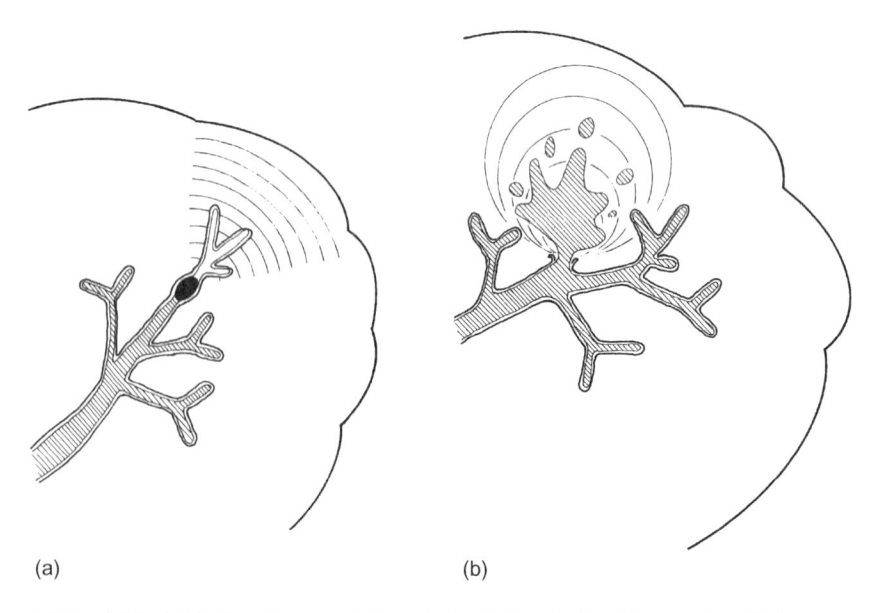

(a) (b)

Figure 8.5 (a) A clot lodged in one of the arteries in the brain; (b) a ruptured blood vessel.

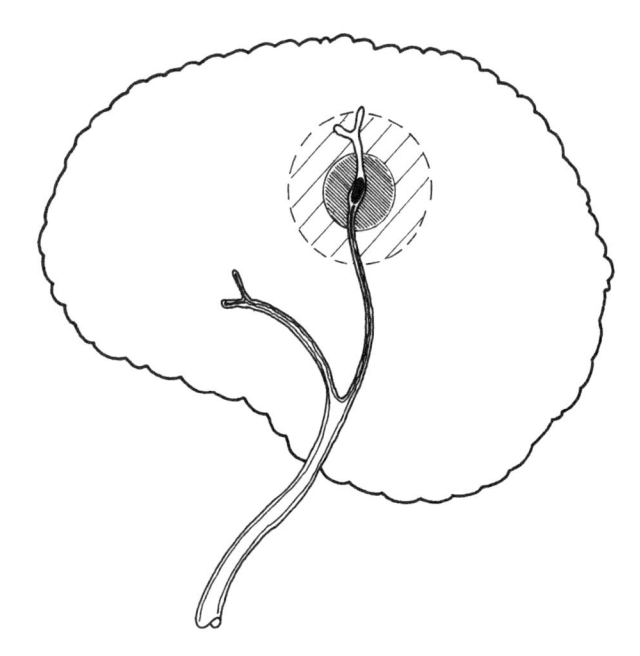

Figure 8.6 The dark shading shows the area of brain tissue which no longer functions because of the stroke. The circled area with diagonal line shading is the brain tissue affected by bruising and swelling. This part of the brain will recover.

wheelchairs and transfer from wheelchair to chair, bed or toilet. You can help people to regain as much independence as possible following a stroke by encouraging them to exercise and to learn how to cope with disability and remain as independent as possible.

Fractures

Older people are more at risk of falling than younger people. Many older people develop osteoporosis; one woman in two and one man in five develops this condition. Osteoporosis leads to the bones becoming thinner, weaker and more likely to break. Figure 2.3 (page 49) shows (a) normal bone and (b) osteoporotic bone. When older people fall, they often break their wrist, thigh bone (femur) or hip.

Nowadays most people who suffer from a fractured femur have surgical treatment. The bone is pulled together and held in place with a metal plate and screws. If the neck of the femur is fractured a screw may be inserted to hold the bone together, or the surgeon may replace the neck of the femur with metal. If the hip is fractured, the surgeon may carry out a hip replacement.

Many older people are admitted to homes following fracture have not regained previous levels of mobility. You should work with senior staff to enable the person to become as mobile as possible. Observe the person for pain and discomfort and inform a senior member of staff if the person is in pain.

Some older people who are in pain do not tell staff. One survey carried out in hospital found that patients who were in pain waited for nursing staff to ask about pain because they did not want to appear to be complaining. The same survey found that nursing staff waited for patients to tell them that they were in pain. You should learn to observe individuals, as often our behaviour shows whether we are in pain. If you think the person may be in pain, ask.

Many older people who have had a severe fall have lost all confidence in walking. They may require encouragement and help in beginning to walk again. Some older people who have had surgery to repair a fractured femur or hip may now have one leg shorter than the other. This can make walking difficult and dangerous. Fortunately, it can easily be corrected by ordering and providing special shoes. One shoe has a slightly higher, built-up heel and this corrects any differences in leg length. Further details are given later in the chapter.

The older person with osteoporosis can also develop fractures of the spinal vertebrae. These can happen spontaneously and may cause height loss and postural changes. Such fractures can cause pain and the presence of several may lead to other problems such as incontinence, digestive problems and breathlessness which can have a significant impact on a person's quality of life.

The older person with new spinal fractures is often treated with painkillers and rest until pain has settled. Because the vertebrae heal in a new shape which can press on nerves and irritate surrounding soft tissues, some people can be left with chronic back pain. This can be managed with painkillers, physiotherapy and other approaches such as TENS machines and heat packs.

Osteoporosis is normally treated with drugs to help slow down bone loss and build up bone. These are usually given weekly. The person is also given calcium and vitamin D supplements.

Vision

Over a half a million Britons over the age of 75 have extremely poor eyesight. Research carried out by experts in London has found that 1 in 10 older people is visually impaired and 1 in 50 is blind. It also showed that more women than men experience poor eyesight, with three out of four women likely to have serious difficulties by the age of 75. Poor vision can make it difficult for older people to move around freely.

Research from the Royal College of Opticians shows that 96% of people over the age of 80 require spectacles. Many older people admitted to care homes wear spectacles but may not have had their eyes tested for many years. New spectacles and an up-to-date prescription for lenses may help them to move around with newfound confidence.

Some older people suffer from cataracts. These affect vision long before they are noticeable to others. Now many older people can benefit from cataract surgery. An eye test will detect the presence of cataracts.

Some older people suffer from eye diseases such as glaucoma. Untreated glaucoma can cause blindness. An eye test will detect the presence of glaucoma and the person's doctor can prescribe eye drops which will prevent vision deteriorating. Recently doctors carried out research to find out why people admitted to hospital with falls had fallen. They found that most of the people who had fallen had very poor vision. Almost all visual problems could be treated.

Some older people suffer from extremely poor vision and little can be done to improve it. If staff are aware that the individual's vision is poor, they can ensure that the environment is as safe as possible. Details of maintaining a safe environment are given in Chapter 2.

Older people should have their eyes tested each year. This enables opticians to detect eye diseases and also to maximise the older person's vision.

Dangers of immobility

When older people lose the ability to move around freely, it has a devastating effect on their physical and mental health. Many older people fear becoming a burden and they wish to carry on caring for themselves. The idea of being dependent on others can be very upsetting. Imagine what it must be like to be unable to walk to the toilet and to have to rely on others to take you. Imagine how it must feel to be unable to get up when you wish or to go to bed when you wish. Many older people become depressed, anxious and upset when they lose the ability to move around.

The physical effects of immobility are also distressing. People who sit for long periods often find that their feet and ankles become swollen. This is because they are not walking. Walking helps the veins to return blood to the heart. People who are sitting for long periods are at risk of developing blood clots in the legs. These are called deep vein thrombosis. A deep vein thrombosis can break away from the vein in the leg and enter the venous circulation. The clot then travels around the body until it becomes stuck either in a heart valve or in the vein entering the lung (pulmonary vein). This condition is known as a pulmonary embolism and can be fatal.

Moving around causes us to breathe more deeply and this deep breathing is one protection against chest infections. People who are immobile are more at risk of developing a chest infection than those who walk around.

Movement causes the bowel to contract. People who do not move around are more at risk of becoming constipated. People who can go to the toilet without help are less likely to suffer from incontinence than those who require help. People who require help are dependent on staff to take them to the toilet. Often staff do not respond quickly enough to an individual's call for assistance (perhaps because they are doing something else) and incontinence can result. People who are not using muscles find that their muscles quickly become smaller and weaker, and strength and ability is rapidly lost.

Movement helps us to digest food and build up an appetite. It also enables us to sleep better.

Helping older people to move around

The role of all staff working in healthcare is to enable the older person to function to capacity, to maximise ability and to minimise the effects of any disability. The role of care assistants in helping individuals to retain or regain independence is important. You can help or hinder the older person who wishes to remain independent.

The care assistant who 'takes over' and offers or insists on doing things for the person who can do it themselves is not helping and making things easier for the person. The care assistant is making life more difficult. Faced with such 'help' some older people can feel that there is little point in trying and that it is better to let the staff 'get on with it'. Care assistants can unintentionally make older people feel useless. If you offer to bring a person downstairs in a wheelchair 'because it's quicker', the person may soon lose the confidence and strength to come down alone. She will also lose independence and may begin to feel that she is a nuisance and a burden to staff. The sensitive carer will provide support and help without robbing the person of her independence (Case Study 8.1).

Case Study 8.1

Mrs Edna Brown has lived in a nursing home for some time.

At the morning report, staff are informed that Mrs Brown fell while walking to bed the night before. The care assistant caring for her, Sarah Easton, asks Mrs Brown how she feels. Mrs Brown confesses that she feels shaken by her fall.

Sarah offers to help her get her clothes ready and asks if she would like any help with washing or dressing. Mrs Brown says she can manage. Later Sarah walks with Mrs Brown to the lounge. This action gives Mrs Brown confidence; help is at hand if needed but Mrs Brown has maintained her independence.

Walking aids

Many older people rely on walking aids to help them move around. Some older people are admitted to homes with aids. Some individuals who do not have aids might be able to move around independently or with less help if they had an aid. There are several different types of walking aid. The commonest is the Zimmer or walking frame.

Zimmer frames

Zimmer frames help older people who are unsteady on their feet or who lack confidence, because when they are used properly people are more stable. Zimmer frames come in a variety of heights and widths; it is possible to adjust the height on some frames. Each person is measured for his or her frame so that it is the right height. Too tall a frame encourages an individual to reach up; this unbalances the person and can cause falls. Too low a frame can lead to a person bending over the frame, which can also cause falls. When an older person has been measured for a frame, it is important to label the frame so that frames do not become mixed up. This is an important safety measure if falls are to be prevented.

Zimmer frames have small rubber ends on each of the four legs, called ferrules. Each ferrule should have a whorl-like pattern on it. These patterns of raised rubber prevent the frame from slipping. You should check every few months that the patterns have not worn off as worn ferrules can lead to the frame slipping and the individual falling. Ferrules can be replaced if this happens, new ones being obtained from the community supplies department of the local PCT.

Some older people, especially those suffering from arthritis, do not have the strength to lift a frame off the ground and are unable to use standard Zimmer frames. They are often supplied with special Zimmer frames that have wheels at the bottom. The individual pushes the wheeled frame along. Wheeled frames are normally supplied after a careful assessment. An older person who tends to move quickly could easily fall or injure themselves using a wheeled frame. The wheels of these frames require oiling from time to time.

Gutter frames

Gutter frames are specialist frames. They are often supplied to individuals who have difficulty in gripping and lifting a normal frame. Such frames are often supplied to individuals who have severe arthritis in the arms and hands. Such individuals may require help to stand up and gain their balance on the gutter frame.

Tripods

Tripods are often used as walking aids by individuals who have suffered from strokes. The stroke may have left the individual with a weakness or paralysis on one side, which means that using a Zimmer frame is not possible. Tripods should be fitted to ensure that they are the correct height. A person with a left-sided weakness will require a right-handed tripod and one with a right-sided weakness a left-handed tripod. Some tripods have a handle that can be swivelled around to accommodate right- and left-handed users. Using a tripod allows the individual to improve balance and regain as much independence as possible. Sometimes people are able to walk alone using a tripod after a stroke; sometimes they need someone to help.

Walking sticks

When older people feel unsteady, they may buy or acquire walking sticks. It is important that walking sticks are the correct height for the individual and do not encourage stretching or stooping, which can lead to falls. Unfortunately, few older people are measured for walking sticks. If an individual enters the home with walking sticks and these appear to be the wrong height, the height should be checked. The stick should have a ferrule and these should be changed when worn. Further details are given later in the chapter.

Obtaining aids

Many older people enter homes with aids. These may have been supplied in hospital or at home; occasionally older people acquire them from friends or relatives. You may feel that an older person might benefit from a walking aid. Sometimes an older person is no longer able to manage with a particular aid. The person who managed well with a Zimmer frame but who has suffered a stroke is no longer able to use her frame. She may benefit from a tripod.

Walking aids are normally supplied by the community physiotherapist. The procedure for obtaining aids varies from area to area. Normally the person's doctor asks the physiotherapist to see the person and assess for a walking aid. The physiotherapist visits and assesses the person and orders any walking aids or equipment that is required.

Walking aids are usually delivered direct to the home. Staff are often asked to call the physiotherapist when the aid arrives. The physiotherapist normally visits, makes any adjustments that are required, and checks that the aid is safe and suitable. The physiotherapist may take the unwanted aid away so that it can be reused.

Helping and encouraging older people to use their aids

Many people are nervous when they first receive a walking aid. You can help individuals gain confidence by encouraging them to use the aids. Older people who are getting used to an aid should be accompanied on walks until staff are sure that they can walk safely and confidently alone.

Some older people who use aids will always require someone to assist them. The use of an aid in such circumstances means that the older person can walk with an aid and one member of staff instead of two. People who depend on aids should always have these placed near them. It is easy to move an aid out of the way when settling someone in bed and forget to place it back within reach of the individual before leaving the room. If someone is unable to reach their walking aid, they may try to get up and walk without it. This can lead to a fall and the older person could suffer from a serious injury.

Using aids enables many older people to become more independent than before. Older people who use aids benefit from the exercise involved in walking. They feel more in control and are less likely to feel depressed. Family and friends may feel more confident about taking the individual on short outings and the individual's quality of life improves. The exercise improves the circulation to the legs and reduces the risk of swollen ankles and legs. Movement helps the bowel to work properly and the individual is less likely to become constipated. Gentle exercise such as walking may give patients who had no interest in food an appetite. Overweight patients benefit from exercise, and the ability to move around and go on outings will help them to lose weight or to avoid gaining more. Staff within the home have more time to spend chatting or taking part in activities with the patient as they no longer have to spend so much time helping the person move around.

Wheelchairs

Helping people in wheelchairs retain and regain independence

Some people, because of disability or disease, are unable to walk even with aids and must use wheelchairs to help them move around. People with diseases such as multiple sclerosis or severe arthritis may need wheelchairs. Some people may be able to walk short distances but rely on a wheelchair when going on outings or when having a bad day or when they are unwell. People who are unable to walk can still retain independence if they are helped and encouraged to do so. Unfortunately, many people are issued with wheelchairs that they cannot use themselves and they must rely on others to push them. This is a great shame as many people are able to learn how to move around in their wheelchairs. There are two different types of (non-electric) wheelchairs. Self-propelling wheelchairs have large wheels, which have circular metal handgrips around them. The person uses the handgrip to turn the wheel and push herself along.

Many people are able to become independent when they get used to their wheelchair. Some people who have suffered from strokes have only one working hand with which to push the wheelchair. Some people who have had a stroke request that the footplate on the side of the body not affected by the stroke is left off. The person then uses the unaffected leg to help steer and move the wheelchair around. This should be noted on the person's care plan as wheelchairs should normally have both footplates attached to prevent accidents. Other wheelchairs are designed for people who are unable to move around themselves. These chairs have smaller wheels.

Keeping wheelchairs in good repair

Older people who rely on wheelchairs to move around need chairs that are kept in good repair. Poorly maintained wheelchairs are at best difficult to use and at worst dangerous. Tyres should be kept firm. It is very difficult to push a wheelchair with flat tyres, and flat tyres can prevent wheelchair brakes from working properly. Wheelchairs that move when someone is transferring can cause falls. All wheelchairs are supplied with a pump and tyres that are becoming soft should be pumped up. You should find out who is responsible for this in your home. Tyres that become soft again shortly after being pumped up may have a puncture. Wheelchair tyres should have a clearly visible tread on them. If the tread has worn away, the tyres need replacing.

Wheelchair brakes can easily become damaged; if the brakes are not working, urgent repairs should be organised.

Organising repairs

Wheelchairs are supplied to individuals. Each wheelchair should have the individual's name on it. When wheelchairs are supplied to individuals in homes, the manager is supplied with a reference number for each chair. Arrangements for repair of wheelchairs vary from area to area. In some areas, the primary care trust (which is responsible for supplying and maintaining the wheelchairs of people living in homes) employs its own staff to repair wheelchairs. In other areas, the primary care trust employs a contractor to carry out repairs. The manager of your home will be able to tell you what the local arrangements are.

In all cases the staff responsible for carrying out repairs are telephoned. Often a message has to be left on an answerphone as staff are out repairing, collecting or delivering wheelchairs. The name of the patient, type of wheelchair and reference number, and if possible details of the fault, are required. The repairer requires these details so that spare parts, which may be required, can be brought along. If possible the chair will be repaired or parts such as tyres replaced at the home. If this is not possible the chair is taken away for repairs and a replacement chair is loaned to the person until the wheelchair can be returned.

Exercise and passive movement

You should encourage residents to exercise and to move their limbs. Sometimes, though, people are unable to do so. A person who has lost all movement and feeling in the legs because of a disease such as multiple sclerosis may not be able to move her legs. An individual who has suffered from a severe stroke may be unable to understand or remember your advice on moving his paralysed hand.

Joints that are not moved quickly stiffen up. The tendons, which connect joints, contract and shorten. Muscles become smaller and waste away. If the legs of an older person who is unable to move them are not moved, they can become fixed. A person who sits for most of the day in a wheelchair can develop legs that are fixed in a permanent sitting position. If the legs are not gently moved and exercised, it will become impossible to straighten them within a few months. These changes are known as flexion contractures. You can prevent such deformities by gently moving limbs that the person is unable to move for himself or herself. If there is any existing deformity or limbs do not move normally, do not attempt to move the limbs. Seek professional advice.

Splints

Sometimes people who have had a stroke are supplied with special aids, known as splints, to prevent deformities and contractures to the hand on the affected side. Splints and exercise or passive movement are used together. The splint prevents the hand from remaining in a closed position when it is not being exercised. If a patient has a splint, it is important to help put it on and encourage its use. There are several different types of hand splint. Each splint is made especially for the individual patient. A registered nurse or physiotherapist can provide advice and information.

Journeys and visits

Assisting people to prepare for journeys and visits

For most of us, home is a cradle from which we spring, not a prison that encloses us. Many older people enjoy going out. Others need support and help to prepare for journeys and visits. Some people have been housebound for years before coming into the home. The outside world can seem a very hostile and threatening place to some older people. Table 8.1 outlines ways in which you can support the person and help prepare for journeys and visits.

Table 8.1 Supporting and enabling people to prepare for journeys and visits.

Method	Reason
Organise local trips to the shops	Enables the person to build up confidence before longer journeys
Help the person to plan the trip	To ensure that she has the skills (such as transferring) or stamina to undertake the trip as planned
Help the person to choose suitable clothing	To ensure the person is comfortable and suitably dressed; to enable the person to feel in control
Increased fluid requirements	Illness

Accompanying residents on visits and journeys

There are many reasons why you might be asked to accompany a resident on a journey. Sometimes you will be escorting the person to a hospital for treatment, or you may be asked to escort the person on an outing or a family celebration (Case Study 8.2).

Case Study 8.2

Sidney Bashford's youngest grandchild Helen was getting married. Sidney, as head of the family, had attended all the family celebrations for over half a century but he was becoming increasingly frail. His family desperately wanted him to attend but were anxious about their ability to look after him during the wedding.

They asked if Adam Odigie could accompany Sidney to the wedding. Adam encouraged Sidney to talk about any fears he had about his granddaughter's big day and did his best to plan for every eventuality.

Adam arrived early, helped Sidney to dress and prepare for the journey. Adam and Sidney travelled to the wedding by car. Adam was on hand to help meet Sidney's care needs.

Summary

Many older people admitted to homes have difficulty in moving around. Your approach and attitude are important in helping older people remain as independent as possible.

Your role is to support older people and help them to retain independence. Many older people rely on aids to move around. Some people use wheelchairs but wheelchair users can still retain independence and freedom. Some people require assistance to move paralysed limbs to prevent deformity developing. Older people living within the home have an enormous range of abilities and care assistants who understand individual needs can work as part of the team to meet those needs.

Key points

- Ageing and illness increase the risk of an older person developing mobility problems.
- Older people may need assistance and encouragement to remain mobile or to regain mobility after illness and accident.
- People with certain long-term conditions may require aids to enable them to remain mobile.
- The older person may require assistance and support when using an aid.
- Ensuring that the older person has regular eye tests and receives treatment to maximise vision helps increase confidence and prevent falls.
- Your role in encouraging people to move around and reporting any problems is of vital importance.

Portfolio preparation

Your assessor must have evidence that you can meet the performance criteria for this unit. Before beginning this unit, discuss assessment strategies with your assessor. Most of the evidence for this unit can be gained by direct observation of your work.

Products: This might be a copy of a care plan that you completed giving details of any assistance the person requires to remain mobile. It could be a note in a resident's notes giving details of any aids that the person uses or details of assistance that the person requires detailed on a care plan. It could be a care plan that you have drawn up or contributed to on how you are contributing to helping the person to remain mobile.

Witness testimony: This is a statement from a senior member of staff. It might be a statement detailing how you have met certain performance criteria.

Written work: You might be asked to prepare a piece of work about how you encourage residents to remain mobile. You might be asked to write a case history about a resident whom you have helped to remain mobile or become more mobile. You may be asked to discuss the difficulties you face in enabling people to move around the home and how you deal with these difficulties. Your assessor may also use other methods to help you gain evidence for this unit. These may include:

- Verbal questioning
- Written questions.

Simulations can be used to increase your awareness of mobility problems. One assessor borrowed wheelchairs and asked her students to spend the morning in town. Students soon found out how inaccessible many buildings are for wheelchair users. Others reported that they were ignored or treated differently because they were in wheelchairs. Students then began to realise why some older people dread leaving the home.

Further information

The Arthritis and Rheumatism Council for Research (ARC)
Copeman House
St Mary's Court
Chesterfield
Derbyshire S41 7TD
Telephone: 01246 558033 or 0870 850 5000
Website: http://www.arc.org.uk

ARC is a charity that provides information for patients, carers, doctors and nurses. It produces a wide range of leaflets and booklets, including *Rheumatoid Arthritis: A handbook for patients* and *Osteo-Arthritis: A booklet for patients*. Information leaflets for patients and a range of materials for healthcare staff can be downloaded from their website. You can also write requesting leaflets and information.

The Stroke Association
CHSA House
240 City Road
London EC1V 2PR
Telephone: 020 7490 2686
Helpline: 0845 3033 100 (Monday to Friday, 9 am to 5 pm)
Website: http://www.stroke.org.uk

The Stroke Association is the only national charity concerned solely with stroke. The association provides telephone helplines and offers support to over 400 stroke clubs. It funds research into the causes of stroke and aims to educate the public in how to remain healthy and reduce the risk of stroke.

Their website has a wealth of information and reports. There are also leaflets for patients. These can be downloaded free and include information on transient ischaemic attacks, physiotherapy and occupational therapy. You can also write requesting these. A number of booklets, books and videos are also available.

Royal National Institute for the Blind
105 Judd Street
London WC1H 9NE
Tel: 020 7388 1266
Helpline: 0845 766 9999 (Monday to Friday, 9 am to 5 pm)
Fax: 020 7388 2034
Website: http://www.rnib.org.uk

The RNIB provides advice and support to people who are blind, carers and professionals. Their website contains a wealth of information including fact sheets and leaflets.

Chapter Nine

Pressure Area Care
HSC217
Undertake agreed pressure area care

This unit consists of two elements:
HSC217a Prepare to carry out pressure area care
HSC217b Carry out pressure area care

This chapter

- Explains how pressure sores develop and why older people are at risk of developing them
- Provides information on how to prevent and treat pressure sores
- Explains who is at risk of developing pressure sores and how to assess risk
- Provides information about aids that can be used to prevent and treat pressure sores

What is a pressure sore?

A pressure sore is an area of localised damage to the skin and tissue and usually occurs over bony prominences such as the base of the spine, hips and heels.

A pressure sore is caused by unrelieved pressure on the skin or shearing forces. These cause the blood supply to the skin to be cut off and tissue dies. Anyone can develop a pressure sore if the blood supply is cut off for long enough. Some groups of people are at greater risk of developing pressure sores than others. Pressure sores are commonly called bedsores. The technical name for them is decubitus ulcers. They will be referred to throughout this chapter as pressure sores.

Why do pressure sores develop?

Three major factors contribute to pressure sores developing: pressure, shear and friction. Table 9.1 gives details.

Pressure is the single most important factor in the development of pressure sores. Capillaries supply oxygen-rich blood to the skin and drain away deoxygenated blood. The pressure in a capillary is 32 mmHg at the arterial end and 12 mmHg at the venous end. Unrelieved pressure reduces the capillary pressure and prevents the skin receiving oxygen and nutrients. Tissues deprived of oxygen and nutrients die and pressure sores develop.

Shear affects the deep tissues. The tissues attached to the bone are pulled in one direction and the skin surface sticks to bed linen or clothing, causing the tissue to distort. Shearing forces may be caused by a person slipping down the bed or chair or by poor handling techniques. The person who keeps sliding down the chair is subjecting her sacrum to shearing forces. Staff who pull the person back up (because it takes too long to use a hoist) are also subjecting the person's tissues to shearing forces. If you put a film or hydrocolloid dressing on a person's sacrum and find that it curls up at the edges this is an indication of shear caused either by the person sliding

Table 9.1 Why pressure sores develop.

Cause	Effect
Pressure	Capillaries supply the skin with oxygen-rich blood and remove deoxygenated blood. Capillaries are very thin (usually only one cell thick). Pressure cuts off capillary circulation and the skin dies.
Shear	If the skin surface sticks to bed linen or clothing while the person is moving, the deep tissues attached to the bone distort and blood supply is cut off.
Friction	This occurs when two surfaces rub against each other. This strips the top layer of skin away and can cause blisters and sores.

down in the chair or poor handling techniques. Shearing and pressure are interlinked. It only needs half the amount of pressure to cause damage if there are high levels of shear. Sacral dressings that curl up and need to be replaced suggest that shear is taking place.

Friction occurs when two surfaces rub against each other. This friction strips the epidermis away and can produce shallow ulcers and blisters.

These three forces work together. A blistered heal is more at risk of further damage than one with intact skin. It only needs half the amount of pressure to cause damage if there are high levels of shear.

Normally when a person begins to develop a pressure sore, the first sign is a red mark on the skin. If you place a finger lightly on the red area and it whitens, this shows that the capillary circulation is undamaged. If you act quickly, you may be able to help prevent a pressure sore developing. If the skin remains red when light finger pressure is applied, capillary circulation has been damaged. There may be a slight sore or blister on the skin. It will worsen if you do not act promptly and seek advice.

At one time, it was recommended that reddened skin should be massaged. It was thought that a firm massage improved the circulation and got the blood flowing back into the reddened skin. However, researchers found that massaging reddened skin did not improve circulation and actually caused further damage and made it more likely that the person would develop pressure sores. Reddened skin should not under any circumstances be massaged.

How common are pressure sores?

The number of people in care homes with pressure sores is not known. Research carried out in 1999 found that 6% of care home residents had pressure sores. The older person admitted to a nursing home may be admitted with an existing sore. Research in Liverpool indicated that 28% of people who experienced pressure sores already had the sore at the time of admission; this means that most people (72% according to this example) acquire their sores within homes. People living in care homes are at high risk of developing pressure sores because of their poor general health.

The goal of skilled professional nursing care is to prevent pressure sores developing and to heal any pressure sores present on admission. Your role is to observe a person's skin and to report any changes that indicate that the person may develop a pressure sore. If the person has a pressure sore your role is to carry out agreed pressure area care and to report any changes.

Who is at risk?

Older people are 20 times more likely to develop pressure sores than people in their 20s and 30s. Women are more likely to develop pressure sores than men, because women have a higher proportion of body fat than men. Fat has poorer blood supply than muscle or lean tissue. People who suffer from a long-standing illness are more likely to develop pressure sores than people in good health. Most older people living in homes have been admitted because of poor health and therefore are at greater risk of developing pressure sores than people who live in their own homes. Some older people are less likely to develop pressure sores because they enjoy good health, while others, who are frail, are at greater risk of developing pressure sores. Box 9.1 gives details of pressure sore risk factors.

Box 9.1 Pressure sore risk factors

- Ageing
- Poor mobility
- Reduced or absent sensation
- Confusion, lack of ability to interpret discomfort
- Long-term conditions
- Poor circulation
- Poor nutrition
- Urinary incontinence
- Poor moving and handling
- Medicines that cause drowsiness

Ageing

Ageing increases the risk of developing pressure sores; 70% of people who develop pressure sores are over 70 years old.

An older person's skin (Fig. 9.1b) is different from a younger person's (Fig. 9.1a). The skin becomes drier and more fragile. The number of collagen fibres is reduced. Collagen supports the skin. Older skin is less firm, more wrinkled, more likely to sag and more vulnerable to damage. The amount of fat under the skin is also reduced and so skin is less protected from damage.

Poor mobility

Normally people who are able to move around will feel stiff and uncomfortable if they are sitting or lying in one position. Getting up and walking or rolling over in bed will relieve pressure and prevent tissue damage. People who are unable to move around without help rely on staff to help them turn over, get up or change position. If an older person at high risk

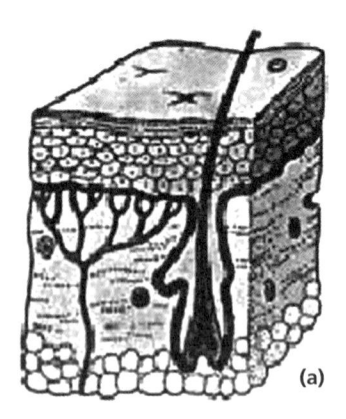

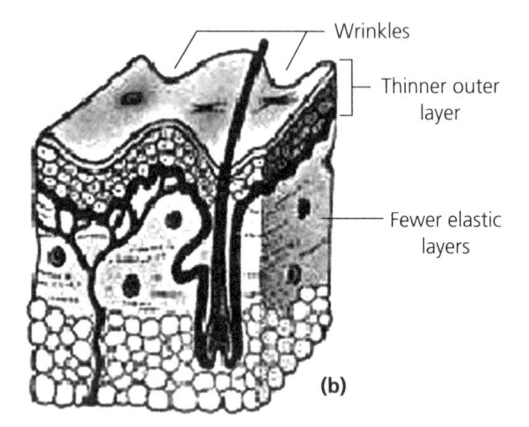

Figure 9.1 (a) Young skin; (b) Older skin.

of developing pressure sores is not moved or helped to move, severe skin damage can occur and a deep pressure sore can develop.

Reduced or absent sensation

People who have certain diseases such as multiple sclerosis, motor neurone disease and stroke may be unable to feel discomfort. This lack of sensation increases the person's risk of developing a pressure sore. People who have diabetes can suffer nerve damage and reduced sensation. Neurological diseases can also affect the ability to interpret sensation and to communicate discomfort. The person with impaired sensation may feel some discomfort but may have difficulty communicating that discomfort to their carer.

Confusion, lack of ability to interpret discomfort

People who are confused are at risk of developing pressure sores. Normally if we are forced to sit still for a long time, perhaps on a car journey, we unconsciously adjust our weight to reduce the effects of pressure. People who are confused are often unable to work out the cause of their discomfort and adjust their position. Some people who are confused sit quietly for hours and staff may be busy attending to the more alert people who are able to ask for help. The confused person may not be aware of the discomfort or pain caused by remaining in one position for a long time. Sometimes the person is aware of the discomfort but is unable to explain.

Sometimes people who are confused are prescribed sedatives. This may be because the person is agitated or wanders around. Sedatives should only be used as a last resort and then with great care. They can cause more problems than they solve. Sedatives can make older people drowsy and less aware. People who are drowsy will be less aware of pain and discomfort.

People with heart disease and high blood pressure

People with heart disease and high blood pressure are at risk of developing pressure sores because they have poor circulation. When circulation is poor, the skin becomes more sensitive to the effects of pressure and is more easily damaged.

People with long-term conditions

People with long-term conditions such as diabetes, heart failure and circulatory problems are at increased risk of developing pressure sores because of the effects of their condition.

Diabetes becomes more common as people age. Approximately 10% of 85-year-olds have diabetes. People from some ethnic backgrounds are more likely to develop diabetes. Approximately 14% of older people from Afro-Caribbean backgrounds develop diabetes; and 20% of people of Indian or Pakistani descent develop diabetes in old age. People with diabetes often suffer from poor circulation. People who have mild diabetes, which is treated with a special diet, are less at risk than diabetics who require tablets to help control diabetes. People who require insulin injections to control diabetes are more likely to suffer from poor circulation than other diabetics.

Some people with diabetes, especially those who require insulin injections, develop loss of feeling in the feet, lower parts of the legs and the hands. This condition is known as peripheral neuropathy, and there is no treatment for it. People with diabetes are at great risk of developing pressure sores on the heels, as they are often unaware of pain or discomfort caused by pressure. Poor circulation and the effects of diabetes, which slow down the rate of wound healing, make it difficult to heal such pressure sores if they develop.

Heart failure and **poor circulation** increase the risks of developing pressure sores because, when circulation is poor, small changes can easily lead to pressure sores developing.

Poor nutrition

Nutrition is a very important factor in the development of pressure sores.

Very thin older people lack a protective layer of fat that protects muscle from the effects of pressure. Bony prominences such as hip bones are unprotected and the person is at extremely high risk of developing pressure sores.

Underweight people are even more likely than overweight people to develop pressure sores. Their lack of protective fat increases the effects of shearing forces because their bones are more prominent.

Very overweight people are also at risk of pressure sores. The obese person can be hot and sticky. The person may have skin folds that become sore and infected and vulnerable to developing sores. Obese people have more fat than people of normal weight and fat has a poorer blood supply than normal tissue. This poor blood supply increases the risk of pressure sores. Many overweight people have a poor diet that is too high in sugars and low in vitamins. A diet low in vitamins affects the health of the skin and increases the risk of pressure sores.

Incontinence

Urinary incontinence if poorly managed can cause skin damage and lead to pressure sores.

People who are incontinent of faeces and urine are at greater risk of developing pressure sores than those who are incontinent of urine only. People who are incontinent can develop skin rashes if pads are not changed frequently or if the skin is not carefully washed after each episode of incontinence. Urine, especially concentrated urine, can burn the skin. People who are incontinent of faeces may wet on a soiled pad. This causes the release of ammonia and can cause the skin to become sore and red very quickly. Skin soreness and rashes cause the skin to become inflamed. Sore, inflamed skin can develop blisters and boils. These can become infected. People who have sore or infected skin are more at risk of developing pressure sores than people who have healthy skin.

Many people who are incontinent wear pads. If pads are not put on properly, ridges from the pad can cause pressure on the skin and this can lead to pressure sores. There are many different types of pad. The quality of pad varies, as does the cost. All pads are made of paper (cellulose) pulp. This is covered by a one-way liner that is designed to draw urine away from the patient's skin and into the pad. Most pads have a plastic backing to prevent urine leaking onto the patient's clothes. Some pads contain more pulp than others. Some pads also contain super-absorbent crystals. The crystals turn into a gel and lock urine into the pad. Good-quality pads draw urine away from the skin quickly and keep the skin drier between changes. Skin that is not soaked in urine is less likely to become sore or infected or develop pressure sores.

Poor handling and positioning

Poor handling and positioning increase the risk of skin damage. Pulling or dragging a person up in bed or a chair can cause friction and shear damage. Clothing made of nylon or synthetic fibres can cause tissue damage. Nylon can make the person more likely to slide down the bed. Synthetic fibres do not absorb perspiration and can lead to moist sticky skin that is easily damaged.

Medication that causes drowsiness

Medication can increase the risk of pressure sores developing. Some medications such as sleeping pills and sedatives can cause drowsiness. The person who is drowsy is less likely to move and may develop a pressure sore because of this.

Other factors

Some types of medication can increase pressure sore risk. Non-steroidal anti-inflammatory drugs (NSAIDs) are often given to treat arthritis and pain. They can lead to slow blood loss and anaemia. NSAIDs can also slow down the rate of healing.

White people are more likely to develop pressure sores than black people. This is because black people have a more robust collagen structure than white people. This is one of the reasons why black skin ages more slowly than fair, white skin.

Other factors that increase risk are infection, pain, stress and lack of sleep.

Where do pressure sores occur?

The areas of the body most at risk of pressure damage are the sacrum, heels, buttocks and greater trochanters. Almost half of all pressure sores develop on the sacrum and almost 20% develop on the heels. Most pressure sores develop between the buttocks on the bony area known as the sacrum. Anyone who is unable to move and who is not helped to move can develop a pressure sore after a few hours. Pressure sores are not caused by bedrest; people sitting in chairs also develop sacral pressure sores.

The heels are also a common site for pressure sores. A person sitting with heels resting on a footstool is just as much at risk as the person whose heels are resting on a mattress in bed.

Pressure sores can develop on any part of the body (Fig. 9.2). They can occur on ears, cheeks, arms, trunk, legs and heels.

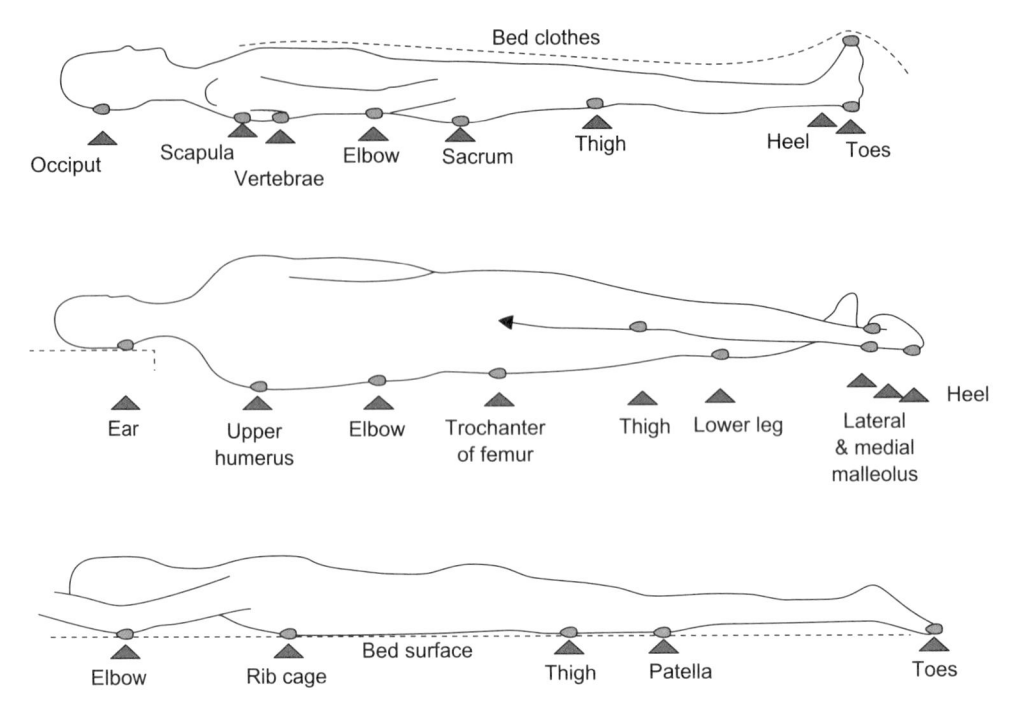

Figure 9.2 Areas where pressure sores can occur.

Pressure sore grading

Pressure sores are difficult to treat. They can easily become infected and can cause pain and discomfort. It is important to assess pressure sores before treating them. In the past there was no standardised way of assessing pressure sores and different scales were used. Pressure sores are now classified throughout Europe using four grades.

In grade 1 pressure sores (Fig. 9.3) the skin is warm and red and may be swollen. There are no breaks in the skin.

In grade 2 pressure sores (Fig. 9.4) the skin is blistered or damaged. This damage may involve the epidermis or the dermis.

In grade 3 pressure sores (Fig. 9.5) skin and the fatty tissue under the skin is damaged.

In grade 4 pressure sores (Fig. 9.6) the damage extends to muscle, bone and supporting structures. The sore may be open or partially closed.

The effects of pressure sores

Pressure sores can cause a great deal of pain and discomfort. If the person develops a pressure sore on a heel it can make walking difficult and painful and can prevent the person walking. Pain can prevent an older

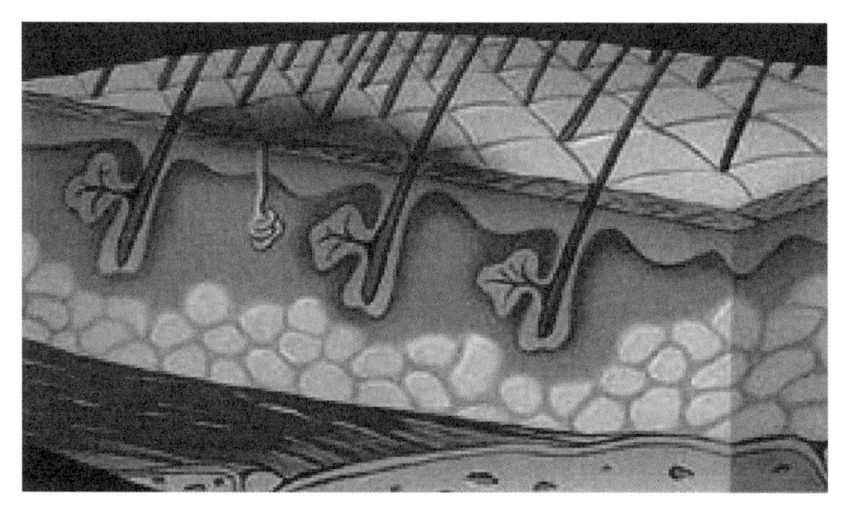

Figure 9.3 Grade 1 pressure sore.

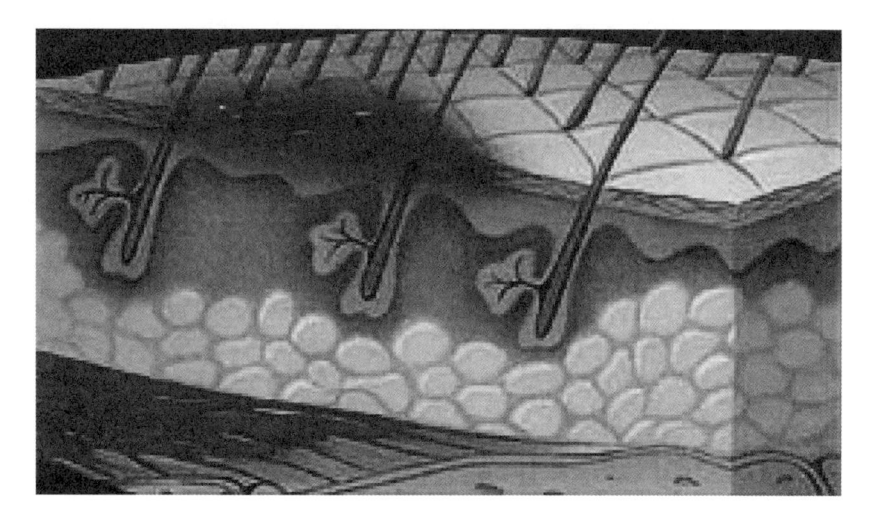

Figure 9.4 Grade 2 pressure sore.

person moving around, chatting and taking part in the activities of the home. Pain can prevent the older person from getting a good night's sleep. Doctors can prescribe painkillers, and people with large or deep pressure sores may require strong painkillers. Unfortunately strong painkillers can make some people feel sick and can cause constipation.

Lack of sleep can make the individual feel unwell. Pressure sores, especially those on the sacrum and the hips, can easily become infected. Infection can cause the person to develop a high temperature and to feel unwell. The individual may feel too unwell to eat, yet a diet full of protein, vitamins and carbohydrates is essential if the wound is to heal. People who

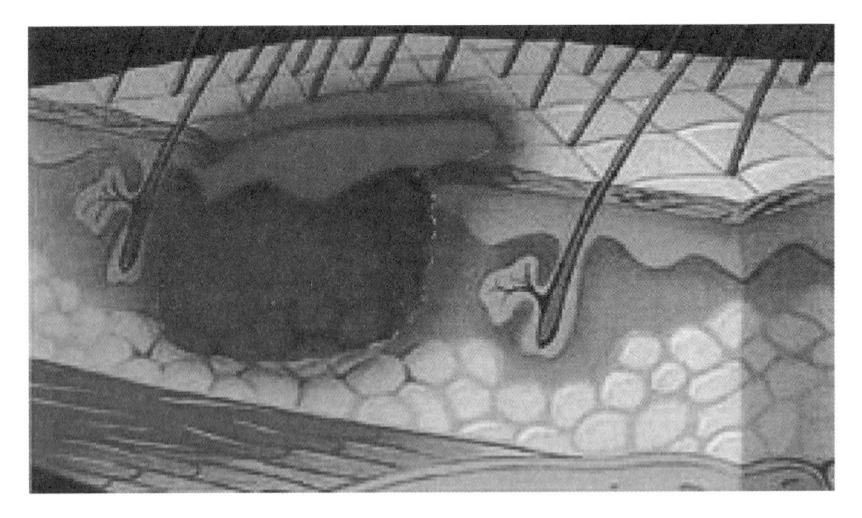

Figure 9.5 Grade 3 pressure sore.

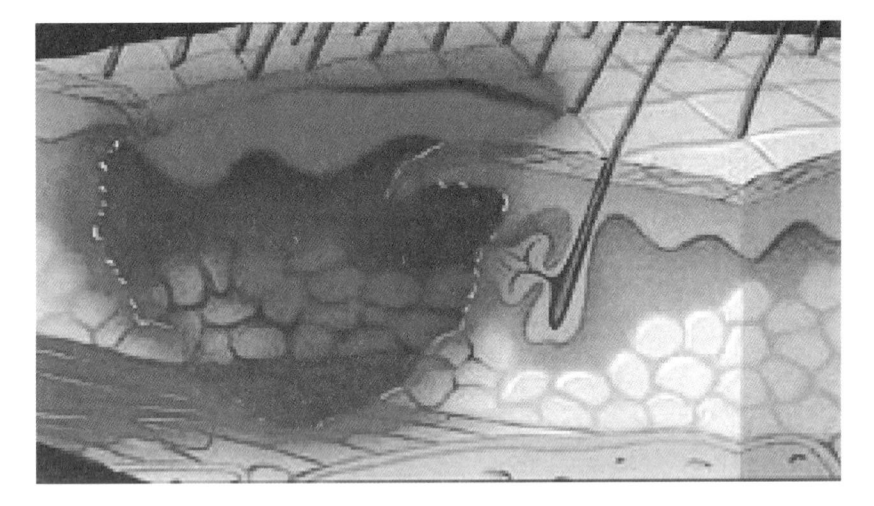

Figure 9.6 Grade 4 pressure sore.

have infected wounds are usually prescribed antibiotics by their doctors. Antibiotics can make some people feel sick and lose their appetites. Some people can also suffer from diarrhoea when prescribed antibiotics.

Infected wounds often smell. Some wounds, because of the bacteria with which they are infected, smell dreadful. This can be very upsetting for the person. Some people who develop deep pressure sores can suffer from infection that infects the bone. They can develop blood poisoning (septicaemia) and, even with hospital treatment, some people will not survive.

Many older people who have developed pressure sores become depressed. Some are so depressed that they feel life is not worth living and require antidepressant tablets.

Assessing and reducing risks

An ounce of prevention is worth a ton of cure. The best way to prevent pressure sores developing is to assess the person's risk and use a problem-solving approach to reduce risk.

Risk assessment scales are commonly used to determine the person's level of risk. We do not yet have enough clinical evidence to work out which risk factors are important under which circumstances. Assessment should be carried out when the person is admitted and whenever there are any significant changes to the person's health. There are a number of risk assessment scales. Each scale scores risk factors and the scores indicate the individual's risk of developing a pressure sore. Assessment scales enable you to assess risk and plan care to prevent pressure sores occurring. The assessment scale should take into account all the risk factors and accurately predict the risk of damage occurring.

The first, the Norton scale, was developed by Doreen Norton in 1962. It assesses the patient's general health, mental state, activity, mobility and continence. People score points based on these categories. An individual in poor health who is confused, immobile and incontinent will have a lower score than an individual who is in poor health but who is alert, walks with help and is continent. The total points are added up and this is known as the Norton score. A score of 16 points or below indicates that the person is at risk of developing a pressure sore. The lower the score the higher the risk of the person developing pressure sores. By the 1980s healthcare changes such as surgery being carried out on the very old and increasing longevity led many nurses to question its accuracy. It is now seldom used.

Many other risk assessment scales were developed but the most commonly used is the Waterlow scale (Fig. 9.7). The Waterlow scale was developed as a result of research carried out in 1985, and is a more detailed assessment scale. It assesses factors such as build, weight, continence, skin type, mobility, sex, age and appetite. The score has special high risk factors such as surgery, medication, age and diseases. Each risk factor carries points and the points are added up. A score of 10 indicates that the person is at risk of developing pressure sores; a score of 15–20 indicates that the person is at high risk; and a score of more than 20 indicates that the person is at very high risk. The higher the score the greater the risk of the person developing pressure sores. You can download the Waterlow scale and other information from the Waterlow website (see Further information).

The Braden scale (Table 9.2) was developed in the United States in the 1980s. It was developed to take account of increased knowledge about the factors that lead to pressure sores. It is an objective scale and eliminates the problem of different nurses assessing an individual's risk differently. The Braden scale has been extensively researched with large numbers of elderly people. Research suggests that the Braden scale is

WATERLOW PRESSURE ULCER PREVENTION/TREATMENT POLICY

RING SCORES IN TABLE, ADD TOTAL. MORE THAN 1 SCORE/CATEGORY CAN BE USED

BUILD/WEIGHT FOR HEIGHT	◆	SKIN TYPE VISUAL RISK AREAS	◆	SEX AGE	◆	MALNUTRITION SCREENING TOOL (MST) (*Nutrition* Vol.15, No.6 1999 – Australia)			
AVERAGE BMI = 20–24.9	0	HEALTHY	0	MALE	1	A – HAS PATIENT LOST WEIGHT RECENTLY		B – WEIGHT LOSS SCORE	
ABOVE AVERAGE BMI = 25–29.9	1	TISSUE PAPER DRY	1 1	FEMALE 14–49	2 1	YES – GO TO B		0.5–5 kg	= 1
OBESE BMI > 30	2	OEDEMATOUS CLAMMY, PYREXIA	1 1	50–64	2	NO – GO TO C UNSURE – GO TO C AND SCORE 2		5–10 kg 10–15 kg > 15 kg unsure	= 2 = 3 = 4 = 2
BELOW AVERAGE BMI < 20	3	DISCOLOURED GRADE 1 BROKEN/SPOTS GRADE 2–4	2 3	65–74 75–80 81+	3 4 5	C – PATIENT EATING POORLY OR LACK OF APPETITE 'NO' = 0; 'YES' SCORE = 1		NUTRITION SCORE If > 2 refer for nutrition assessment/intervention	
BMI = Wt (kg)/Ht (m)²									

CONTINENCE	◆	MOBILITY	◆	SPECIAL RISKS			
COMPLETE/ CATHETERISED	0	FULLY RESTLESS/FIDGETY	0 1	TISSUE MALNUTRITION	◆	NEUROLOGICAL DEFICIT	◆
URINE INCONT.	1	APATHETIC	2	TERMINAL CACHEXIA	8	DIABETES, MS, CVA	4–6
FAECAL INCONT.	2	RESTRICTED	3	MULTIPLE ORGAN FAILURE	8	MOTOR/SENSORY	4–6
URINARY + FAECAL INCONTINENCE	3	BEDBOUND e.g. TRACTION CHAIRBOUND e.g. WHEELCHAIR	4 5	SINGLE ORGAN FAILURE (RESP, RENAL, CARDIAC) PERIPHERAL VASCULAR DISEASE	5 5	PARAPLEGIA (MAX OF 6) MAJOR SURGERY or TRAUMA	4–6
				ANAEMIA (Hb < 8)	2	ORTHOPAEDIC/SPINAL	5
				SMOKING	1	ON TABLE > 2 hr#	5
						ON TABLE > 6 hr#	8

SCORE	
10+ AT RISK	
15+ HIGH RISK	
20+ VERY HIGH RISK	

MEDICATION – CYTOTOXICS, LONG-TERM/HIGH-DOSE STEROIDS, ANTI-INFLAMMATORY MAX OF 4

\# Scores can be discounted after 48 hours provided patient is recovering normally

© J Waterlow 1985 Revised 2005*
Obtainable from the Nook, Stoke Road, Henlade TAUNTON TA3 5LX
* The 2005 revision incorporates the research undertaken by Queensland Health.

www.judy-waterlow.co.uk

REMEMBER TISSUE DAMAGE MAY START PRIOR TO ADMISSION, IN CASUALTY. A SEATED PATIENT IS AT RISK.
ASSESSMENT: IF THE PATIENT FALLS INTO ANY OF THE RISK CATEGORIES, THEN PREVENTIVE NURSING IS REQUIRED. A COMBINATION OF GOOD NURSING TECHNIQUES AND PREVENTIVE AIDS WILL BE NECESSARY.
ALL ACTIONS MUST BE DOCUMENTED

	PREVENTION	Skin Care	
PRESSURE-REDUCING AIDS Special Mattress/beds:	10+ Overlays or specialist foam mattresses. 15+ Alternating pressure overlays, mattresses and bed systems 20+ Bed systems: Fluidised bead, low air loss and alternating pressure mattresses Note: Preventive aids cover a wide spectrum of specialist features. Efficacy should be judged, if possible, on the basis of independent evidence.		General hygiene, NO rubbing, cover with an appropriate dressing
		Assessment	**WOUND GUIDELINES** Odour, exudate, measure/photograph position
Cushions:	No person should sit in a wheelchair without some form of cushioning. If nothing else is available, use the person's own pillow. (Consider infection risk) 10+ 100 mm foam cushion 15+ Specialist gel and/or foam cushion 20+ Specialised cushion, adjustable to individual person.	GRADE 1	**WOUND CLASSIFICATION – EPUAP** Discolouration of intact skin not affected by light finger pressure (non-blanching erythema) This may be difficult to identify in darkly pigmented skin
		GRADE 2	Partial-thickness skin loss or damage involving epidermis and/or dermis The pressure ulcer is superficial and presents clinically as an abrasion, blister or shallow crater
Bed clothing:	Avoid plastic draw sheets, inco pads and tightly tucked-in sheet/sheet covers, especially when using specialist bed and mattress overlay systems Use duvet plus vapour-permeable membrane	GRADE 3	Full-thickness skin loss involving damage of subcutaneous tissue but not extending to the underlying fascia The pressure ulcer presents clinically as a deep crater with or without undermining of adjacent tissue
General	**NURSING CARE** HAND WASHING, frequent changes of position, lying, sitting. Use of pillows	GRADE 4	Full-thickness skin loss with extensive destruction and necrosis extending to underlying tissue
Pain	Appropriate pain control		
Nutrition	High protein, vitamins and minerals		
Patient handling	Correct lifting technique – hoists – monkey poles Transfer devices		
Patient comfort aids	Real sheepskin – bed cradle	Dressing guide	Use local dressings formulary and/or www.worldwidewounds
Operating table Theatre/A&E trolley	100 mm (4 in) cover plus adequate protection		IF TREATMENT IS REQUIRED, FIRST REMOVE PRESSURE

Figure 9.7 Waterlow pressure ulcer risk scale. Reproduced by permission of Judy Waterlow, www.judy-waterlow.co.uk.

Table 9.2 The Braden scale.

	1	2	3	4
SENSORY PERCEPTION ability to respond meaningfully to pressure-related discomfort	**1. Completely limited** Unresponsive (does not moan, flinch, or grasp) to painful stimuli, due to diminished level of consciousness or sedation OR limited ability to feel pain over most body surfaces	**2. Very limited** Responds only to painful stimuli. Cannot communicate discomfort except by moaning or restlessness OR has a sensory impairment which limits the ability to feel pain or discomfort over half of body	**3. Slightly limited** Responds to verbal commands but cannot always communicate discomfort or need to be turned OR has some sensory impairment which limits ability to feel pain or discomfort in one or two extremities	**4. No impairment** Responds to verbal commands. Has no sensory deficit which would affect ability to feel or voice pain or discomfort
MOISTURE degree to which skin is exposed to moisture	**1. Constantly moist** Skin is kept moist almost constantly by perspiration, urine, etc. Dampness is detected every time patient is moved or turned	**2. Very moist** Skin is often, but not always, moist. Linen must be changed at least once a shift	**3. Occasionally moist** Skin is occasionally moist, requiring an extra linen change approximately once a day	**4. Rarely moist** Skin is usually dry. Linen only requires changing at routine intervals
ACTIVITY degree of physical activity	**1. Bedfast** Confined to bed	**2. Chairfast** Ability to walk severely limited or non-existent. Cannot bear own weight and/or must be assisted into chair or wheelchair	**3. Walks occasionally** Walks occasionally during day, but for very short distances, with or without assistance. Spends majority of each shift in bed or chair	**4. Walks frequently** Walks outside the room at least twice a day and inside room at least once every two hours during waking hours
MOBILITY ability to change and control body position	**1. Completely immobile** Does not make even slight changes in body or extremity position without assistance	**2. Very limited** Makes occasional slight changes in body or extremity position but unable to make frequent or significant changes independently	**3. Slightly limited** Makes frequent though slight changes in body or extremity position independently	**4. No limitation** Makes major and frequent changes in position without assistance

NUTRITION
usual food intake pattern

1. Very poor
Never eats a complete meal. Rarely eats more than one-third of any food offered. Eats two servings or less of protein (meat or dairy products) per day. Fluids taken poorly. Does not take a liquid dietary supplement
OR
is NBM and/or maintained on clear liquids or IVs for more than five days

2. Probably inadequate
Rarely eats a complete meal and generally eats only half of any food offered. Protein intake includes only three servings of meat or dairy products per day. Occasionally will take a dietary supplement
OR
receives less than optimum amount of liquid diet or tube feeding

3. Adequate
Eats over half of most meals. Eats a total of four servings of protein (meat, dairy products) each day. Occasionally will refuse a meal, but will usually take a supplement if offered
OR
is on a tube-feeding or TPN regimen which probably meets most of nutritional needs

4. Excellent
Eats most of every meal. Never refuses a meal. Usually eats a total four or more servings of meat and dairy products. Occasionally eats between meals. Does not require supplementation

FRICTION AND SHEAR

1. Problem
Requires moderate to maximum assistance in moving. Complete lifting without sliding against sheets is impossible. Frequently slides down in bed or chair, requiring frequent repositioning with maximum assistance. Spasticity, contractures or agitation leads to almost constant friction

2. Potential problem
Moves freely or requires minimum assistance. During a move skin probably slides to some extent against sheets, chair restraints or other devices. Maintains relatively good position in chair or bed most of the time but occasionally slides down

3. No apparent problem
Moves in bed and in chair independently and has sufficient muscle strength to lift up completely during move. Maintains good position in bed or chair at all times

more accurate than any other risk assessment scale. You can download the Braden scale and other information from the Braden website (see Further information).

The benefits of assessment scales

Accurate, research-based assessment scales enable staff to predict an individual's risk of developing a pressure sore more accurately. This is invaluable. The individual at low risk can sleep on foam or hollow fibre overlay or replacement mattress rather than a specialist overlay or mattress replacement. Most older people would prefer this to an unnecessary specialist product. The individual at low risk can sleep undisturbed. The individual at high risk of developing pressure sores will benefit from increased staff interventions to reduce risk and prevent pressure sores developing. Nursing workload is reduced when risk is accurately assessed and equipment and care can be targeted accurately.

The benefits of observation and communication

Assessment tools are tools. Assessment tools can never replace observation and experience. If you notice that a person's skin is becoming sore or red you must report these changes so that action can be taken. If you are concerned that the person's skin condition is worsening, seek professional advice.

Preventing pressure sores

Pressure sore prevention is not simply a matter of putting people at risk on pressure-relieving mattresses and overlays. It is about caring for the whole person. It is a team effort and when working out how to prevent pressure sores you will be working with registered nurses to plan and carry out care. When you have identified who is at risk and why the person is at risk, the next step is to identify which risk factors you can change. Table 9.3 gives details of modifiable and non-modifiable risk factors.

Table 9.3 Modifiable and non-modifiable risk factors.

Modifiable	Non-modifiable
Poor mobility	Age
Poor nutrition	Lack of sensation
Poor moving and handling practice	Poor circulation
Medicines that cause drowsiness	Lack of awareness
Medicines that slow down healing	
Poorly managed long-term conditions	

The next stage is to work out a plan of care that reduces the risks that can be changed. If the person is very thin then you will aim to improve nutrition and help the person to gain weight. The best way to do this is to encourage the person to eat a diet high in calories, vitamins and minerals. If this is not successful the person may be prescribed supplements to help weight gain.

Most pressure sores can be prevented. The development of a pressure sore, in most cases, is a sign that care is not of a high standard and that staff failed to take action to prevent the sore developing. Staff who understand why pressure sores develop can act to prevent them occurring. Pressure sores are caused by unrelieved pressure that affects blood flow and causes sores to develop. Relieving the pressure and moving people allows blood to flow normally to the tissues and prevents pressure sores developing. People who are sitting in a chair all day are just as much at risk of developing pressure sores as people who are nursed in bed.

People who are sitting in chairs and who are able to walk should be encouraged to do so. Encouraging and helping an older person to walk to the dining room for lunch will help prevent a pressure sore. Serving lunch on a tray may mean the individual continues to sit and pressure on the bottom is unrelieved. Many people need help and encouragement to walk. You should encourage residents to walk, walking with them and encouraging them to walk at their own pace.

Offering to wheel a person, who is capable of walking, to the dining area does little to relieve pressure and help circulation. People who are unable to walk can be encouraged to stand. The person can use a Zimmer frame, grab rails or standing hoist or be helped by staff. Encouraging people to stand, even with help, not only helps prevent pressure sores but also prevents joints becoming stiff and reduces the risk of the patient's legs developing deformities such as flexion contractures. People who are unable to walk or stand are at risk of pressure sores and should not sit all day in the same chair, as this will almost certainly cause pressure sores.

Older people require less sleep than younger people do and tire more easily than when they were young. Older people are more likely to have a nap in the afternoon and often sleep for an hour after lunch. In some homes, older people fall asleep in their chairs after lunch. They may waken feeling stiff, uncomfortable and not refreshed by their sleep.

Encouraging frail older people who feel tired to go to bed for a nap will help prevent pressure sores. You can assist the individual to bed and can help the person to lie on one side, which will relieve pressure on the bottom. The older person will sleep comfortably and awake refreshed, ready for a cup of tea, a visit from family or friends or activities in the home. People normally turn over in bed while they are asleep. Moving around in bed prevents us from developing pressure sores while we sleep.

Many frail older people who are at risk of pressure sores are unable to turn over in bed. All people who are at risk should be turned every two hours. The person is normally nursed on their back for two hours, then turned onto perhaps the left side. Two hours later the person is turned onto the right side. If a patient's sacrum is becoming red, they may lie on one hip and then the other, avoiding wherever possible any pressure on the sacrum. If one of the hips is becoming red, the person may lie only on the other hip or on the sacrum. If a person is lying on their side there is a risk that they will roll back onto their back. A soft pillow is often placed either under the mattress or at the back of the patient, to prevent this.

Some risk factors cannot be changed. If the person is incontinent and cannot be helped to regain continence, you must work out ways to minimise the risk of damage. You may use a barrier cream to protect skin. You may need to change pads more often to prevent skin becoming soggy.

Pressure-relieving mattresses and overlays are part of these harm reduction measures. There are many different types of pressure-relieving mattresses and overlays. They all act in the same way, though some are more effective than others. All pressure-relieving devices work by reducing the pressure on vulnerable areas of the skin. It is important to ensure that, if the person is sitting out in a chair, the chair has a pressure-relieving cushion.

Pressure-relieving devices reduce pressure but they do not eliminate it. It is important to encourage the person to change position every few hours. If the person is unable to change position you must do this for her.

Older people who are at risk of developing pressure sores may still develop pressure sores even if turned every two hours. It can be difficult to turn people more frequently. Often two staff are needed to turn the person. If two staff work together the person is at less risk of shearing forces that can cause pressure sores, and care assistants reduce the risk of developing a back injury. Details on moving and handling people are given in Chapter 12. People who are turned every hour have little opportunity to rest or sleep.

Many different types of mattresses and mattress overlays have been designed to reduce the risk of pressure sores developing. Pressure-relieving equipment usually either replaces the existing mattress or lies on top of the existing mattress.

Pressure-relieving mattresses and overlays

These aim to relieve the pressure that can lead to pressure sores developing or as part of the treatment of existing pressure sores. The choice of mattress or overlay should be related to the level of risk. Tables 9.4 and 9.5 show interventions that should be used if using the Waterlow or Braden scales.

Overlays or foam mattresses can be made of foam that aims to reduce pressure. Increasingly visco-elastic foam is being used. This foam moulds to the person's body to evenly distribute weight and reduce pressure (Fig. 9.8). Some foam and fibre pressure-relieving mattresses/overlays have a special vapour-permeable multi-stretch cover. This vapour permeability

Table 9.4 Interventions based on Waterlow scale.

Score	Equipment
Waterlow score 10+	Overlays or specialist foam mattresses
Waterlow score 15+	Alternating pressure overlays, mattresses and bed systems
Waterlow score 20+	Bed systems: fluidised bead, low air loss and alternating pressure mattresses

Table 9.5 Interventions based on Braden scale.

Score	Equipment
Braden scale 15–18	Overlays or specialist foam mattresses if bed- or chair-bound
Braden scale 13–14	Overlays or specialist foam mattresses
Braden scale 10–12	Alternating pressure overlays, mattresses and bed systems
Braden scale 9 or below	Bed systems: fluidised bead, low air loss and alternating pressure mattresses

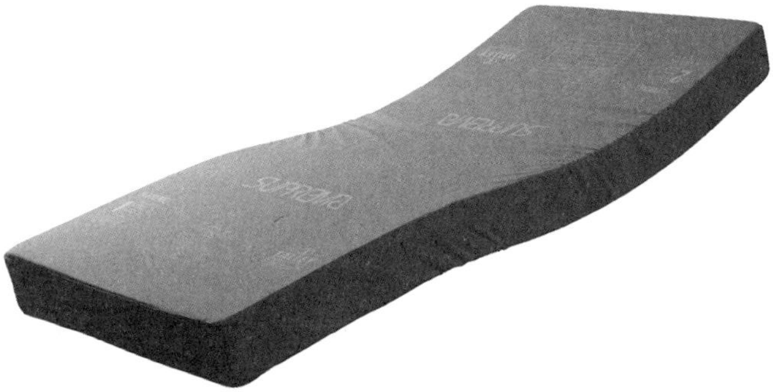

Figure 9.8 Suprema overlay mattress.

allows the patient's skin to breathe and prevents the person from becoming hot and sweaty. This means that the skin is less likely to become macerated. The covers are water-resistant and the multi-stretch properties help to prevent the cover wrinkling and bunching up and reduce friction. Manufacturers recommend that the covers are washed with soap and water. Disinfectants, detergents and deodorisers should not be sprayed onto the covers. If you are unsure, ask your manager who will check the manufacturer's cleaning guidance.

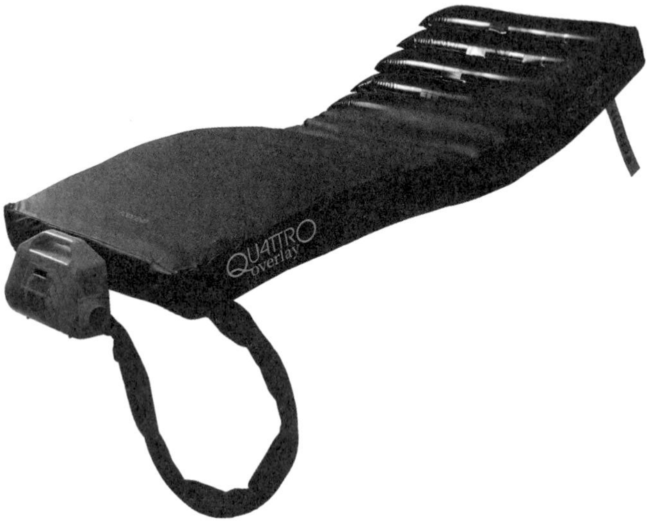

Figure 9.9 Quattro pressure-relieving overlay.

Alternating pressure overlays, mattresses and bed systems are normally made of horizontal cells of air, which inflate and deflate on a cycle. This cycle is controlled by an electrical pump. The alternate cells that are inflated support the patient, while the deflated cells are relieving the pressure to that area of the patient's body. Alternating pressure mattresses/overlays are sometimes referred to as ripple mattresses. Pressure-relieving mattresses are used for the prevention of pressure sores and also the treatment of any existing sores.

Some pressure-relieving mattresses/overlays automatically adjust the amount of air in the cells. They are able to adjust to the weight and position of the individual. Others, however, have a small dial that needs to be set according to the weight of the patient. There is normally a printed table on the electronic pump giving details about which settings should be used for people within certain weight ranges.

Pressure-relieving mattresses and overlays (Figs 9.8, 9.9 and 9.10) are used for different levels of risk and grade of pressure sore. It is important that you seek advice from a registered nurse if you are unsure which product is suitable for an individual.

When using a pressure-relieving mattress/overlay, the sheet should not be tucked in tightly and Kylie-type bed sheets, draw sheets and incontinence pads should be kept to a minimum as they may reduce the effectiveness of pressure-relieving mattresses. It is best to leave the pressure-relieving mattress/overlay switched on even when not in use. The motor has to work harder to reinflate than to maintain the inflated pressure. Deflating the mattress means that the individual cannot go back to bed if tired, as the mattress/overlay should be inflated before the person uses it.

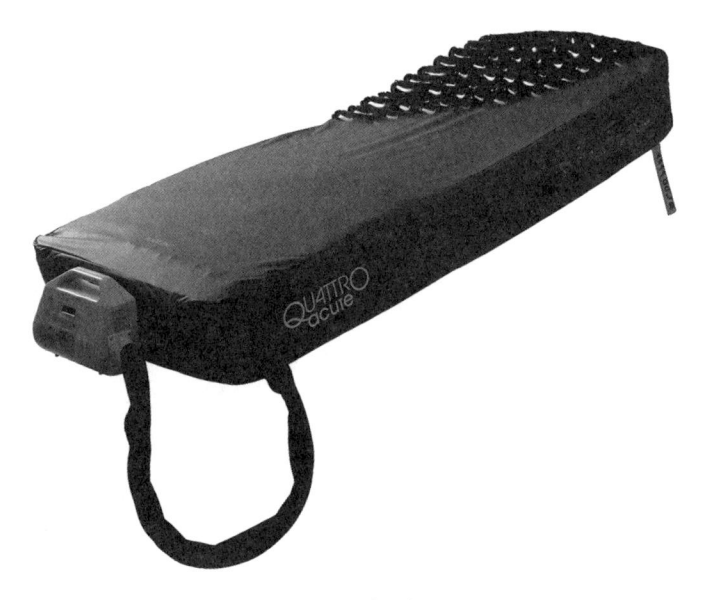

Figure 9.10 Quattro Acute pressure-relieving mattress.

In some nursing homes, hospices and hospitals, specialised beds such as low air loss and fluidised bead beds are sometimes used for people who are very ill, have existing pressure sores and cannot easily be moved. If you require any further information on these specialised beds, ask a registered nurse or obtain details from the manufacturer (details are given at the end of the chapter).

Cushions and pressure-relieving aids

People who are at risk of developing pressure sores are at even greater risk when they are sitting in a chair. A range of cushions should be available within the home to help prevent and treat pressure sores. In nursing homes, the type of cushion on which the individual sits during the day should be written in the care plan.

Cushions

Cushions can be made of a variety of materials including Silicore, foam, gel, fluid and air (Figs 9.11 and 9.12). Depending on the material used and their construction, cushions will be suitable for different levels of risk. Seek professional advice if you are unsure about what type of cushions to use.

Silicore cushions are padded cushions covered in fabric. They are used for comfort only. They can be machine washed and dried. Some have a waterproof side or seat that can be wiped clean. Special Silicore cushions

218   NVQs in Nursing and Residential Care Homes

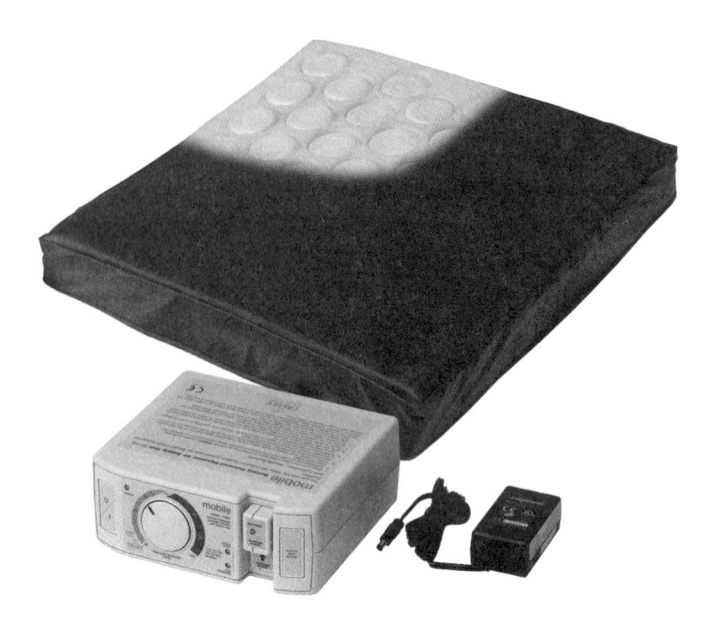

Figure 9.11   Mobile pressure-relieving cushion.

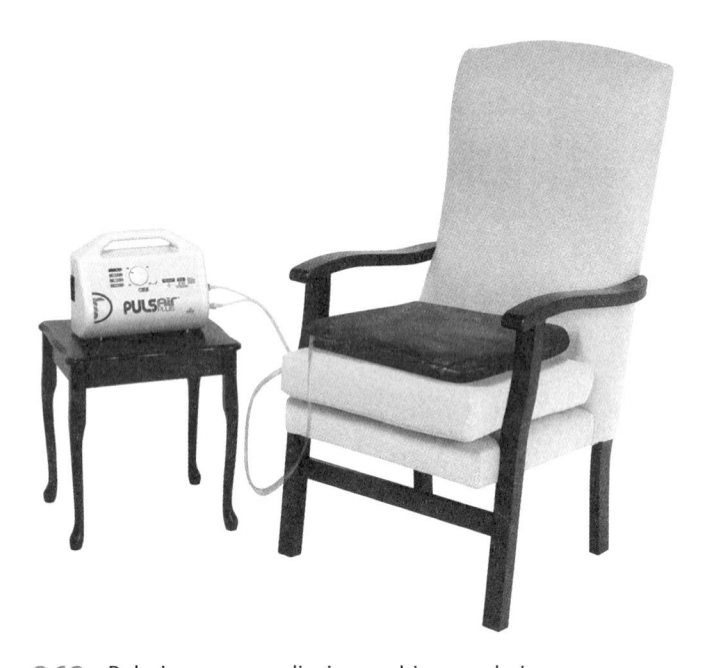

Figure 9.12   Pulsair pressure-relieving cushion on chair.

are designed to fit into wheelchairs. Armchairs with integral pressure-reducing cushions are now available.

Foam cushions come in varying densities and can be made of different kinds of foam. They are light and simple to use. Some have a moulded surface that helps the cushion conform better to body shape and reduces shear. Some have a special core that allows air to circulate and prevents heat building up. Gel cushions may be solid or fluid and are sometimes combined with foam to make them lighter. Fluid cushions can also be filled with foam in a way that has a dampening effect on the flow of fluid or to provide support for a fluid-filled pad.

Alternating air cushions are designed to relieve pressure from the seating surface. Like pressure-relieving mattresses, their cells inflate and deflate in sequence to either support or relieve pressure from this area. They are either mains-operated or powered by battery packs.

Heel protectors

Heel protectors are aids used to protect the heels of people who are very frail and at high risk of developing pressure sores. They are made of either sheepskin (real or synthetic) or Silicore fibre, and are held in place with Velcro straps. They help reduce and relieve pressure. Heel blocks are made of soft foam and have a U shape in the middle. The ankle fits into the U shape and the heels are held up and do not touch the mattress. Heel blocks can only be used when the person is sitting up or lying on their back. Heel protectors are used when the person is lying on their side.

Elbow protectors

Elbow protectors are designed to protect elbows. They are also made of sheepskin or Silicore and are held in place with Velcro straps.

Treating pressure sores

Treatment aims are:

1 To reduce pressure and prevent further damage
2 To improve the person's condition to enable healing to take place
3 To dress the wound and encourage healing
4 To prevent infection whenever possible.

If you fear that a person is developing a pressure sore, you should always seek professional help and advice. In most cases, nurses will be responsible for treating the pressure sore. The nurse will assess the sore and plan treatment and care. This will include changing the person's position regularly; special mattresses, cushions and pressure-relieving aids may be used. The pressure sore will be covered with a protective dressing to keep the wound clean and prevent it from drying out. Wounds of all types, including pressure sores, are now known to heal more quickly if they are kept warm and moist. You will be involved in helping carry out the plan of care.

Caring for the whole person

People develop pressure sores because they are unable to move and relieve pressure. Illness can make a person more at risk of developing a pressure sore and the patient's doctor will treat any illness that could contribute to the development of a pressure sore.

If pressure sores are to be prevented it is important that the individual eats a healthy diet and has sufficient food and vitamins to prevent the skin breaking down. Older people who feel unwell may be reluctant to eat. It is important that you inform senior staff if an individual has gone off their food. You can also find out what food the older person is fond of and inform other members of staff about their likes and dislikes.

It is important that the individual drinks enough fluid. You can encourage the older person to drink and can ensure that they have drinks that they like. You can inform other members of staff about the individual's likes and dislikes. Further details on diet and fluids are given in Chapter 7.

Summary

Older people are more at risk of developing pressure sores than younger people. People living in homes are more at risk than those who live in their own homes. Pressure sores are at best uncomfortable and painful; at their worst they can be life threatening. Most pressure sores can be prevented. Some people living in homes are more frail than others. Assessment enables nurses to work out the individual's degree of risk of developing pressure sores, and to develop a plan of care. This enables the nurse to decide which type of mattresses, cushions and aids are required. The nurse should discuss the plan of care with the individual and obtain their consent and cooperation. You are an important part of the team. You need to be aware of the plan of care and should work with senior staff to prevent individuals developing pressure sores.

Key points

- Ageing and illness increase the risk of an older person developing a pressure sore.
- Pressure sores are caused by pressure, shear and friction.
- Risk assessment tools help to assess a person's risk of developing pressure sores.
- Risk assessment tools are a guide, not a substitute for observation.

- Adopting a problem-solving approach reduces pressure risk.
- Pressure sores can lead to infection, illness and even death.
- Your role in encouraging people to move around, assisting people to change position and reporting any problems is of vital importance.

Portfolio preparation

Your assessor must have evidence that you can meet the performance criteria for this unit. Before beginning this unit discuss assessment strategies with your assessor. Most of the evidence for this unit can be gained by direct observation of your work.

Products: This might include a copy of progress notes or a care plan on pressure area care that you have completed. It could be a note in a resident's notes giving details of any aids that the person uses or details of assistance that the person requires, detailed on a care plan. It could be a care plan that you have drawn up or contributed to on how you are helping to reduce risk factors.

Witness testimony: This is a statement from a senior member of staff. It might be a statement detailing how you have met certain performance criteria.

Written work: You might be asked to prepare a piece of work about the factors that increase the risk of pressure sores developing. You might be asked to write a case history about a resident at risk of pressure sores and how you have supported and enabled the person to reduce risk factors. You may be asked to discuss the difficulties you face in preventing pressure sores and how you deal with these difficulties. Your assessor may also use other methods to help you gain evidence for this unit. These may include:

- Verbal questioning
- Written questions.

Simulations can be used if it is not possible to obtain evidence by direct observation.

Further information

Braden scale: One of the authors of the Braden scale has a website (http://www.bradenscale.com). You can download copies of the scale and obtain other information from the site.

Waterlow scale: Judy Waterlow, the author of the Waterlow scale, has a website (http://www.judy-waterlow.co.uk/). You can download copies of the scale and obtain other information from the site.

You can obtain leaflets and further information on wound care and preventing pressure sores from the companies listed below.

Convatec
Harrington House
Milton Road
Ickenham
Uxbridge UB10 8PU
Helpline: 0800 289738
Website: http://www.convatec.com/UK/

Coloplast
Peterborough Business Park
Peterborough
Cambs PE2 6FX
Telephone: 01733 392000
Website: http://www.coloplast.co.uk

Smith & Nephew Healthcare
S&N Healthcare House
Goulton Street
Hull HU3 4DJ
Telephone: 01482 222200
Website: http://www.smith-nephew.com

Talley Group Limited
Premier Way
Abbey Park Industrial Estate
Romsey
Hampshire SO51 9DQ
Telephone: 01794 503500
Website: http://www.talleygroup.com

Huntleigh Healthcare
310–312 Dallow Road
Luton
Bedfordshire LU1 1TD
Telephone: 01582 413104
Website: http://www.huntleigh-healthcare.com

Further reading

National Institute for Clinical Excellence (2003) *Pressure Ulcer Risk Assessment and Prevention*. NICE, London. This can be downloaded from http://www.nice.org.uk.

Chapter Ten

Personal Care and Hygiene

HSC218 Support individuals with their personal care needs

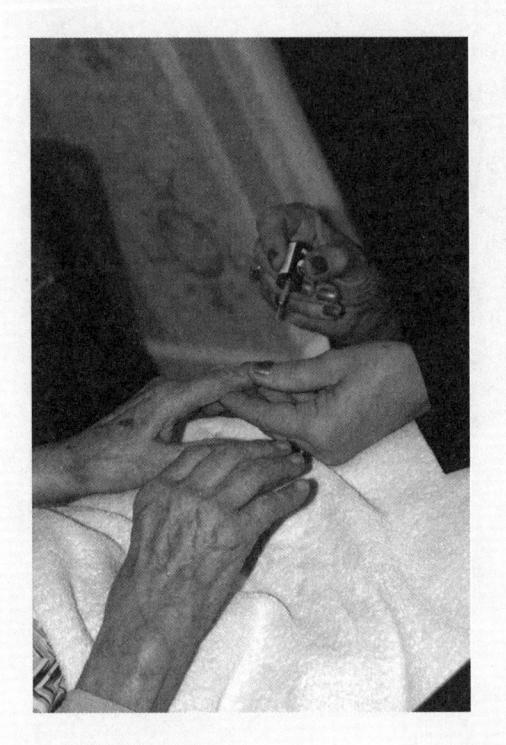

This unit consists of three elements:
HSC218a Support individuals to go to the toilet
HSC218b Enable individuals to maintain their personal hygiene
HSC218c Support individuals in personal grooming and dressing

Please note this unit cannot be used in combination with HSC219: *Support individuals to manage continence.*

This chapter

- Provides information on normal elimination of urine and faeces
- Explains how ageing affects bowel and bladder function
- Provides information on how to enable the older person to use the toilet independently
- Explains how to enable the older person to maintain dignity and privacy at all times
- Discusses health and safety issues
- Explains why older people may have difficulty meeting their personal care needs independently
- Provides information on how to encourage and enable older people to bath, shower and wash
- Explains how you can help the older person to bath and wash
- Explains how ageing affects skin and how to care for older skin
- Provides details on shaving, caring for hair and nails
- Gives information on dressing and assisting people to dress

Understanding elimination

Figure 10.1 shows the urinary system. The urinary system in men and women consists of the kidneys, the ureters, the bladder and the urethra. Let's look at the urinary system in detail.

Urine is produced by the kidneys. The kidneys have three main functions. These are:

1. To remove waste products and drugs from the blood
2. To conserve water and salt
3. To maintain the balance of chemicals (electrolytes) in the blood.

The amount of urine produced varies, depending on the time of day, the amount of fluid consumed and the amount of fluid lost. Normally the kidneys concentrate urine at night while we are asleep so the first urine passed in the morning is concentrated. If a person drinks a lot of fluid, the urine is lighter coloured and more dilute. In hot weather or if a person is not drinking very much, the urine becomes darker and more concentrated.

The average person should drink eight mugs or 2 litres of fluid a day. If a person drinks 2 litres of fluid 500 ml of this fluid is normally lost in the moisture in breath, in sweating and in faeces. This is known as 'insensible loss'. The person will then pass around 1500 ml of urine in 24 hours.

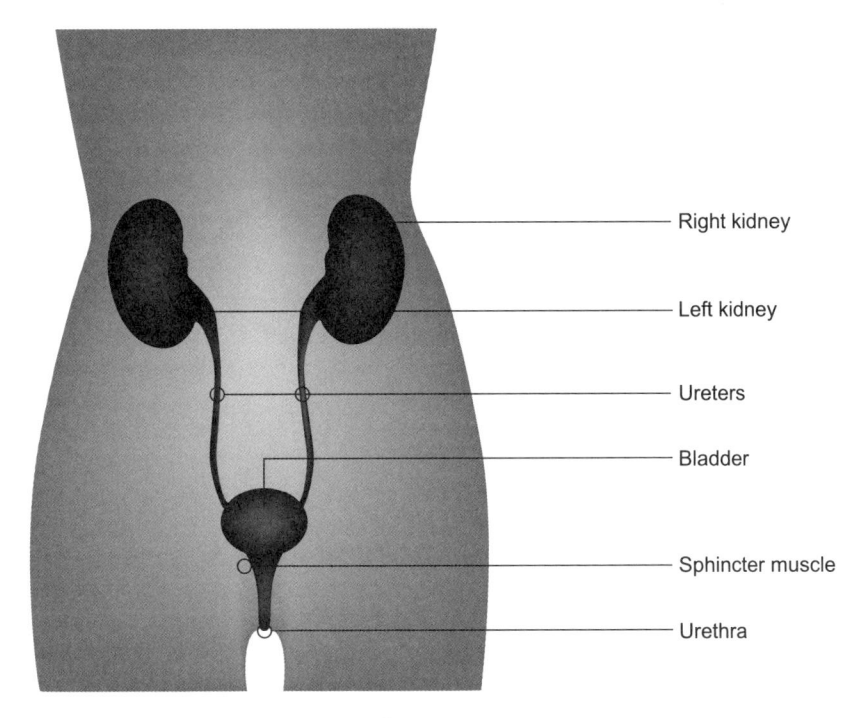

Figure 10.1 The urinary system.[1]

Brain

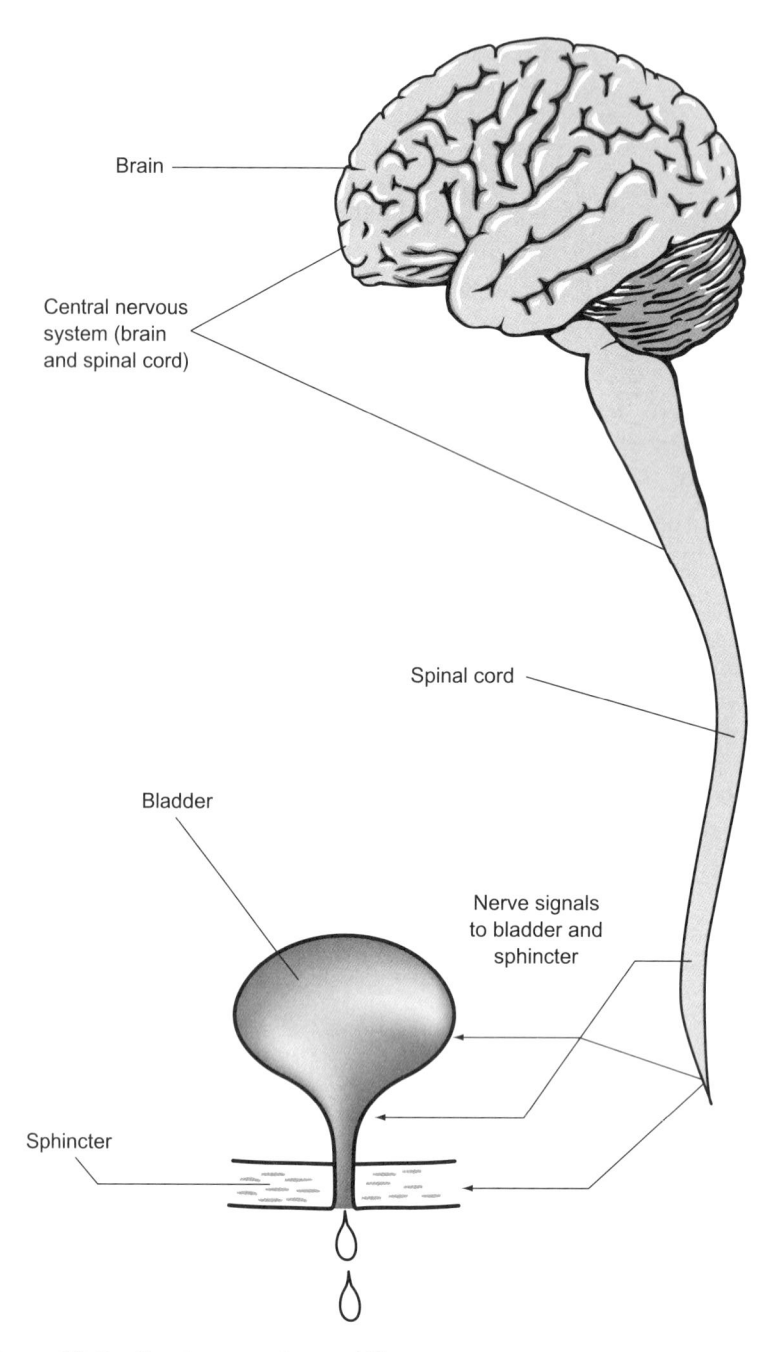

Central nervous system (brain and spinal cord)

Spinal cord

Bladder

Nerve signals to bladder and sphincter

Sphincter

Figure 10.2 Continence, a learnt skill.

If a person is sweating a lot or has loose stools or a wound that is losing a lot of fluid, then the amount of insensible loss will rise and the urine output will fall.

Urine drains from the kidneys into the ureters. It is collected in the bladder, shown in Fig. 10.2. The bladder muscle (detrusor) stretches in all directions to allow it to fill with urine. The urethra keeps the bladder closed so that we do not pass urine while the bladder is filling. The bladder contains special nerves known as stretch receptors. These stretch receptors send messages to the brain so that we know when the bladder is becoming full. When the bladder is becoming full we find a convenient place to pass urine. When we are ready to pass urine the urethra relaxes to allow urine to drain. The bladder muscle contracts to squeeze urine from the bladder.

Bladder capacity varies. Male bladders normally hold more than female bladders but some people have larger bladders than others; tall, big-boned people have big bladders and small people have smaller bladders.

Continence: a learnt skill

The ability to hold urine until we can find a suitable place to empty our bladders is one that we probably take for granted but it's important to remember that we are all born incontinent. Continence is a skill that we learnt as our bodies and brains matured.

In babies the kidneys produce urine and this is stored in the bladder. When the bladder is full a signal goes to the spinal cord and the bladder automatically empties. This is known as 'reflex bladder emptying'.

In adults the mechanism is different.

The bladder fills while the detrusor (bladder) muscle is relaxed and the urethra is closed. When the bladder is partially full the stretch receptors in the bladder send a message up the spinal cord to the brain and we realise that our bladder is filling up. We are not normally aware of any sensation of bladder fullness until the bladder contains about 300 ml of urine. The frontal lobe of the brain contains an area known as the micturition centre. This enables us to hold on until it is convenient to pass urine. When we hold on the urethra remains tightly closed and the bladder continues to fill. The fuller the bladder becomes, the harder it is to hold on.

As adults we can control our bladders and hold on to urine until it is convenient to pass urine.

How ageing affects the urinary system

The body has plenty of reserve capacity when people are young. Ageing affects all aspects of bodily function and reduces the level of reserve capacity.

The kidneys become less efficient with age. They become less effective at concentrating urine. This means that older people produce larger amounts of more dilute urine than younger people do. Older people are more at risk of dehydrating than younger people because when they are losing a lot of fluid they cannot concentrate urine to preserve fluid. If we are becoming dehydrated we get very thirsty. Ageing affects the thirst mechanism; so dehydrated older people may not feel thirsty. Adults do not normally have to get up in the night to pass urine because only 25% of our urine output is produced at night. This can easily be stored in the healthy adult bladder. Older people usually have to get up twice a night to pass urine because the ageing kidneys do not concentrate urine effectively at night.

The bladder muscle becomes stiffer and less stretchy with age. This means that bladder capacity is reduced and bladder emptying is less efficient. When young adults pass urine only a small amount of urine is left in the bladder. Ageing affects the ability to empty the bladder efficiently and older people may have up to 150 ml of urine left in the bladder after passing urine. This stale urine can increase the risk of infection.

The stretch receptors in the bladder are also less efficient so older people get less warning of the need to pass urine. Most older people are only aware that they need to pass urine when the bladder is 80–90% full.

How illness affects the ability to remain continent

Often relatives tell us that the older person was continent at home but has just become incontinent because of illness, hospitalisation or because of moving to the home. Illness and moving to a new environment can easily affect a person's ability to remain continent. Continence is a complex skill. In order to remain continent we have to be able to:

1 Recognise that the bladder is full
2 Hold on until we can find a toilet
3 Be able to find a toilet
4 Be able to get to the toilet and adjust clothing or communicate the need to use a toilet and get help.

Your actions in helping the older person can enable the person to remain continent.

Recognising bladder fullness

Illness can lead to a normally lucid older person becoming confused. If the older person develops a chest infection the major signs are often confusion and falls. If the person is confused then she may not be able to recognise the signs of a full bladder. A hacking cough may cause the bladder pressure to rise and the person to leak urine. Diabetes can affect the function of every nerve in the body, sometimes people with diabetes may be unaware of the sensation of bladder fullness.

Sometimes older people can become involved in a pleasurable activity and may put off going to the toilet or asking for help. The older person may then find she does not have enough time to get to the toilet and may be incontinent.

Holding on

Older people have a reduced bladder capacity and are not able to hold on for long periods. Some diseases such as stroke and Parkinson's disease make the bladder more irritable and the person finds it more difficult to hold on. If the person has a chest infection and is coughing the cough may increase the bladder pressure and lead to urine leakage while holding on.

Finding the toilet

Ageing and diseases such as diabetes may affect vision. The older person may find it difficult to identify the toilet when faced with a corridor full of doors with small signs. Locating the right room takes time and the person may move slowly and require a toilet urgently.

Getting to the toilet

Older people need to be able to get to the toilet faster than younger people. They have less warning than the younger person and are less able to hold on. Illness can affect a person's ability to get to the toilet. The person who has had a stroke may be paralysed down one side and may be unable to get to the toilet unaided. The person with Parkinson's disease may be unable to walk well enough or steadily enough to get to the toilet unaided. If the person is unable to get to the toilet unaided she will depend on you to help her maintain continence. Research suggests that the ability to get to the toilet and use it unaided is the single most important factor in maintaining continence.

Communicating the need to use the toilet

If a person is unable to use the toilet unaided she needs to be able to communicate her need to you. Illness can affect this ability. Stroke can make it difficult for people to speak and communicate. Parkinson's disease can affect the ability to speak and the person may only be able to speak very quietly.

Examining and testing urine

If you help people to use the toilet or commode you need to know what normal urine looks like and what is abnormal.

Normal urine is clear. Urine that is cloudy or thick or has bits floating in it should be saved and professional advice sought. Fresh urine does not smell. Urine which has been standing or which has been collecting in a catheter bag may smell because bacteria break down urine and produce ammonia.

Urine should be golden or straw coloured. The first specimen of the day is usually darker. Dark urine is more concentrated than light urine and is normally a sign that the individual is not drinking enough.

Some drugs and foods can cause the urine to change colour. Eating beetroot can produce red or pink urine. Some people who are prescribed the antibiotic nitrofurantoin produce turquoise urine. If the urine looks abnormal in colour you should save the specimen and seek professional advice.

Blood may cause the urine to appear red or pink. If you suspect that the urine contains blood, professional advice should be obtained immediately.

Urine testing

Urine is normally tested when an older person is admitted to the home. Testing urine enables staff to detect abnormalities. Urine is normally tested with a Multi-stick. This is a plastic strip that has a number of pads on it. Each pad has chemicals on it and changes colour when it is dipped into fresh urine and an abnormality is present. Urine is normally checked for a number of substances.

Blood

Blood in the urine can be caused by infection, kidney stones or other conditions.

Ketones

Ketones are substances produced when the body is burning up fat. This occurs if the person is diabetic and the diabetes is poorly controlled. Ketones are also present in the urine of people who are losing weight. The overweight person who is on a diet may have ketones in the urine. Undernourished people and people who have been vomiting (and are therefore not eating) may have ketones in their urine.

Glucose

Glucose is a form of sugar. It may be present in the urine of people who have diabetes.

Protein

Protein may be present in the urine of people who have kidney disease or who have a urine infection.

pH

pH indicates whether the urine is acid or alkaline. Normally urine is slightly acid and has a pH of between 5 and 7. A pH above 7 may indicate that the person has an infection. Vegetarians normally have a urine pH of above 7 and this is normal for people who do not eat meat.

Specific gravity

Some urine testing sticks also measure the specific gravity. This enables staff to check how concentrated urine is. The normal specific gravity of urine is 1002–1030. A specific gravity of more than 1030 indicates that the urine is very concentrated.

Nitrite

Some sticks also test for nitrite. Nitrite is produced when there are bacteria in the bladder. This may indicate that an infection is present.

Storing urine test sticks

Urine test sticks will give inaccurate results if they are not stored properly. It is important to close the container tightly and not to remove the small packet which is in the bottle with the sticks. The packet contains crystals that prevent the sticks becoming damp and giving a false reading.

Bowel function

The gastrointestinal tract stretches from the mouth to the anus (Fig. 10.3). When we eat food we chew it and mix it with saliva and swallow the bolus. The food goes down the oesophagus and enters the stomach via the cardiac sphincter. There it is bathed in hydrochloric acid, churned and released into the small bowel. Nutrients and fluid are absorbed from the small bowel and passed into the colon.

The colon has four basic functions: reabsorption, manufacture of vitamins and biotin, elimination, and formation and storage of faeces.

The colon reabsorbs around 1 litre of water each day. It also reabsorbs bile salts that have been secreted from the liver to enable digestion to take place.

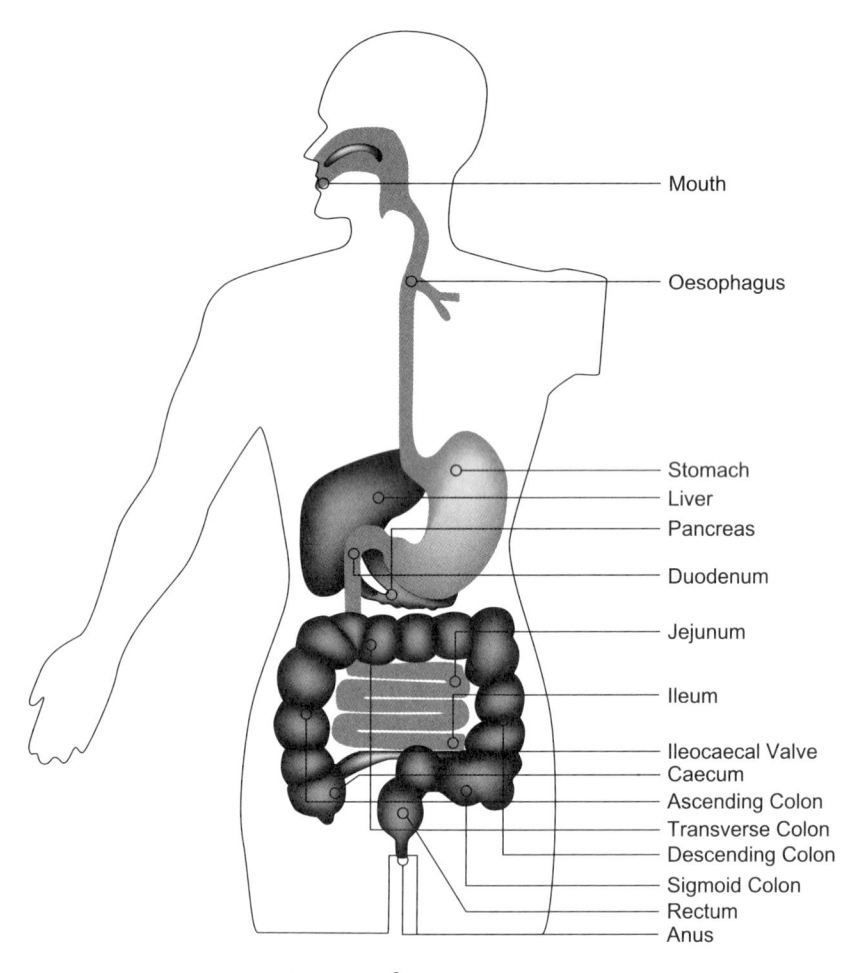

Figure 10.3 The digestive system[2].

Bacteria in the colon are involved in producing three substances: vitamin K, necessary for blood clotting; vitamin B_5, required for nerve function and hormones; and biotin, a substance that enables us to use glucose.

The colon eliminates toxins and the indigestible residue of food. As the end products of digestion pass through the colon they become thicker and more formed. The colon's end product, faeces, is stored in the colon until it can be eliminated. Normal bowel frequency varies (see Box 10.1).

Normal defecation

Food moves through the large bowel in waves known as peristalsis. Peristalsis deposits faeces in the rectum. This is called the gastrocolic reflex. Exercise, eating and drinking hot drinks stimulate this reflex. The gastrocolic

> **Box 10.1** Normal bowel frequency
>
> - 7% of men and 4% of women defecate two or three times daily.
> - 40% of men and 30% of women defecate once daily.
> - The normal bowel habit varies from three times a day to three times a week.
> - Women of childbearing age are more likely to be constipated than older women. This is thought to be because oestrogen and progesterone, the female sex hormones, reduce colonic motility.

reflex is strongest in the morning after breakfast. People who do not eat breakfast or who delay defecating are at increased risk of constipation.

When faeces move into the rectum the internal sphincter relaxes and the anal pressure drops. The anorectal angle increases and faeces move into the anal canal. When we defecate the external sphincter relaxes and stool is passed.

If it is not convenient we can tighten our anal sphincters and hold on. If we hold on long enough all desire to defecate vanishes and we can sometimes push the faeces back up into the sigmoid colon. If we do not find the time and the place to defecate, the faeces will dry out and become hard and difficult to pass.

Does ageing affect bowel function?

Older people are seven times more likely to complain of constipation than young people.

Ageing affects all aspects of the body. Ageing affects the sense of taste. Things don't taste as good when people are old because the taste buds become less efficient. Ageing affects dentition. Older people are more likely to have missing teeth or to wear dentures. Ageing affects the ability to chew food. Ageing also slows peristalsis. This means that older people have more difficulty swallowing than do younger people. These changes may affect the food that people eat and the amount of food that they eat. The stomach empties more slowly in old age. This means that older people digest more slowly and feel less hungry. Stomach acid is reduced in old age. This increases the time taken to digest food. The thirst mechanism is less sensitive in old age so older people may drink less fluid.

Ageing leads to reduced absorption. Older people are less able to extract vitamins and nutrients from food. Ageing leads to reduced peristalsis in the large bowel and reduced ability to absorb fluid from the colon. The nerves in the rectum become less sensitive and older people have greater difficulty in distinguishing between flatus (wind), fluid and solid matter.

The anal squeeze pressure is reduced in old age. This is more common in women and may be related to damage to the pudendal nerve caused by childbirth. Those who are 'too posh to push' during childbirth may have a point!

Despite these changes the healthy older person's bowel functions normally. Older people are however more likely to complain of constipation and to take laxatives. This may be because of illness, dietary changes, reduced activity and the effects of medication.

What is constipation?

The word constipation is based on the Latin word *constipare* and means to crowd together. Any person who defines themselves as constipated is making a judgement on how often they expect to have a bowel action, how easy that bowel action is to pass, the volume of the bowel action and the consistency of stool. The Rome diagnostic criteria (Box 10.2) provides a tool to diagnose constipation.

Box 10.2 Rome diagnostic criteria[3]

Two or more of the following for at least 12 weeks in the last 12 months:

1 Straining in more than half of all defecations
2 Lumpy or hard stools in more than a quarter of all defecations
3 Sensations of incomplete evacuation in more than half of defecations
4 Sensation of anorectal obstruction or blockage in more than half of defecations
5 Manual manoeuvres to facilitate more than half of defecations (e.g. digital evacuation or perineal support)
6 Bowel frequency of less than three times a week.

Loose stools are not present and there are insufficient criteria for irritable bowel syndrome.

Why constipation occurs

Disorders of propulsion

The length of time it takes for food to move from mouth to anus is known as gut transit time. Transit times vary according to the amount of exercise, fluid and fibre a person takes. In people eating a typical British diet, transit times of 5 days are considered normal. Frail older people living in care homes can have transit times of 14 days. Propulsion disorders are thought to be caused by degeneration of the nerve supply to the gut. This may be the result of prolonged use of stimulant laxatives.

Defecatory difficulty

Some people with constipation have normal transit times but have difficulty expelling stools.

The character of the stool can contribute to defecatory difficulty. Hard stools are more difficult to pass than soft stools. The Bristol stool chart (Fig. 10.4) can be used to assess and record the type of stool a person is passing.

People with defecatory difficulty need to push down using their abdominal muscles. If these are weak, defecation is made more difficult.

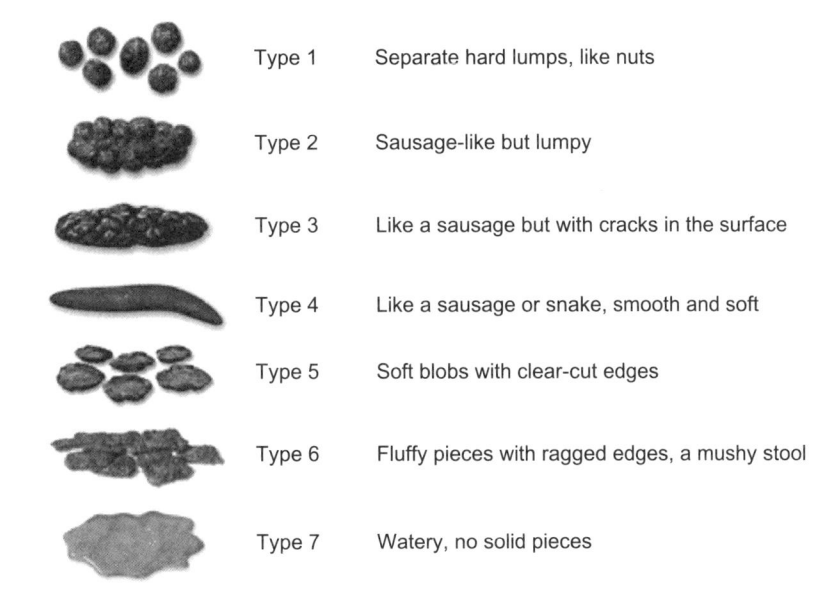

	Type 1	Separate hard lumps, like nuts
	Type 2	Sausage-like but lumpy
	Type 3	Like a sausage but with cracks in the surface
	Type 4	Like a sausage or snake, smooth and soft
	Type 5	Soft blobs with clear-cut edges
	Type 6	Fluffy pieces with ragged edges, a mushy stool
	Type 7	Watery, no solid pieces

Figure 10.4 Bristol stool chart[4].

Disorders of sensation

Some people postpone having their bowels open. This can in time lead to the rectum being less sensitive to fullness. The person may be unaware of the need to defecate. Some conditions such as multiple sclerosis and spinal cord injury may lead to a person losing sensation.

Promoting a healthy bowel habit

Common causes of constipation are insufficient fluids and fibre, poor mobility, medication and poor toileting habits.

Fluid and fibre

The average adult requires 1.5 litres of fluid daily. Ageing affects the thirst mechanism and many older people do not drink sufficient fluids. Improving fluid intake helps prevent and treat constipation.

Increasing the amount of fibre in the diet improves propulsion times. The fibre helps speed up the passage of faeces through the colon. It also improves defecatory difficulty because the stools are softer and easier to pass. This improves bowel habit and reduces discomfort. It is possible to offer even the frailest older person an appetising diet rich in fibre. Fruit can be cut up into small pieces, poached, puréed or juiced. Vegetables can be added to soups, casseroles and stews. Oats, wheat and dried fruit can be added to puddings, cakes and flapjacks.

Mobility

Walking and moving stimulate peristaltic waves in the colon. Illness and nursing practice can reduce mobility. Encouraging older people to remain as mobile as possible encourages normal bowel function, improves appetite and contributes to well-being.

Care practice

The care you give can either prevent or contribute to constipation. Encouraging the older person to defecate after breakfast when the gastrocolic reflex is strongest encourages normal bowel activity. Defecation is an intensely private activity. Most people would prefer to defecate in a locked toilet rather than perched precariously on a bedpan or being expected to use a commode. Helping people to the toilet and providing a private, unrushed environment enables them to retain normal bowel activity.

Medication

Medication can cause constipation and is an important factor in 50% of people admitted to hospital with constipation. If you notice that a person you are caring for is developing problems with constipation, inform a senior member of staff. Medication can be checked and whenever possible changed to avoid constipation. If it is not possible to change medication and constipation is becoming a problem, the prescriber will normally advise that the person should receive more fluids and fibre. If these changes are ineffective a laxative may be prescribed.

Laxatives

The NHS spends more than £43 million a year on laxatives. In the past people were treated with laxatives without first being assessed. Bowel assessment is now considered good practice.

Table 10.1 Laxatives.

Type of laxative	Example	Indication
Bulk forming	Fybogel, Normacol, Celevac	Low intake of dietary fibre
Stimulant	Senna, bisacodyl	Short-term relief of acute constipation
Osmotic	Lactulose, Movicol, Idrolax	Chronic constipation
Stool softeners	Docusate sodium	Chronic constipation

Laxatives may be required to treat people who do not respond to measures to promote a healthy bowel. Laxatives can help people with disorders of propulsion or defecatory difficulty; however, they are often unhelpful in people with sensory disorder, who benefit from suppositories or enemas. Laxatives can be divided into four groups (see Table 10.1).

If a person has short-term constipation a stimulant laxative is often prescribed. Stimulant laxatives stimulate the nerves in the myenteric nerve plexus. This causes the bowel to contract. They work within 8–12 hours. These should not be used on a long-term basis because they can lead to *atonic colon*. The bowel becomes inactive and dependent on ever larger amounts of stimulant laxatives. Side effects include cramp and loose stool. If an individual has been taking stimulant laxatives for a long time the prescriber may have little alternative but to continue to prescribe them.

Bulk-forming laxatives provide fibre that is missing from the diet. They take some days to work and must be given with plenty of fluids. Osmotic laxatives work by retaining fluid in the stool as it passes through the bowel or changing the way water is distributed in faeces. Lactulose is normally prescribed and macrogols such as Movicol and Idrolax are reserved for constipation that does not respond to lactulose.

Faeces

Faeces contain waste products and food such as fibre that cannot be digested by the body. Faeces are normally brown and soft. Bile salts give faeces their brown colour. The normal stool is produced without straining.

Some drugs can alter the appearance of faeces. Iron tablets cause the faeces to become black, sticky and tar-like in appearance. Some drugs can cause the individual to bleed either from the stomach or the bowel.

Blood in faeces can also make them appear black and tar-like. If the individual bleeds from the lower bowel, blood can be seen clearly. If a resident passes faeces that appear abnormal, save the specimen or leave the toilet unflushed and obtain professional advice.

Enabling older people to use the toilet

Some older people living in homes will have difficulty walking. Often with help, encouragement, physiotherapy and walking aids they can regain the ability to walk to the toilet independently. Details on mobility are given in Chapter 8.

Some older people may have difficulty in identifying the toilets. If the toilets are in a corridor and all the doors look the same, it can be difficult to find the toilet. The older person with poor eyesight may be unable to read the small signs that say 'toilet'. In some homes, all toilet doors have been painted a special colour, perhaps yellow, so that they stand out from all other doors. In other homes, staff have made up large posters with pictures of toilets on them (Fig. 10.5). Other homes have large signs saying 'toilet' in letters six inches high. These measures help older people to find toilets quickly and enable them to use the toilet independently.

Older men who have poor eyesight may find it difficult to see the toilet. If the toilet and the floor are the same colour, a poorly sighted man can find this difficult. In some homes, a toilet seat in a contrasting colour such as black on a white toilet helps the person to see the toilet. This method works unless the male resident is in the habit of lifting the toilet seat, as many men do. In some homes, a coloured toilet cleanser is put in the cistern; each time the toilet is flushed, it refills with blue-coloured water. The poorly sighted male resident can then aim for the blue water.

People who suffer from arthritis, especially arthritis of the hips and knees, may manage to sit on the toilet but find it difficult to get up because the seat is too low. Providing raised toilet seats that fit over the toilet can help people with arthritis to use the toilet independently.

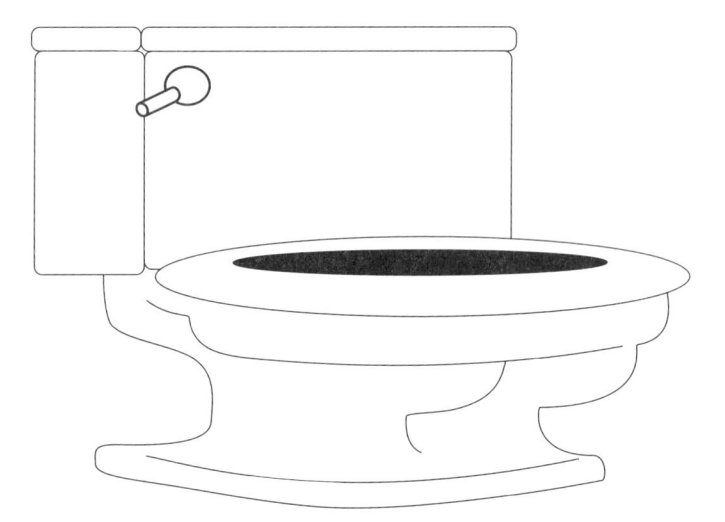

Figure 10.5 A picture to identify the toilet door.

Some people may find it difficult to pull down or adjust their clothing without help. You can suggest clothing that is easier to remove and adjust. Trousers with elastic waistbands are easier to manage than those with zips and buttons. Some male residents find jogging pants comfortable, but these seldom have zips in the front. Placing a zip in the front helps many older men to use the toilet without help. Some men's trousers have short zips; if these are replaced with longer zips many male residents find it easier to use the toilet.

Female residents may have difficulty pulling up dresses or skirts that are tightly fitted around the legs and hips. Wearing skirts and dresses that are flared or have pleats makes it easier to hitch up clothing and use the toilet. Male and female residents should be advised not to wear pants that are too tight. Tight pants are not only uncomfortable but are difficult to pull down. People who have difficulty dressing and undressing can be encouraged to practise. There are many ways of learning to dress and undress which take disability into account.

Some older people become forgetful and may lose track of time. You can help by reminding forgetful residents to use the toilet. Reminding the older person to use the toilet may help the older person to remain continent.

Dignity and privacy

Using the toilet is a private activity. Older people who are using the toilet should be able to do so without fearing that staff or other residents will burst in on them. Toilets should have locks and residents should be encouraged to lock the toilet door. If the older person is using a commode or bedpan in a shared bedroom, the bed curtains should be drawn carefully to protect the individual's privacy and dignity.

Health and safety

Although the older person has the right to privacy and dignity when using the toilet, staff may need to enter the toilet in the case of an emergency. The individual may have fallen or collapsed and requires urgent help. Many homes have toilets that can be opened by staff in an emergency. Some homes have doors which open if the edge of a coin is inserted in a slot on the outside of the door, and turned. Other homes use a master key system; the key is placed in the outside of the lock and turned.

Most toilets have vinyl floors. Many floors are made of special vinyl which is non-slip even when wet. There is a danger, though, that people will slip over if walking on a wet floor. If the toilet floor is wet it should be cleaned and dried at once to prevent falls occurring.

Most toilets have special rails that people can use to pull themselves up and hold on to when using the toilet. If these work loose, this should be reported at once. Normally the toilet should not be used until grab rails are made safe. If it is not possible to stop using the toilet, staff should accompany residents requiring help until repairs have been completed. Toilets should have call bells fitted in case a person requires urgent help. Call bells should be within easy reach.

Assisting people to use toilets

Research shows that people are more likely to suffer from incontinence if they have to depend on someone else to take them to the toilet. It is easy to understand the reasons for this. An older person asks, 'Can you take me to the toilet please?' But the care assistant is busy laying the tables for lunch and says, 'Just a minute, Mrs Johnston, I'll just finish laying the table.' The care assistant finishes laying the table and helps Mrs Johnston to the toilet. Mrs Johnston walks very slowly because she has had a stroke, her balance is poor and she uses a tripod. The toilet is some distance away. Just as they enter the toilet Mrs Johnston wets herself.

The section on the effects of ageing on the bladder at the beginning of this chapter explained how older people have less warning about the need to empty their bladders than younger people do. Mrs Johnston only became aware of the need to use the toilet when her bladder was almost full. She may have noticed that the staff were busy and waited until it seemed convenient; by then she was bursting to go.

The well-educated care assistant who is aware of how ageing and illness affect the bladder would have reacted differently. When Mrs Johnston asked to go to the toilet the care assistant would have come over at once and asked, 'Are you desperate or have we got time to walk there?' Mrs Johnston would have replied, 'No, I'm not desperate, we have plenty of time.' Because the care assistant responded promptly, Mrs Johnston had plenty of time to walk to the toilet. Had her need been more urgent, the care assistant could have wheeled her to the toilet and walked her back. The episode of incontinence would have been avoided.

If the older person is desperate to use the toilet but staff are encouraging the person to walk, wheeling her to the toilet and helping her to walk back will help the person to exercise and provide sensitive care. If the person requires help to use the toilet, you should help the person to sit on the toilet, ensure that the individual can reach the call bell and offer to wait outside. The individual can call when she has finished. It is important to help the person to wash her hands after using the toilet. You should wash your hands every time you take an individual to the toilet. This is very important as it prevents the spread of infection.

Commodes

Commodes are sometimes used in homes. Often people who need to use the toilet at night are helped on and off commodes. If the person is sharing a room, ensure that you draw bed curtains so that there are no gaps.

Bedpans

Bedpans are sometimes offered when the individual is in bed. It can be very difficult to sit comfortably on a bedpan and some people are unable to pass urine in them because they fear that the urine will splash on the bed. It is important to find out if the individual prefers to use a commode or a bedpan.

Enabling individuals to maintain personal hygiene

People of all ages like to feel and look good. Many older people who have been in hospital arrive in homes wearing night-clothes and looking ill and tired. When the person is dressed in her normal clothes, has her hair set and is wearing make-up, she feels and looks much better (Fig. 10.6).

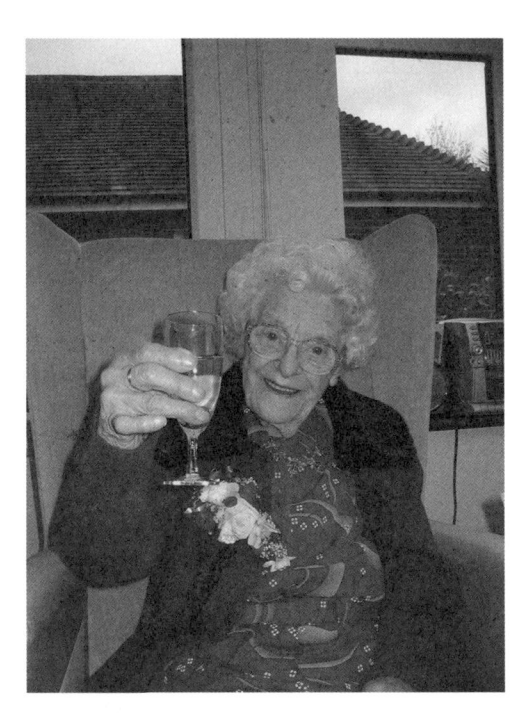

Figure 10.6 Looking good.

When we feel dirty, untidy and under the weather, bathing and making the effort to look good make us feel so much better.

Many older people who have just undergone surgery, for example for a fractured femur, feel worn out and fed up. Often they are unable to wash, dress and care for themselves without help. The care assistant can make a real difference to the person's quality of life. You can encourage and assist the older person to bath, to care for her hair and nails and to dress. This can make a real difference to the individual's morale. Suddenly the experience of coming into a home is not as bad as the individual feared. She is being helped to care for herself and is beginning to feel human again.

It has been said that the role of the nurse is to do for the patient what they would do for themselves if they had the strength and the will. Helping people to care for their personal appearance is not about helping residents to look or appear as we would wish, but as they would wish.

Bathing

Nowadays most of us take bathrooms and their supply of constant hot water for granted. Many older people, though, grew up without such luxuries. They grew up in homes without bathrooms, central heating or hot water. People who did not have bathrooms either heated up water and bathed in a tin bath in front of a fire in the living room, or they visited the public baths. This involved much more effort than going upstairs and running a bath and so many older people bathed much less frequently than we do now.

How often a person baths is a personal choice. Some older people prefer to bath each day, while others feel that bathing twice a week is adequate. Bathing every day can help some residents to feel fresh and clean, for example those who perspire heavily or who suffer from incontinence. No harm, however, will come to most people if they do not bath every day. The decision on how often to bath should be the older person's. While you can persuade an older person to bath, no older person should be bullied into bathing if they do not wish to do so. Bathing should be a pleasure and not a hurried chore. If you take the time and trouble to make the person's bath a pleasant experience you will find that the older person will look forward to the next bath.

Making bathing a pleasure

Many older people living in homes require help to bath. Even people who can bath without help depend on us to ensure that the bathroom is safe, warm and comfortable. In some homes bathrooms become used as storerooms and fill up with boxes, broken chairs, commodes and other equipment. You should do everything you can to make sure that the bathroom is not used as a storeroom. Imagine how you would feel bathing in a room full of junk. Ask senior staff if equipment can be stored elsewhere. Keeping the bathroom clear makes it less likely that residents or staff will have an accident in the bathroom.

Often the bathroom window is left open and the room becomes cold. You should check that the window is closed before running the bath. The bathroom radiator should be turned on. If you find the bathroom hot, remember that the person who has just got out of the bath will find it much cooler. The bath water should be the correct temperature. You should ask the individual how they like the water. Hot water is usually stored at 60 °C to prevent bacteria growing in the tank. Water of this temperature will scald people so thermostatic valves are used to reduce water temperature to safe levels. It is always best to check the water temperature by dipping your elbow into it. Valves can become defective. It is better to be safe than sorry. People who are confused may be unable to tell you if the water is too hot. The water should be deep enough to wash in and not just a few inches deep.

Bubble baths and bath oils

Many people like to use scented bubble bath or bath oils in the bath. Bubble bath adds a touch of luxury and many people enjoy using it. Some bubble baths, though, can make an older person's skin very dry; moisturising cream bubble bath can prevent this. Some older people have very sensitive skin and bubble bath can make it itch. It is now possible to buy bubble baths especially for people with sensitive skin. These avoid using agents such as lanolin, which can cause allergies. Most supermarkets sell their own brand of sensitive skin bubble bath and many other companies make them too. You can either ask relatives to buy these, or buy them for the older person who can pay from their personal allowance, or take the older person shopping. This will depend on the policy of the home. Some older people continue to suffer from dry or sensitive skin despite these measures and you should seek professional advice. The person's doctor may prescribe bath additives designed for people with very sensitive skin.

Bath oils should be used with caution. Some make the skin very slippery. This does not normally cause a problem if the older person is helped in and out of the bath by using a hoist. If the individual only requires a hand to step out of the bath then bath oils that can make the skin, the bath and even a bath mat slippery should be used with care.

Soap

Some older people prefer to wash with soap instead of using bubble bath, shower gel and foam washes. Most people can use soap without any ill effects. Some older people who have dry skin find that soap makes it even drier. It is now possible to buy soaps that have moisturising cream in them; using these prevents the skin becoming dry. Dove soap, for example, is a superfatted emulsion that moisturises skin. There are two types – blue for people with normal skin and green for people with sensitive skin. Simple soap is also useful for people with sensitive skin as it is unperfumed and made specially for sensitive skins. Some older people, especially those with eczema, may, on doctor's advice, wash using emulsifying ointment instead of soap.

Talcum powder

Many older people like to use talcum powder after drying their skin. Some older people may find that heavily perfumed talc makes their skin itch. Using either baby powder or unscented talcum powder can prevent this problem.

Persuading the reluctant resident to bath

Some older people may be reluctant to bath. They may have found that the bath was rushed and was an ordeal rather than a pleasure. Male residents may be embarrassed to appear naked in front of a young female care assistant. Some older people need help to get in and out of the bath but may not like to ask as they do not want to 'appear a nuisance' or 'trouble the staff'.

Some older people may be in pain and may fear that getting in and out of the bath will make it worse. Others may feel that there is no opportunity to bath in private. You should take the time and trouble to find out why the older person is reluctant (Case Study 10.1) and should try to make bathing as pleasant an experience as possible.

If the person likes a long leisurely soak but the bathrooms are busy in the morning, perhaps you could suggest a bath in the afternoon or evening

Case Study 10.1

Mrs Eltringham was admitted to The Hollies from hospital. She had refused to bath in hospital and was described as 'difficult'.

Mrs Eltringham's key worker, Joanne Davies, spent time with Mrs Eltringham. She discovered that Mrs Eltringham was terrified of bathing. A year earlier she had slipped in the bath at home. She broke her arm, was unable to get out of the bath and spent several hours alone and afraid before her daughter visited and found her.

Joanne suggested that Mrs Eltringham try a shower and Mrs Eltringham agreed.

when the home is not so busy. If the individual does not wish to bath, you should respect the person's wishes.

Using hoists: legal requirements

Hoists are often used to help frail older people get in and out of the bath safely. Many people living in homes need help to get in and out of the bath. Some people merely require a steadying hand; others are unable to stand, bend or get into the bath unless they are lifted. In such circumstances hoists are used. Chapter 12 gives details.

Safety and privacy in the bathroom

Most people expect to enjoy a bath in peace without interruptions. Most people lock the bathroom door and enjoy a relaxing bath. How many residents in homes can enjoy peace and privacy while bathing? In some homes staff leave the bathroom door ajar so that they can 'keep an eye on' the older person. In other homes staff have strict instructions that residents must not be left alone in the bathroom, 'in the interests of safety'. Yet the nursing or residential home is the person's home and all over the country older people bath without being watched.

Some people, though, are very frail and it would not be safe to leave them alone. Some individuals who suffer from dementia and are confused could try to get up and could fall, or could slip over and drown.

How can staff respect the person's privacy and dignity and yet prevent accidents? It is important to assess the person's risk of injuring themselves while bathing. Staff have a duty of care and any member of staff who left a resident unattended in the bath knowing that the resident was at risk of injury would have failed in that duty of care.

Older people living in homes have differing abilities. An older person who lives in a home and who requires assistance to get in and out of the bath has the same right to privacy as a person living in their own home. If the older person can be safely left in the bath then everyone should respect the individual's right to privacy.

However, if the older person is confused and in danger of injuring herself, you would be failing to provide proper care if you failed to remain with the person. If the person suffers from a disease that may cause her to faint or lose consciousness, you should remain with the person to ensure that she is safe.

In homes, the care plan should include details of how much assistance the individual requires and what measures are required to maintain safety. If you are not sure, check with senior staff. The charity Counsel and Care has produced a book about balancing resident safety and providing dignity and privacy.[5]

Showers

Many new homes have specially designed shower rooms. In some homes these shower rooms are seldom used. Many older people are reluctant to use showers because they have not used them before. Many staff who have worked in older homes without showers prefer not to use showers. Showers can be refreshing. Modern specially designed showers enable older people to wash themselves. Some showers are in specially designed rooms with slightly sloping floors.

Special shower seats are provided so that the individual can shower sitting down. Often shower controls have been placed at sitting height and the showers have thermostatic valves to prevent scalding. Shower chairs with wheels are available so that the person who cannot walk can be wheeled into the shower room where she can shower or be helped to shower. Some showers are not purpose-built and resemble ordinary shower cubicles. Placing a plastic chair in the cubicle, such as the type of stacking chair homes often provide for visitors, can enable people who are unable to stand to use the shower.

Showers should have non-slip flooring; however, some 'non-slip' floors can become quite slippery when wet. You should help older people who are in danger of slipping, when they are going in and out of the shower.

Soap can be difficult to keep hold of in the shower, especially for older people who may have suffered from strokes or have arthritic hands. Soap on a rope can be hooked around the shower control (if at sitting height) or on a hook, to make washing easier.

Some residents prefer to use shower gels or body washes that can also be used as shampoos. These are available in sensitive skin and non-perfumed versions for people who have dry and sensitive skin. People who have difficulty gripping a flannel can find it difficult to wash independently using soap and a flannel. One solution is to squeeze shower gel onto a nylon beauty buff (such as that made by Oil of Olay) as this can be used one-handed.

Assisted washes

Individuals who do not wish to bath or shower each day may need help to wash. They may need help to get soap, flannels, talc, deodorant and clothing ready. If everything is ready before the wash, the water will not get cold. You can help the person to the wash basin and help them to wash. It is safer for most older people to wash sitting in a chair.

The wash basin may be too high to allow the person to use it comfortably when seated. In this case, you can bring a bowl of warm water. The person remains seated in the chair and the water is placed on a bed table. It is important to make sure that the person is able to wash in private. If the person shares a room with another person, curtains should be drawn.

If the room is overlooked, the window curtains should be drawn. If the person has a single room it may have a 'do not disturb' or 'engaged' sign on the outside; this should be used so that visitors do not enter and embarrass the person who is washing.

The individual may require help to undress. You should encourage the person to wash as much of the body as they can manage. Often older people who require assisted washes find it difficult to wash the back, bottom, lower legs and feet. You can wash these areas, dry them thoroughly, and apply powder if the person uses it. Then help put on any clothing that the individual is unable to manage.

Bed baths

People who are very frail and ill may require a bed bath. This is simply a name for a wash that is carried out in bed. It may be carried out by one or two members of staff depending on the home's policies, staffing levels and how much care the resident requires.

Towels, flannels, soap, talcum powder, deodorant and any other toiletries are removed from the person's locker, with the person's permission, and placed on the bed table. A bowl of water is brought to the bedside. The bed curtains are drawn in a shared room, the room door closed and window curtains drawn if the room is overlooked. You must explain that you intend to wash the person and make her more comfortable.

The bedclothes or duvet are removed and the person is covered with a sheet, blanket or large towel depending on the home's policy and the temperature. If it is a hot, sticky summer's day, a blanket could be hot and uncomfortable. On a chilly winter's morning, a sheet would not be warm enough. Two flannels are used for washing. One, usually a light colour, is used for the face. Another, usually a darker colour, is used for the body. Many people, especially women, do not use soap on their faces and only wash the face with plain water. You should ask the person if she normally washes her face with soap.

You then fold the cover back and wash the neck, arms, chest and abdomen. The flannel is soaped and an area of the body washed. The flannel is then rinsed and the area of the body rinsed and dried. Apply deodorant or antiperspirant if the person wishes. Apply talcum powder if the person wishes. It is easy to use too much talcum powder if using it directly from the container. This can be uncomfortable and can cause skin irritation. If too much talcum powder is used in skin folds, such as under the arms or under the breasts, the powder can cake. Placing talcum powder on a powder puff and then applying it to the skin prevents this, as it is easier to avoid putting too much on. Supermarkets and chemists sell powder puffs designed for applying talc.

If the person can sit forward, ask her to do so and wash her back. People who are able to do so should be encouraged to wash their own genital area. If the person is unable to assist by sitting up, a second member of staff can help lie the person down and roll her over onto her side. Staff should explain what they are going to do and obtain consent before moving her. The front of the body is covered and the back, buttocks and the area between the legs (perineum) is washed and dried.

The person may like to have powder on her back. It is not advisable to put powder on the perineal area or the groin as the powder can cake. This is a particular problem with people who are incontinent and people who sweat a lot. If the person is incontinent, a barrier cream may be applied lightly to the buttocks and perineum. Too much cream interferes with the action of incontinence pads. Further details on caring for the skin of incontinent residents is given in Chapter 11.

The water should then be changed. This is important because the water will have become cooler and full of soap suds. The backs of the legs are then washed and the person is rolled over onto her back. The top half of the person's body is covered and the remaining parts of the lower front of the body washed and dried and powder applied if the person wishes.

Some staff prefer to turn the person onto her back before changing the water. This practice will vary depending on the person's condition. A person with breathing difficulties will find it easier to breathe if sat up, while other people may be safer left on their sides. Some staff prefer to lift and wash the front of the leg and then lift it to wash the back. This again will depend on the person's condition, as this can be uncomfortable for people who have arthritis. Although techniques vary, the basic principles remain the same. It is important to protect the person's dignity at all times. You must ensure that the person's body remains covered and that only the part being washed is exposed. The person is then dressed or helped to dress in clean clothes. If the person is well enough she can be helped to sit in a chair while bed linen is changed and the bed made. You can then help the person to clean their teeth or dentures, to comb and style their hair, and to apply make-up if she wishes. Male residents may require help with shaving.

In some homes, you may find that the bed-bathing technique varies. Some staff use two bowls of water to carry out a bed bath, one for washing and the other for rinsing. Both bowls of water will still require changing, as the water will become cooler.

It is important to remember that although bed-bathing techniques differ, the aims remain the same. The person's dignity and privacy should be protected at all times. The person should be covered to prevent her from becoming cold. The person's own preferences should be sought. One important part of bed bathing is sometimes forgotten – the person being bed bathed. Bed bathing a person gives you the opportunity to get to know the person and to communicate with her. Often people confide their worries and fears during a bed bath. A resident may tell you that her arthritis seems to be getting worse and that the painkillers do not seem to be doing so much good these days.

Another might confide that the new tablets make her feel sick. It is important that you share such information with senior staff. The doctor may be able to change the painkillers or increase the dose so that the person is no longer in pain. The person whose tablets are making her feel sick may be able to have a different type of tablet.

Skin care

Skin is a waterproof protective covering. It is sensitive to heat, cold, touch and pressure. Skin is elastic and stretches, and it grows and contracts as a person becomes fatter or thinner. Healthy skin protects the body against infection. As people age, their skin becomes less elastic and tends to wrinkle. The skin becomes drier and thinner and can be more easily damaged than the skin of younger people. Certain medicines, such as steroids and anti-inflammatory drugs given to treat arthritis, affect the skin. These medicines can cause the skin to be very easily damaged.

When the skin is damaged, it is no longer able to prevent infection. Dry skin can become damaged more easily than healthy skin. Many older people suffer from very dry skin, and it is usually worst on the legs and arms. Older people's skin is often more sensitive than younger people's. You should advise older people with sensitive and dry skin to avoid using heavily perfumed soaps and bubble baths. Special moisturising bubble baths and soaps can now be bought in most supermarkets and chemists.

Caring for dry skin

People who have dry skin may have found their own solutions. Some people have their own favourite moisturisers that they have been using for years. Sometimes the older person is no longer able to bend down and apply moisturiser to the legs or another part of the body. You should offer to do this if the older person can no longer manage.

Sometimes the skin is so dry that normal moisturisers and oils are not effective. In this case, seek professional advice. The person's doctor may prescribe special moisturising creams. These should normally be applied after a bath. Some creams are more effective if applied to damp skin. Registered nurses will be able to offer advice and show you how to apply these moisturising creams. People who require specially prescribed creams should have this noted in their care plan in nursing homes. A record should also be kept in residential homes. Care assistants who are applying these creams will soon see if the prescribed cream is effective. You should inform professional staff and colleagues about the condition of the person's skin. If the skin is not improving the doctor will visit again and may prescribe a different cream. In very severe cases, the person's doctor may ask a skin specialist or dermatologist to see the person.

Mouth care

Mouth care is an area of caring that is often forgotten, carried out poorly or thought to be of little importance. Mouth care, though, is very important. The person who has a toothache, sore gums because dentures are rubbing or a sore tongue because a broken tooth is catching on it may not wish to eat or drink. Without sufficient food and fluids, the person will become weaker and less able to fight off illness. A sore mouth can make a person feel miserable and depressed. It has been said that the best way of judging the quality of care is to check the mouths of residents.

Caring for natural teeth

Many older people living in homes no longer have any natural teeth. Some older people, though, have some or all of their own teeth. People admitted to nursing homes will have a nursing history taken before they are admitted. This will have information about the person's teeth, dentures or partial dentures written on it. In residential homes, you may have to enquire.

People who have their own teeth should care for them normally. The teeth should be brushed morning and evening; some forgetful residents may need reminding. People who are unable to walk to the wash basin will require a tooth mug with water, a dish to rinse their mouths into, and their toothbrush and toothpaste. Some older people are unable to brush their teeth and you may have to do it for them.

People who have their natural teeth should continue to have six-monthly dental check-ups and may require dental treatment such as fillings and crowns. Dental check-ups can be carried out either at the dental surgery or at the home. Dentists who provide dental care to the home may be either dentists who practise locally or part of the community dental service. Find out what the dental arrangements are in your home.

As people age, their teeth are more at risk of breaking or cracking. People who have their own teeth should be advised not to eat hard sweets such as boiled sweets and sugared almonds, as crunching on these can cause teeth to break. Toffees and eclairs can sometimes cause loose fillings to come out.

Reflect on practice

Try practising by brushing a colleague's teeth. You can then swap roles and discuss it when you have finished. Some of the mistakes that people make when brushing other people's teeth are rubbing too hard (especially on sensitive gums) and failing to brush the area where the gum meets the tooth. Discuss with your colleague what it feels like to have your teeth brushed, so you can improve your technique.

Caring for dentures

Caring for dentures is as important as caring for natural teeth. Food debris will build up under dentures that are not cleaned. This can cause gums to become sore and inflamed. Some older people do not remove dentures but clean them while they are in the mouth. It is not possible to clean the inner part of the dentures or the top palate without removing them. Individuals should be advised to remove dentures so that they can be cleaned properly.

Dentures should be cleaned with a soft toothbrush and toothpaste to remove debris, then soaked overnight. Recent research has found that dentures can become heavily contaminated with bacteria. These bacteria can cause sore mouths, gums and throats. Using denture-cleaning tablets after thorough cleaning destroys these harmful bacteria. The denture pot is filled with warm water and the denture-cleaning tablet is added. Denture-cleaning tablets contain a mild bleach and this removes stains such as coffee and tea. It can be difficult to remove such stains by brushing. Badly stained dentures or dentures with a visible build-up of tartar can be professionally cleaned by the dentist.

If an older person who wears dentures complains of sore gums, professional advice should be sought. The denture may have become ill fitting and is rubbing. The dentist can treat this and adjust, alter or make new dentures if required.

Mouth care for the frail older person

People who are very ill or frail may depend on staff to clean their mouths. Many older people who are unwell are unable to tolerate their dentures. The person who feels sick may feel more comfortable without their dentures. Other people prefer to continue to wear their dentures. Denture care is as given above.

The frail person should be offered mouthwashes. There are many different types available. Dentists now recommend that plain water is offered as a mouthwash. Mouthwashes, research has discovered, can kill off bacteria in the mouth that keep the mouth healthy. Using mouthwashes can cause sore mouths and some individuals can develop oral thrush if they are used. Normally, unless a mouthwash has been especially prescribed by the person's doctor or dentist, the mouth is only rinsed with plain water.

Some people are so ill and frail that they are unable to rinse their mouths with water. Some homes have mouth care trays, which have special swabs to clean out the mouth. These are sticks with a piece of pink foam on top. The foam is dipped into water and then inserted into the person's mouth. Some homes no longer use these. There have been cases where the foam has come off the stick or has been bitten off. The foam has been inhaled in a few cases and emergency hospital treatment required to remove the foam from the lung. In some homes pre-moistened swabs that resemble giant cotton buds are available. There have been no reports of problems with their use.

The aim of mouth care is to remove food debris and traces of milky fluids from the mouth. Dentists now recommend that gauze moistened in water is wrapped around a gloved finger and used to gently clean the mouth. The inside of the mouth can be wiped with glycerine after cleaning. This keeps the mouth moist and prevents soreness. Lips can become dry, sore and cracked when people are very ill. Petroleum jelly or lip salve prevents this and keeps the individual feeling comfortable.

Nail care

Many older people have difficulty in caring for their nails. People who suffer from arthritis can find it difficult to use scissors or nail clippers because their hands can no longer manage fine movements. People with poor eyesight cannot see well enough to cut or file their nails. People suffering from Parkinson's disease often suffer from fine tremors that make nail care difficult. People who have suffered from strokes and can only use one hand find it impossible to care for their nails. One survey of fit and healthy people over the age of 85 found that few people of this age could manage to bend down and cut their own toenails.

Uncared-for fingernails can become dirty and torn and people with nails like this look uncared for and dishevelled. Many people prefer to have their nails cut with nail scissors or clippers and kept short. Some women though prefer to keep their nails longer and have them filed, manicured and painted with nail varnish. You should ask individuals how they prefer to have their fingernails (Case Study 10.2) and should not assume that all older women like short nails.

Toenails

Many older people are unable to cut their own toenails and many are admitted to homes with nails that have become so long they are curling over and cutting into the toes. Some older people have toenails that are very thick and difficult to cut. Toenails become thicker when circulation to the feet is poor. It is almost impossible to cut thickened toenails with ordinary nail scissors. Older people who do not have thickened toenails can have their toenails cut with ordinary nail scissors. You should check what the policy is for cutting the nails of people who have thickened toenails. In some homes, these nails are cut by registered nurses. The home should have strong nail scissors, clippers and files so that these nails can be cut. In other homes, registered nurses do not cut nails but arrange for the chiropodist to call and do it.

> **Case Study 10.2**
>
> Grace Adams felt depressed when she had to give up her home and enter a nursing home. Her key worker noticed that her nails were long and dirty and offered to attend to them. Grace explained that she had always been proud of her hands and nails and had kept her nails long, manicured and painted red all of her adult life. Having attractive hands and nails made her feel feminine and attractive. One of the things that had upset her most was that she was unable to care for her hands and paint her nails after having a stroke.
>
> Her key worker, June Adair, soaked her hands in a bowl of water, scrubbed the dirt from beneath her nails, and pushed back the ragged cuticles surrounding the nails with a Cutipen. She applied hand cream to the hands, painted Grace's nails with two coats of nail varnish, and applied a top coat of varnish. Grace felt like an attractive woman again and not a 'dishevelled old dear with dirty nails'. Caring for the person's nails can have an important effect on morale. You get a great sense of satisfaction from making a person feel better.

Podiatrists

Chiropodists are increasingly known as podiatrists. Many podiatrists work with foot care assistants and will often arrange for a foot care assistant to come to the home and cut nails. Chiropodists will call and treat residents who have foot problems such as ingrowing toenails, corns and bunions. The chiropodist who visits the home may be either a private chiropodist or one employed by the local NHS primary care trust. Private chiropodists charge either by the session (usually three quarters of an hour) or charge for each resident seen. If your home uses a private chiropodist, find out how much each treatment costs. In most homes individuals pay these charges as they are seldom included in home fees except in the most expensive of private homes. There is no charge for NHS chiropody but some areas do not have enough chiropody staff and it can be difficult to arrange regular visits.

Hair care

As people age, the hair loses the pigment that gives us our hair colour. Hair becomes grey or white. White hair is coarser in texture and drier. Hair thins with age. Men may lose all their hair and become bald. The scalp becomes drier and more sensitive with age. Older people very rarely have greasy hair and usually a shampoo once or twice each week will keep the hair clean. Washing the hair daily will make dry hair and a dry scalp even drier. Older people should be encouraged or helped to wash their hair once or twice a week. If the hair is dry, a mild shampoo for dry hair should be used.

Many older women have their hair permed regularly. Perming makes the hair dry. Residents who have perms should use a conditioner after shampooing, to prevent the hair becoming dry and brittle and make it easier to comb and style. Some people prefer to use a shampoo and conditioner in one. If this is used then one specially for dry hair should be chosen.

If a person is unwell and unable to have a shampoo, a dry shampoo can be used to freshen up the hair. Dry shampoos can be purchased in chemists and are powders that are puffed onto the hair through an applicator and then brushed out. They remove dirt and debris from the hair but do not tire a person out when she is feeling unwell. Dry shampoos are not intended to be used long term. They can be useful if someone is feeling under the weather, perhaps because of a chest infection or an illness.

Some older people develop dry, flaking and itching scalps; in extreme cases, sores can form on the scalp and these can bleed. If an individual develops a dry, flaking, itchy scalp, professional advice should be sought. The person's doctor will normally prescribe a shampoo containing coal tar (to prevent the flaking and treat the itching) and coconut oil (to treat the dryness). The hair is normally shampooed daily and the shampoo left on for 10–15 minutes; as the condition improves the hair is washed less frequently, until it is washed once or twice each week. These shampoos can dry the hair terribly and a rich conditioner should be applied after use. Perming lotions, tints and setting lotions should not be used until the doctor has agreed that the scalp is normal. The hairdresser should be informed about any problems with a person's scalp and will test each lotion on the individual's forearm to make sure that the person is not allergic to it, before using it on the person's hair.

Hairdressing

For many women a trip to the hairdressers is a treat. Women feel good when their hair looks good. Having a hairdo is important to many older women. Most homes have a hairdresser who visits once or twice a week and washes, cuts, perms, shampoos and sets hair for female residents. Male residents have their hair cut. It is important to realise that women do not stop caring about their appearance as they age. You can help residents keep their hair looking nice between styles. Some people have fine hair and find that wearing a hairnet helps keep a set looking good for longer. You can help the individual put on her hairnet before going to sleep if she can no longer manage this. When you are helping the individual to wash and dress remember to help comb and style their hair if the person has difficulty.

Shaving

Men, especially older men, often feel dirty and scruffy if they are unshaven. Many male residents have difficulty shaving. A stroke can cause an older person to lose the use of one hand. Parkinson's disease can cause tremor. Poor eyesight can make it difficult to see well enough to shave.

Wet shaves

Many older men prefer to use a shaving stick and brush to make shaving foam. This is applied to the bristles to soften the hair. Shaving foam may contain perfume and people with sensitive skin can react to this and suffer from red and itchy skin. It is now possible to buy shaving sticks, foam and gel for sensitive skin. A razor is then used to remove hair.

Using a foam and a razor gives a closer shave than using an electric razor, and many older men prefer a wet shave. Many care assistants fear cutting the person's skin and encourage the individual (or his relatives) to buy an electric razor. Wet shaving is not difficult (half of the adult population do it daily). It is a skill that is easily learnt. If a male resident prefers to have a wet shave, respect the individual's wishes. Senior staff can help and advise you in learning how to shave a male resident.

Electric razors

Many male residents, including those who have a tremor or can only use one hand, find it possible to shave using an electric razor. Electric razors can help an older person retain his independence. Each male resident should have his own razor. You should not 'borrow' another resident's electric razor for someone whose own shaver is broken. Electric razors can cause very small cuts on the skin. If two people share a razor, there is a risk of both developing a skin infection.

After-shave

Many men like to use after-shave, but it contains perfume, alcohol and colourings and these can inflame the skin of some people. Special after-shave made for people with sensitive skin can be used if ordinary after-shave irritates the skin.

Cosmetics

Some women living in nursing homes have been wearing cosmetics all their adult lives and feel naked without 'a touch of powder, rouge and lipstick'. Others prefer 'not to paint my face'. You should respect the individual's wishes. Some people find it difficult to apply make-up because of failing eyesight. Using a magnifying mirror can make it easier for the person to see more clearly. Some people may require help in putting on make-up, especially lipstick which can be difficult to apply if hands are not steady. People with sensitive skins can buy hypo-allergenic make-up that is less likely to cause allergies and skin reactions.

Key points

- Ageing affects bladder function.
- It is more difficult for older people to maintain continence than younger people.
- Your help is often essential to enable the older person to remain continent.
- Ageing affects the skin.
- Older people may have skin that is dry and more sensitive.
- Older people may have difficulty bathing, showering or washing independently.
- You should offer appropriate assistance.
- Grooming is important to older people.
- Helping the older person to maintain personal hygiene and to look their best improves morale and well-being.
- Care assistants can make very valuable contributions to the older person's well-being by offering appropriate support and assistance.

Portfolio preparation

Your assessor must have evidence that you can meet the performance criteria for this unit. Before beginning this unit, discuss assessment strategies with your assessor. Most of the evidence for this unit can be gained by direct observation of your work. You may be asked to provide the following types of evidence:

Products: This might be a copy of a care plan you completed showing how you met an individual's personal care needs. It could be a note in a resident's notes giving details of how you provided individualised care. It could be details of a person's life preferences and needs for assistance with personal care.

Witness testimony: This is a statement from a senior member of staff. It might be a statement detailing how you have met certain performance criteria.

Written work: You might be asked to prepare a piece of work about how ageing affects the ability to remain continent or to meet personal care needs.

Your assessor may also use other methods to help you gain evidence for this unit. These may include:

- Verbal questioning
- Written questions
- **Simulations** to demonstrate that you have the skills to work effectively in situations when a resident is reluctant to accept care.

Notes

1. Coloplast (2000) *An Introduction to Stoma Care*. Coloplast.
2. Coloplast (2000) *An Introduction to Stoma Care*. Coloplast.
3. Drossman DA (1999) The functional gastrointestinal disorders and the Rome II process. *Gut* **45** (Suppl 2: II1–II5.
4. Lewis SJ & Heaton KW (1997) Stool form scale as a useful guide to intestinal transit time. *Scandinavian Journal of Gastroenterology* **32**: 920–924.
5. Counsel and Care (1993) *The Right to Take Risks*. Counsel and Care, London.

Further reading

Jenkins J (1992) *The Clothes in Question*. Scutari Press, Harrow, UK. This book gives advice and information on choosing, adapting and caring for people's clothes when they are living in homes.

Disabled Living Foundation (1994) *All Dressed Up*. Disabled Living Foundation, London. This book is full of practical advice and tips on choosing and adapting clothes. It also provides elderly people with advice on how to dress. There is a section on how to dress people who are unable to dress themselves.

Chapter Eleven
Continence
HSC219
Support individuals to manage continence

This unit consists of two elements:
HSC219a Support individuals to maintain continence
HSC219b Support individuals to use equipment to manage continence

Please note that this unit cannot be used in combination with HSC218: *Support individuals with their personal care needs.*

In my view it is a shame that units HSC218 and 219 cannot be combined because although there are overlaps there are also key differences. I have interpreted the key elements of these units to be about continence promotion and the management of incontinence. The first part of this chapter will explain why older people may develop continence problems and how these can be treated. The second part will deal with the management of incontinence. Please see Chapter 10 for information about how ageing and illness can make it more difficult to remain continent and for information about body waste.

This chapter

- Explains why older people develop continence problems
- Explains the different types of continence problems
- Provides information on investigation and treatment
- Explains when it is appropriate to manage incontinence
- Provides information about pads and aids used to manage incontinence
- Informs you of the advantages and disadvantages of each method
- Provides information to enable you to recognise problems

Continence problems

Incontinence is the inability to control bladder or bowels. Urinary incontinence, the inability to control the bladder, is much more common. Most people feel that such a problem is shameful and are very embarrassed and upset by it. They fear that others may feel that they are dirty or lazy. Some older people who have problems controlling their bladders go to great lengths to conceal it. The older person living in a home may ask her family to bring in sanitary towels. She may use serviettes or toilet paper to line her pants. If her pants become wet she may wash them out and try to dry them on the radiator to prevent staff finding out.

General measures to promote continence

Ageing and difficulties with communicating or using the toilet independently can increase a person's risk of developing continence problems. General measures that take account of the difficulties older people have can often enable the older person to remain continent or to regain continence (see Table 11.1).

If these general measures are ineffective the person should have a continence assessment.

Table 11.1 General measures to improve continence.

Change and consequences	Action
Increased amount of urine produced	Be aware that older person needs to use toilet more often
Reduced ability to concentrate urine, increased risk of dehydration	Provide extra fluids in hot weather, to reduce risk of dehydration
Reduced ability to concentrate urine at night	Be aware that it is normal to get up to the toilet twice in an eight-hour night at the age of 85, and provide appropriate support
Bladder becomes stiff and less stretchy; bladder capacity is reduced	Recognise that older people need to pass smaller amounts of urine more often
Residual urine increases; working capacity of the bladder is reduced	Recognise that older people may need to go more frequently
Residual urine increases; the reservoir of stale urine provides breeding ground for bacteria; risk of infection increases	Encourage fluids. Reinforce good hygiene, such as wiping top to bottom. Ensure infection treated. Recommend cranberry juice 200 ml twice a day if recurring infection a problem
Bladder less sensitive; there is less warning of the need to urinate	Respond promptly to requests for the toilet

Continence assessments

Incontinence is not a disease, it is a symptom, and like any other symptom should be investigated to find out the reasons why it has developed. When we know the reasons for incontinence developing we can begin to treat the problem. Every person who has a continence problem should be seen and investigated. There are four different levels of assessment (Table 11.2).

The aim of assessment is to find out why the person has bladder or bowel problems and to treat problems and restore continence whenever possible. If it is not possible to restore continence, the aim of care is to contain incontinence and to enable the person to maintain dignity at all times.

Table 11.2 Assessment of continence.

Level	Details
1	This consists of a few simple questions and aims to identify people who have continence problems. It can be carried out by people who do not have a healthcare background
2	This consists of taking a history, a simple physical examination and some investigations. This can be carried out by a Registered Nurse who has training in continence care. It aims to identify some of the causes of incontinence
3	This consists of taking a more detailed history, physical examination and more complex investigations. It can be carried out by a continence adviser (a Registered Nurse specially trained in continence care) or a doctor with specialist training
4	This consists of detailed history taking, physical examination and detailed tests and investigation. It may be carried out by a nurse consultant or more usually by a doctor with specialist training and qualifications

Normal bladder function

We are unaware of any sensation of bladder fullness until the bladder contains around 300 ml of urine. Then, we can postpone the need to void until it is convenient. The micturition centre in the brain informs us that our bladder is filling up and allows us to hold on until it's convenient to go. The bladder muscle relaxes and capacity is increased. The urethra remains tightly closed, preventing leakage. When it is convenient to urinate the urethra relaxes and the bladder muscle contracts to expel urine. Figure 11.1 illustrates this process.

Causes of incontinence

There are several types of urinary incontinence. These include:

- Overactive bladder
- Underactive bladder

Continence 263

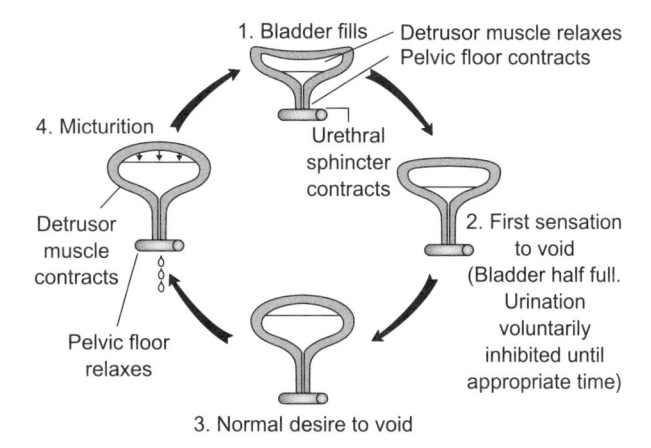

Figure 11.1 Normal urination.

- Stress incontinence
- Mixed incontinence
- Functional incontinence
- Transient incontinence.

Overactive bladder

Overactive bladder is common in women. Research indicates that 16–45% of adults have this problem and most of them are postmenopausal women. People suffering from urgency suffer from uncontrolled bladder contractions. The bladder contracts while it is filling up. This means that although the bladder might have a capacity of 500 ml, contractions might start to occur at 250 ml. The working capacity of the bladder is reduced and the person finds it difficult to hold on. This condition is also known as detrusor overactivity (DO). Figures 11.2 and 11.3 illustrate the overactive bladder.

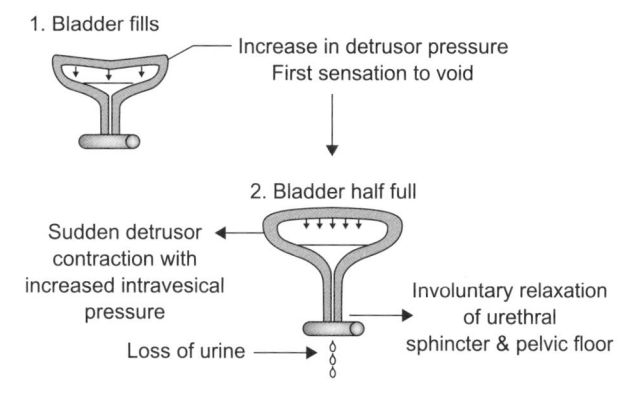

Figure 11.2 The overactive bladder.

OVERACTIVE BLADDER QUESTIONNAIRE
HOW BOTHERED HAVE YOU BEEN BY...

0 – NOT AT ALL 1 – A LITTLE BIT 2 – SOMEWHAT 3 – QUITE A BIT 4 – A GREAT DEAL 5 – A VERY GREAT DEAL

- Frequent urination during the day?
- Uncomfortable urge to urinate?
- Sudden urge to urinate with little or no warning?
- Accidental leakage of small amounts of urine?
- Night time urination?
- Waking up at night because of the need to urinate?
- Uncontrollable urge to urinate?
- Urine leakage associated with a strong desire to urinate?

ARE YOU MALE? If so, add 2 to your overall score

Total score

There are several symptoms that make up what doctors call Overactive Bladder (OAB). Think about each of the symptoms and give yourself a score out of 5 corresponding to how much you feel you are bothered by the symptom, with 0 meaning that you are not bothered at all and 5 meaning that you are bothered a great deal. Then add them up and place your total in the box at the bottom of the page.

If your score is 8 or greater, you may have OAB. Please give your completed questionnaire to your doctor, and he or she will advise you on your condition. There are effective medical treatments for the condition and the result may be that you will be prescribed some medicine that could help you.

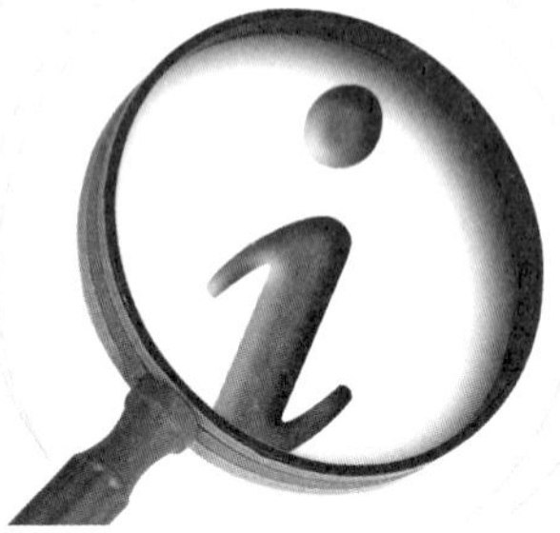

Figure 11.3 Overactive bladder questionnaire.

Certain conditions such as stroke and Parkinson's disease affect the brain and can cause the bladder to become overactive. We do not know why people develop overactive bladders. It is well known, though, that worry and nerves can make the bladder more likely to develop urgency. Some people find that when they are anxious they develop a headache or diarrhoea, while others find that they keep needing to go to the toilet. If the older person is worried about wetting herself, this makes the situation worse. Box 11.1 gives the clinical features of overactive bladder.

> **Box 11.1**   Features of overactive bladder
>
> - Frequency – passing urine often
> - Passing small amounts of urine
> - Urgency – having to rush to use the toilet
> - Urge incontinence
> - Nocturnal enuresis

How can overactive bladder be treated?

There are three ways to treat the person with an overactive bladder. These are to treat the factors that are making the urgency worse, to enable the person to respond to the demands of the bladder, and to treat overactive bladder.

Treating contributory factors

If the person is **constipated**, a large mass of hard faeces can press on the bladder. This makes the bladder even more irritable and makes the problem worse. Treating constipation helps resolve the problem.

Infection makes the irritable bladder more irritable. Treating the infection can often restore continence. It is important to be aware that many older people have bacteria in their bladder and this does not mean that the person has an infection. Infection should be diagnosed on the basis of clinical symptoms (see Box 11.2). If the person suffers repeated infections, investigations are required to determine the cause of infection.

Reinforcing good hygiene and ensuring that the person has a good fluid intake prevents recurrence. If recurrent infection is a problem, offer cranberry juice 200 ml twice a day.

Medication can make urgency worse. If you think that urgency is worsening, inform a senior member of staff.

Treatment of overactive bladder

There are two methods of treating urgency: bladder retraining and medication.

> **Box 11.2** Clinical features of urinary tract infection
>
> - Unusually frequent urination
> - An intense urge to urinate
> - Dysuria – pain, discomfort or a burning sensation during urination
> - Pain, pressure or tenderness in the area of the bladder (midline, above or near the pubic area)
> - Urine that looks cloudy, or smells foul or unusually strong
> - Fever, with or without chills
> - Nausea and vomiting
> - Pain in the side or mid to upper back
> - Nocturia – awakening from sleep to pass urine
> - Onset of enuresis (bedwetting) in a person who has usually been dry at night

Bladder retraining

People who suffer from urgency often get into the habit of using the toilet very frequently to avoid accidents. Over time the bladder becomes smaller and smaller and the problem worsens. Bladder retraining aims to enable the person to take control of the bladder. Bladder retraining aims to teach the patient to 'hold on' for longer periods and gradually increase the time between voiding *without incontinence occurring*.

If the person holds on then bladder capacity increases and the person learns how to dampen down bladder contractions. Bladder capacity becomes larger and the person spends less time thinking about the toilet. As the individual becomes less anxious and begins to enjoy life, bladder control improves. It's important to start slowly; ask the person to hold on for five minutes at first and then build up the time between using the toilet. Give the person something to do or something else to think about.

Medication

If bladder retraining is unsuccessful or only partially successful, drug therapy can be considered. These drugs dampen down bladder contractions and allow the bladder to hold more urine.

Underactive bladder

Underactive (hypotonic) bladder is a common condition in older men and people who have diabetes, have had a stroke or who have Parkinson's disease. An underactive bladder fails to contract and empty properly. The individual may leak small amounts of urine on movement. This condition can easily be confused with stress incontinence. There are several reasons why the bladder fails to empty properly.

Normally the bladder stretches in all directions. When the bladder is reaching normal capacity, the stretch receptors send a signal to the brain that the bladder is becoming full. We can then delay urination for a while. When the bladder becomes underactive, this signalling mechanism fails to work and the bladder becomes overstretched, big and floppy. A hypotonic bladder can hold between 500 ml and 2 litres. The causes of hypotonic bladder include:

- Severe constipation with faeces loaded in the lower bowel.
- An enlarged prostate gland that prevents the bladder emptying fully.
- Brain damage after stroke or head injury.
- Spinal cord damage. This can be caused by injury or diseases such as cancer and osteoporosis.
- Diabetes if poorly controlled can lead to nerve damage including damage to the bladder nerves.
- Multiple sclerosis and Parkinson's disease can lead to bladder emptying problems.

Treatment of underactive bladder

Sometimes it's easy to treat the underactive bladder. If the person is very constipated faeces can press on the urethra, making it difficult for the person to empty the bladder fully. Treating constipation (usually with suppositories or enemas) resolves the problem. Sometimes the person will use an intermittent catheter. This may be used once or twice a day or more frequently to drain the bladder. Sometimes a permanent catheter is required.

Stress incontinence

Stress incontinence is common in women and rare in men. This is because men have two valves to hold urine in the bladder and women only have one. This valve is called the urethral sphincter. The urethra may become less effective in women after menopause due to a shortage of the hormone oestrogen. The bladder is supported by muscles known as the pelvic floor. These muscles can become weakened after childbirth and with ageing. When the muscles are weak they support the bladder less effectively and the bladder leaks when the individual coughs, sneezes or walks around.

Treatment of stress incontinence

Treatment will vary according to the cause. Weak muscles may be treated with pelvic floor exercises. If the muscles are very weak, surgery to repair the muscles and lift them back in place may be carried out. Many older women who have other health problems are not well enough to have surgery. A special ring (known as a ring pessary) may be inserted by a doctor or nurse specialist to hold up the womb if it is dropping down and pressing on the bladder. Sometimes these rings are coated with the female hormone oestrogen, as this can help treat stress incontinence. These are usually changed by a doctor or nurse specialist every year. Sometimes a cream containing oestrogen is prescribed. This is applied to the genital region and helps treat women who suffer from stress incontinence.

Mixed incontinence

Mixed incontinence is a combination of stress and urge incontinence. Usually the person is treated for both stress incontinence and overactive bladder.

Functional incontinence

Functional incontinence is incontinence that occurs in people with normal bladder function. It is common in people with advanced dementia and head injury. People who suffer from functional incontinence are often unaware that they have passed urine or that they are wet.

Managing functional incontinence

People who have functional incontinence are not able to interpret bladder signals or respond appropriately to a full bladder. People with functional incontinence are the most disabled of care home residents. It is not possible to treat functional incontinence but, with careful management, you can keep some people with functional incontinence dry.

Use a chart to identify the times that the person is wet. If you keep the chart for four days you can, with luck, identify a pattern. Take the person to the toilet before the incontinence occurs and you will be able to keep the person dry. Keeping the person dry is totally dependent on staff taking the person to the toilet. If you forget, the person will be incontinent. In my experience around two thirds of people with functional incontinence will display a pattern and can be kept dry if you use an *individual* toileting pattern. Routine two-hourly toileting will not work. You may find that the person uses the toilet twice in two hours in the morning and three-hourly in the afternoon. Only an individual schedule will enable you to keep the person dry.

A third of people with functional incontinence do not display a pattern and you need to work out other ways to manage the incontinence.

Other factors causing incontinence

Many problems that cause incontinence are not bladder problems. Often the older person has been managing to control his or her bladder until a change in circumstances tips the individual over the edge into incontinence. Many things can cause incontinence, including the attitude of staff. The commonest reasons older people develop continence problems are given below.

Moving to a new place

Often when the older person is to be admitted to the home, staff ask if the person has a continence problem. The answer is often no, yet when the person arrives at the home she is incontinent. Leaving his or her own home where a person has lived for many years and entering a residential or nursing home is a stressful experience. The older person is usually admitted from hospital and may dread entering the home. She may have been transferred from an acute ward to an elderly care ward and then finally to the home. This makes older people anxious and worried. Stress and worry can affect the bladder and cause incontinence. Helping the person settle into the home, making her feel welcome and providing sensitive care can help clear up the incontinence quickly.

Medicines

Medicines can cause incontinence. They can act in a number of ways, either working directly on the bladder or affecting the person's general health.

Diuretics are often referred to as water tablets. Diuretics stimulate the kidneys and increase the amount of urine produced. Diuretics are given to treat heart failure, to lower blood pressure or to treat swollen legs. There are many different types of diuretics. Some act slowly and gently, causing a little more urine to be produced throughout the day. Others have a more drastic action and cause the kidneys to produce large amounts of urine for a few hours. Diuretics are usually given in the morning. This can cause problems if the older person requires help to go to the toilet as staff are busiest in the morning, and a delay in responding to the person's request for help can lead to incontinence.

In some homes, older people have sleeping tablets every night. Sleeping tablets cause people to be less alert and drowsier, not just at night but also during the day. They can lead to incontinence. Some older people are anxious and upset when they enter homes. Some are prescribed sedatives and these can cause the person to become less alert and to become incontinent. Other medicines can also cause incontinence.

A continence assessment by a trained professional will include checking the person's medication. If medication is causing incontinence this may be discontinued or changed by the prescriber.

Difficulty with walking

The older person who is unable to use the toilet without help is more likely to suffer from incontinence. Chapter 10 gives details of how you can help older people regain independence. Chapter 8 gives information on helping the older person to move. It is important to respond promptly to calls for help to use the toilet.

Confusion

The person who is confused or forgetful may have problems remembering to go to the toilet. Reminding the person to go to the toilet at set times often helps to prevent incontinence.

How you can help

Don't take incontinence for granted. If an older person is developing bladder problems, seek professional advice. A continence assessment will usually be carried out to find out why the person has become incontinent. You may be asked to help by keeping a fluid balance chart or a frequency volume chart. This involves keeping a record of everything a person drinks and all urine passed. The fluid chart is normally recorded for three to seven days. The registered nurse or continence adviser may ask for a bladder chart to be used. An example is shown in Fig. 11.4. This chart is used to work out what type of continence problem a person has and to monitor the person's progress and to help decide on further treatment. This will vary from person to person and will depend on the nature of the problem.

It's important that you record and report the continence status of the people you are caring for. Senior staff who have less contact with residents depend on you to inform and advise them about residents' well-being.

Caring for people who are incontinent

Some older people are able to remain continent until the end of life. Some older people develop continence problems because of the effects of illness. Older people who are unwell or suffer from the end stage of many diseases often develop continence problems. Sometimes continence promotion strategies are inappropriate or unlikely to be successful. In such circumstances the aims of care are to contain incontinence, to avoid the complications of poorly managed incontinence and to enable the person to maintain dignity.

Choosing the right method to contain incontinence

Continence assessment is important because it enables staff to find out what the person's problems are and to choose a suitable method to contain

Continence 271

BLADDER RECORD CHART –
FREQUENCY AND VOLUME

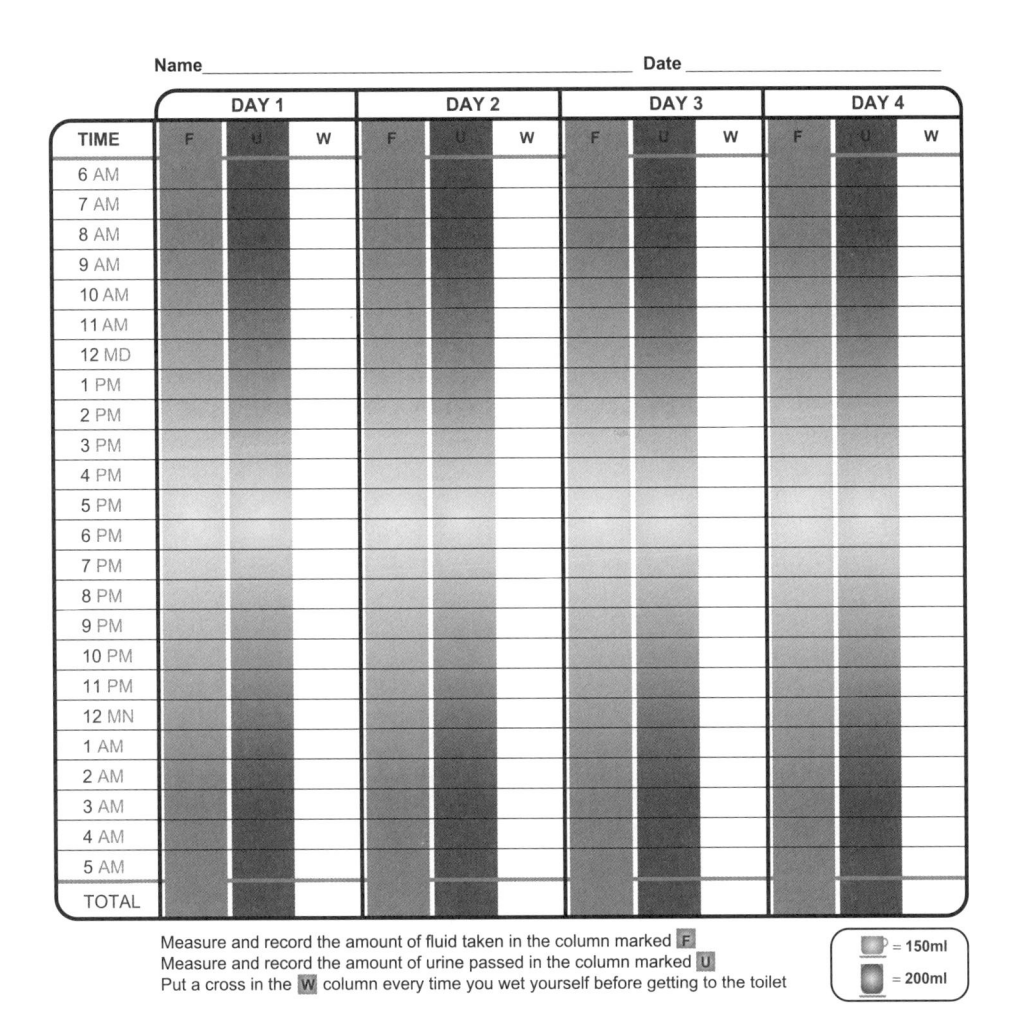

Name_____   Date_____

TIME	DAY 1 F	DAY 1 U	DAY 1 W	DAY 2 F	DAY 2 U	DAY 2 W	DAY 3 F	DAY 3 U	DAY 3 W	DAY 4 F	DAY 4 U	DAY 4 W
6 AM												
7 AM												
8 AM												
9 AM												
10 AM												
11 AM												
12 MD												
1 PM												
2 PM												
3 PM												
4 PM												
5 PM												
6 PM												
7 PM												
8 PM												
9 PM												
10 PM												
11 PM												
12 MN												
1 AM												
2 AM												
3 AM												
4 AM												
5 AM												
TOTAL												

Measure and record the amount of fluid taken in the column marked F
Measure and record the amount of urine passed in the column marked U
Put a cross in the W column every time you wet yourself before getting to the toilet

= 150ml
= 200ml

Figure 11.4 Bladder record chart.

incontinence. Every collection device has advantages and disadvantages. It is important to choose the right collection device for the right person. Registered nurses will normally choose the appropriate collection device but your feedback on how effective a product is and how acceptable it is to the older person is valuable.

There are three main methods of containing urinary incontinence. These are:

1. Incontinence pads
2. Urinary sheaths (for men)
3. Urinary catheters.

Incontinence pads

There are many different types of incontinence pads. There are disposable pads, reusable pads and body-worn aids that incorporate an incontinence pad.

Disposable pads

These consist of:

- a plastic backing
- paper fluff pulp
- a one-way liner.

Good-quality pads contain absorbent powder or crystals. The absorbent material gels on contact with urine and 'locks' urine into the core of the pad, keeping the person's skin dry. Incontinence pads are used to collect urine. They normally have a plastic backing and are filled with cellulose pulp and granules that swell up and form a gel when wet. This gel locks the urine into the pad and helps keep the person's skin dry. Many pads have a liner that draws urine away from the skin.

Some pads have a wetness indicator in the plastic outer covering of the pad. The wetness indicator changes colour when the pad needs changing. If the person has been incontinent of faeces, the pad should be changed immediately to maintain comfort and prevent skin problems.

Pads work more effectively and are less likely to leak if they are fitted closely to the body. Most pad manufacturers recommend that the person wears a pair of specially designed briefs made of nylon to hold the pad in place.

Disposable pads come in a variety of absorbencies. There are mini-pads that are attached to pants with an adhesive strip. These hold 50–80 ml of urine and are suitable for people with stress incontinence. There are also pads suitable for normal and heavy volumes of urine produced during the day. There are also night pads that contain larger volumes of urine and

> **Box 11.3** Features of effective pads
>
> - Shaped pads are more effective in reducing leakage.
> - Pads with elasticated sections around the legs reduce leakage.
> - Pads fitted closely to the body, e.g. using net pants, reduces leakage.
> - Rapid absorption of liquid into core of pad reduces skin problems and leakage.
> - Adequate absorbent material in the central section of the pad reduces leakage.
> - Absorbent crystals or powder reduces leakage and skin problems.

allow the person to remain dry and to sleep undisturbed. Pads should reduce leakage and keep skin healthy. Box 11.3 outlines research findings on the features of effective pads.

The pads that you use may be supplied by the home or by the local primary care trust. No one pad is right for all people. If you find that a particular resident is developing skin problems or that the pads leak although they are changed at appropriate times, you must inform a senior member of staff. The person may require a different type of pad, different absorbencies or a different method of containing incontinence. The advantages of disposable pads are that there are no infection control risks, every pad is new and there are no laundry costs. The main disadvantages are that they take up a lot of space and are not environmentally friendly.

Reusable pads

Reusable pads are not commonly used in care homes but are used by some people in community and other care settings. Each person is provided with named pads. The pads are laundered at high temperatures and reused. They are not recommended for people who are doubly incontinent. The advantage of reusable pads is that they do not take up a great deal of space. The disadvantages are the time and cost of laundry, and higher infection risks.

Incontinence pads are suitable for people who have urge, stress, mixed, functional and transient incontinence. They are not an ideal method of containing incontinence in people who have overflow incontinence because they do not help the bladder to fully empty. If the person has a large pressure sore and their skin is inflamed and sore, another method may be more suitable until the skin has recovered.

Dribble pads

These are small pads which fit over the penis and collect small drips or dribbles. Their use can preserve dignity, protect clothing and prevent odour.

Disposing of incontinence pads

Used incontinence pads cannot be disposed of with normal household waste. Homes have a duty under the Environmental Protection Act 1990 to ensure that pads are disposed of properly. Homes use different systems to dispose of incontinence pads. Some homes use a macerator; the pads are placed in the macerator and are reduced to a pulp and washed away into the drain. Other homes use a yellow bag system. All body waste, which is to be taken away from the home and disposed of, should be collected in a yellow plastic bag. These bags are stored in special sack holders in the sluice room. The bags are collected either by the local council or by a private firm. Homes are charged for each sack of clinical waste removed. The waste is then incinerated at high temperature.

Body-worn aids

Incontinence pads can be bulky. The plastic backing can rustle and they can be sweaty and uncomfortable. An alternative is a normal type of underwear that incorporates a washable incontinence pad. The supplier companies make ladies underwear in lace, patterns and pastel colours in different styles and sizes. There is also a male range. The underwear has an absorbent pad sewn in. This underwear is available in a range of absorbencies from 50 ml to 250 ml. These pants are suitable for people with stress incontinence or minor urge incontinence. They are not suitable for people who are heavily incontinent or doubly incontinent.

Urinary sheaths and collection devices

Disposable urinary sheaths are rolled over the penis and held in place by adhesive. Urine drains from the sheath into a catheter leg bag. Sheaths are made of either latex or silicone. Latex sheaths are brown and silicone sheaths are transparent. Many older men suffer from retraction of the penis and the sheath is difficult to apply and may be difficult to keep in place. Some men may be allergic to the sheath or to the adhesive used to hold the sheath in place. One researcher found that 40% of men using urinary sheaths developed allergic reactions. People are more likely to be allergic to latex than silicone.

It is important to use the correct sheath width. If the sheath is not wide enough a ring of sheath material can compress the shaft of the penis. This can cause tissue damage and in extreme cases pressure sores.

It is important that the sheath is the correct length and is made of materials that do not twist too easily. Sheaths that are too long can easily twist at the tip of the penis and can prevent urine draining.

Wearing a urinary sheath increases the risk of developing a urinary tract infection. One study found that 87% of older men who wore urinary sheaths over a five-month period developed urine infections.

Urinary sheaths are most suitable for men who have mixed and functional incontinence. They are less suitable for men who are circumcised because urine comes into direct contact with the tip of the penis and may irritate this delicate skin. Men who are at high risk of developing infections may find incontinence pads more suitable. Sheaths are not suitable for men who have overflow incontinence. Box 11.4 outlines how to care for a person who uses a sheath.

> **Box 11.4** Caring for a person with a urinary sheath
>
> - Ensure that fluid intake is adequate – concentrated urine will cause skin damage.
> - Remove sheath at least once daily to wash the genital area with soap and water.
> - Ensure that foreskin is retracted and tip of penis is cleaned. This reduces the risks of infection, inflammation of the foreskin and stricture (narrowing) of the urethra.
> - Replace the sheath with a new one.
> - Report any problems such as skin irritation, blisters, redness or swelling to a senior member of staff.

Indwelling urinary catheters

Sometimes care assistants wonder why nurses use pads and sheaths to contain incontinence when they can use catheters. Catheters can at first sight appear to be the answer to all continence problems. This is seldom the case: catheters are not suitable for all patients and have costs as well as benefits.

Problems associated with catheter use

The major problems associated with catheter use are:

- leakage
- pain
- infection.

Let's examine the problems associated with urinary catheters, the reasons they occur and how we can minimise their occurrence.

Leakage

Sometimes catheters leak. If a catheter leaks, check that the catheter bag does not need emptying. If it full, empty the bag. The leakage may stop.

Check that the catheter is lower than the person's bladder. If the person is lying in bed the catheter bag should be suspended on a stand on the floor so that urine can drain out of the bladder. Check that the person has not rolled over and is lying on the catheter. This will block the catheter and cause leakage. Check that the catheter is not twisted and kinked. If the catheter continues to leak it is important that you inform a senior member of staff so that a registered nurse can find out why the catheter has leaked and deal with the problem.

Why do catheters leak?

When a person is catheterised the bladder becomes colonised with bacteria within ten days. These bacteria are often harmless but cause the urine to become cloudy and smelly. The bacteria release substances from urine that lead to crystals forming on the catheter. The catheter furs up in the same way that hard water furs a kettle. This process is known as encrustation. The encrustation can block the catheter and then urine is unable to escape from the bladder through the catheter so it leaks.

If a catheter becomes encrusted the registered nurse may use a bladder washout to dissolve the encrustation and flush the catheter. The nurse may remove the catheter and inspect it. The encrusted catheter will have fur on the tip and if you roll your gloved fingers around the tube you can feel gritty bits in the catheter. If you cut the catheter open you can see the encrustations. Bladder washouts are used less frequently than before. The nurse may choose to use a catheter made of a different material such as silicone to reduce the risk of encrustation. The nurse may also change the catheter more often to prevent blockage.

The nurse may ask you to encourage fluids. This aims to dilute the urine, as concentrated urine is more likely to cause blockage than dilute urine. You may be asked to ensure that the person drinks 200 ml of cranberry juice twice a day. Cranberry juice prevents bacteria sticking to the bladder wall and makes cloudy urine clear, reduces odour and reduces the risks of blockage.

Sometimes catheters leak because the body is trying to expel the catheter. The catheter is a foreign object that has been placed in the bladder. The catheter may irritate the bladder and cause bladder contractions. Urine leaks when this happens. Sometimes the bladder contractions are so strong that the catheter is forced out of the body.

If the person has a large catheter the nurse may change this for a smaller one. A smaller catheter may cause less irritation and prevent leakage. Sometimes the nurse may use a different type of catheter made from a different material to reduce irritation. Silicone catheters can be hard. Changing the catheter to a latex catheter coated with a slippery substance called hydrogel may reduce the irritation. If this is ineffective then the nurse prescriber or doctor may prescribe a drug such as oxybutinin to calm the bladder down and stop contractions.

Pain

Some people find that catheters are mildly uncomfortable; other people find that they are painful. The catheter may be painful because it is causing the bladder to contract. This can be treated by using a smaller catheter, a different type of catheter, using medication to reduce contractions or choosing a different method of containing incontinence.

The catheter may be painful because it is tugging and dragging on the delicate internal tissues. You can help reduce the risks of pain by ensuring that the person does not have an overfull leg bag dragging the catheter down. It is important that the home's routine includes checking and emptying leg bags at regular intervals. Some people will produce more urine than others and care plans and care provided should take individual variations into account.

The female urethra is approximately 5 cm long and the male 20 cm long. Female and male catheters designed to take account of these anatomical differences are more effective and comfortable. If a female resident has a long catheter in place this may kink, block and cause pain and discomfort. Very obese ladies may find that a short female catheter is uncomfortable and may require a male-length catheter.

The catheter may cause pain if it is blocked. If the catheter is blocked you should report this so that a registered nurse can deal with the problem.

Sometimes people who are constipated find that their catheter becomes uncomfortable. It may also leak. If a person has a bowel full of faeces this can press on the internal tissues and cause pain. If the constipation is treated the pain often resolves.

Infection

The person who has a catheter is more vulnerable to infection than a person who is not catheterised. The catheter provides an entry point for infection. Urine bags rapidly become colonised by bacteria. These bacteria form a film known as a biofilm that enables bacteria to enter the catheter and the bladder. Bladder infection is unavoidable if a person is catheterised. This infection is known as bactinuria and means that the bladder is full of bacteria. These bacteria are often harmless unless the person develops a systemic infection that causes the person to become unwell. If the person is unwell and has a high temperature this condition is known as bacteraemia and requires antibiotic treatment.

You can reduce the risks of the person with a catheter becoming unwell by offering cranberry juice 200 ml twice a day. This prevents bacteria sticking to the bladder wall. You can encourage the person to drink sufficient fluid. People who have catheters should drink 1500–2000 ml every 24 hours. You should change the leg bag twice weekly and if it becomes contaminated. Night drainage bags should be attached at night and discarded in the morning. They should not be reused under any circumstances. If a night drainage bag is used overnight, emptied and left it will grow bacteria in the warmth of the home. If you reattach the bag the bacteria will enter the bladder and can cause life-threatening infection. You should use gloves and wash your hands each time you empty a catheter bag.

Catheter hygiene

Antiseptics should not be used to clean a person's genitals or the catheter tubing. Antiseptics can lead to infection with organisms that are resistant to antibiotics. It is important to ensure that dependent male catheterised patients have the foreskin retracted and the glans cleaned at least daily. The person can bath and shower normally.

Catheters are best avoided in people who have transient incontinence as they lead to the bladder becoming smaller and lead to infections. This can make it more difficult for the person to regain continence.

Catheter bags

Urine drains from the catheter into a catheter bag. There are two different types of catheter bag, for night and day use. Night drainage bags are large bags. They are supported on stands which are suspended on the bed or sit on the floor beside the bed. Leg bags are worn during the day. These are strapped to the person's leg and hidden by either a skirt or trousers. It is important to support catheter bags by using either a stand or strapping them to the leg. Catheter bags fill with urine and can become very heavy. If the bag is not supported the weight of urine can pull the catheter and cause the neck of the bladder, where the balloon sits, to become bruised and swollen. This can cause pain and bleeding.

Emptying catheter bags

Catheter bags should be emptied every four hours. If the person is passing a lot of urine, you may need to empty the bag more frequently. The bag should be emptied before it is completely full to avoid pulling on the delicate tissues at the neck of the bladder. Hands are washed and disposable gloves put on. Urine should be drained into a jug which has been sterilised in the bedpan washer. The urine is then tipped down the bedpan washer and the jug resterilised. Gloves should be removed and hands washed.

How often should catheter bags be changed?

The Department of Health recommends that catheter bags are changed twice each week. It can be difficult for staff to keep track of when a catheter bag was last changed as one person may change the bag before going off duty for a few days. The person returning from days off may be unaware of this and may change the bag again. In some homes when a bag is changed the date of the change is written discreetly on the inner side of the bag with a marking pen, as well as recorded on the care plan.

Preventing skin problems in incontinence

Individuals who suffer from urinary incontinence are at risk of developing infection, macerated skin and even sores. The person's skin should be washed gently with soap and water when a pad is changed, when a person has been incontinent and at least once daily if the person has a catheter or sheath. If the skin looks red or sore, report this and seek advice. Many staff use barrier creams to prevent a person's skin becoming sore. Barrier creams can protect the skin but should be used with care. If you apply cream too thickly and a person is wearing a pad the cream can clog up the pad and lead to leakage. Some people are allergic to the ingredients in some creams. If a person's skin is not improving seek advice.

Bowel function

You'll find information on normal bowel function in Chapter 10.

Diarrhoea

Diarrhoea is the frequent passage of loose or liquid stools. The commonest causes of diarrhoea are laxatives, antibiotics, food poisoning and a rectum loaded with stool.

Antibiotics

Antibiotics given to treat an infection can often cause diarrhoea. The most effective way of preventing infection and reducing antibiotic use is careful handwashing.

Food poisoning

Food poisoning can cause diarrhoea. Staff who do not carefully wash their hands after attending to each resident, and do not maintain resident hygiene and carefully dispose of body fluids according to the home's policy, can contribute to an outbreak of diarrhoea within the home.

Constipation

Constipation can also lead to diarrhoea. Hard, dried faeces build up in the rectum and cannot be passed. Further faeces gather behind this and can leak around the blockage. Although it appears that the person has diarrhoea, severe constipation is the real problem.

Caring for the person with diarrhoea

If the older person develops diarrhoea, seek professional advice. Treatment will depend on the cause of the diarrhoea. The older person may no longer require laxatives if they are causing the problem. It may be possible for the doctor to change the antibiotic the person is taking if this is causing the diarrhoea. The person with food poisoning may require treatment if the diarrhoea is severe. The person with severe constipation will require treatment to clear the bowel. It is important to encourage people with diarrhoea to drink plenty of fluids as extra fluid is being lost through the faeces and this must be replaced. The person who has diarrhoea may need assistance to get to the toilet in time. In some cases, a commode by the bed will be required. The person's privacy and dignity should be maintained at all times and air fresheners should be used to ensure the room does not smell, as this could embarrass the individual.

Soiled linen

Every home should have a policy for dealing with soiled linen. Normally it is placed in red plastic bags with an alginate strip. This is taken to the laundry where it is laundered separately from all other linen. The bag is normally placed in the washing machine and placed on sluice cycle. The alginate strip then dissolves and the bag opens. The laundry is rinsed and the bag is then disposed of. The linen is then washed normally.

Stoma care

A stoma is a piece of bowel that has been brought to the surface of the abdomen. The stoma normally looks pink or red. The stoma takes the place of the anus and faeces pass through the stoma. The person with a stoma has no control over when the faeces will come out and must wear a bag to collect faeces (Fig. 11.5). The stoma is made from the large bowel. The large bowel absorbs water so the stool of a person with a colostomy will resemble a normal stool. The person with a colostomy uses a closed bag. When the person has passed a stool the bag is removed and replaced with a new bag.

A person who has a stoma formed from the small intestine (known as an ileostomy) will pass a liquid stool. The amount of stool will be greater and people who have ileostomies will need to drink extra fluid because of this. People who have ileostomies normally wear a drainage bag and the stool is drained into a jug.

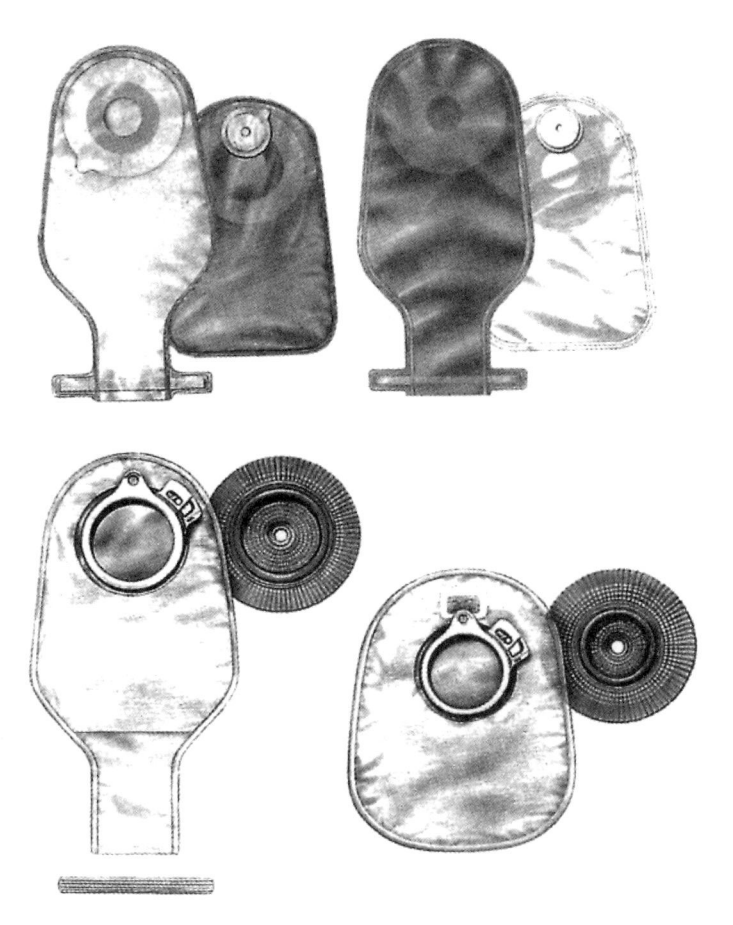

Figure 11.5 A selection of stoma bags.

Disposing of body waste

If the older person has a stoma, there are normally two different methods of disposing of the body waste. All stoma bags come with a small bag with two handles. The bag is designed to hold the stoma bag and then tie up. This sealed bag is then placed in the yellow clinical waste container. In some homes faeces are tipped out of the bag and disposed of in the bedpan washer. The empty bag is then placed in a bag, sealed and placed in the yellow clinical waste bag. If the older person has an ileostomy, the faecal fluid is normally drained into a special jug that is usually named, e.g. 'Mrs Jones, stomal effluent only'. The fluid is disposed of in the bedpan washer. The jug is then resterilised for future use. This jug is kept separate from others and is never used to drain urine from catheter bags.

🔑 Key points

- Ageing and illness increase the risk of developing a continence problem.
- Incontinence is a symptom that should be investigated.
- Incontinence can often be successfully treated.
- When it is not possible or appropriate to treat, the aim is to manage incontinence well, to maintain dignity and skin health.
- A range of products are available; the aim is to choose the right product for the right person.
- Skilled, knowledgeable care assistants can make a real difference to continence care.

📖 Portfolio preparation

Your assessor must have evidence that you can meet the performance criteria for this unit. Before beginning this unit, discuss assessment strategies with your assessor. Most of the evidence for this unit can be gained by direct observation of your work. If two people are required to assist a resident your assessor may take on both the role of assistant and also assessor. You may be asked to provide the following types of evidence:

Products: This might be a copy of a frequency volume chart that you completed. It could be a note in a resident's notes giving details of how you assisted the person to remain continent, or care detailed on a care plan. It could be a care plan that you have drawn up or contributed to on how you are contributing to meeting the assessed need of an individual.

Witness testimony: This is a statement from a senior member of staff. It might be a statement detailing how you have met certain performance criteria.

Written work: You might be asked to prepare a piece of work on how you assessed needs, drew up a plan of care and evaluated the care you delivered.

Your assessor may also use other methods to help you gain evidence for this unit. These may include:

- Verbal questioning
- Written questions.

Simulations may be used to help gain evidence if it cannot be gained by direct observation.

Further information

The Continence Foundation
307 Hatton Square
16 Baldwin Gardens
London EC1N 7RL
Helpline: 0845 345 0165 (Monday to Friday, 9.30 am to 1 pm)
E-mail: continence.foundation@dial.pipex.com
Website: http://www.continence-foundation.org.uk

The Continence Foundation provides information and advice on continence problems and produces a range of useful leaflets. You can download these from their website or write enclosing a stamped self-addressed envelope.

Incontact
United House
North Road
London N7 9DP
Telephone: 020 7700 7035
Fax: 020 7700 7045
E-mail: info@incontact.org
Website: http://www.incontact.org

Incontact is a charity that provides information and support for people affected by bowel and bladder problems. It is an organisation of people affected by continence problems and their carers.

British Colostomy Association
15 Station Road
Reading RG1 1LG
Telephone: 0118 939 1537
Helpline: 0800 328 4257

This charity offers information and advice to people who have colostomies, and produces a number of useful leaflets. It also provides a network of volunteers who are themselves colostomists. The volunteers will visit and provide advice and support to residents who have colostomies.

A number of organisations and companies who supply incontinence products have a telephone service. People suffering from incontinence, care assistants or registered nurses can telephone and ask for advice.

The Bard helpline: 0800 591 783 (Monday to Friday, 12.30 pm to 4.30 pm)

Coloplast Service helpline: 0800 22 06 22 (Monday to Friday, 9 am to 5 pm)

Hollister Incare helpline: 0800 521 377 (Monday to Friday, 9 am to 5 pm)

Further reading

There are a number of books dealing with the subject of continence promotion and the management of incontinence. The books listed are suitable for care assistants. You may be able to obtain these either from the library of the college where you are studying or from the local library.

Fader M & Norton C (1994) *Caring for Continence*. Hawker Publications, London. This book has been written specially for care assistants studying for NVQ qualifications. This book is available from either Hawker Publications or Amazon (http://www.amazon.co.uk).

Norton C (1996) *Nursing for Continence*, 2nd edition. Beaconsfield Publishers Ltd, 20 Chiltern Hills Road, Beaconsfield, Buckinghamshire HP9 1PL. This is a more detailed book that has been written for the registered nurse with an interest in continence care. If you wish to study the subject in greater depth, this is the best book to start with. Although it is written for registered nurses, it is easy to read and a full explanation of all terms is given.

Chapter Twelve
Moving and Handling
HSC223
Contribute to moving and handling individuals

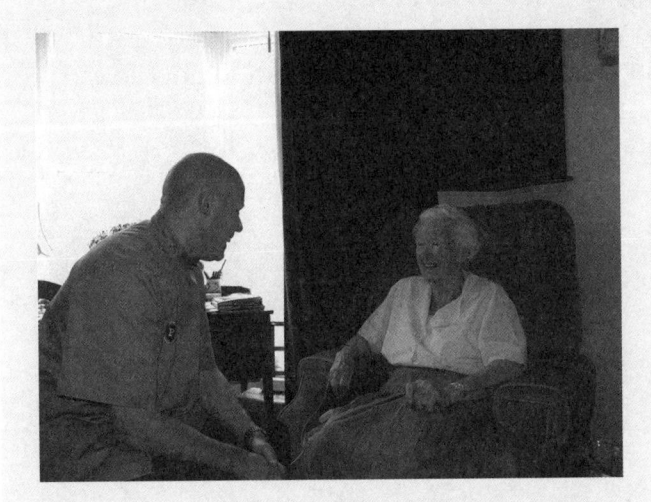

This unit consists of two elements:
HSC223a Prepare individuals, environments and equipment for moving and handling
HSC223b Enable individuals to move from one position to another

This chapter

- Explains legal requirements and policies relating to moving and handling
- Provides information on how moving and handling can cause back injury
- Explains how aids can be used to reduce the risk of staff and resident injury
- Provides information about aids that can be used to enable the older person to move independently
- Provides information about hoists and slings

Legal issues

Moving and handling can injure staff and patients. In 1996, 80 000 nurses injured their backs. Although the rate of back injuries is now falling they still account for half of all work-related injuries. Many staff still do not understand or comply with health and safety legislation.

Legislation aims to prevent injury. The two relevant pieces of legislation are the Health and Safety at Work Act 1974 and the Manual Handling Operations Regulations 1992.

The Health and Safety at Work Act 1974 outlined the responsibilities of employers to provide a safe working environment for staff. The Manual Handling Operations Regulations of 1992 became law on 1 January 1993. They aim to prevent back and other injury by making sure manual handling tasks are evaluated and reducing or eliminating the need for manual handling, wherever possible. Employers and staff have responsibilities under the legislation, outlined in Table 12.1.

Employers have legal duties to:

> So far as is reasonably practical, avoid the need for employees to undertake any manual handling operations at work which involve the risk of their being injured. Undertake an adequate risk assessment for those tasks that cannot reasonably and practicably be avoided.

Table 12.1 Legal responsibilities of staff and employer.

Employer	Staff
Eliminate manual handling whenever possible	Comply with moving and handling policies
Assess all manual handing risks	Inform employer of risks identified
Reduce risk of injury when no alternative to lifting	Inform employer if problems identified
Ensure that staff are physically capable	Inform employer of health problems
Ensure staff receive regular and appropriate training	Attend training sessions
Provide, maintain and monitor equipment	Use equipment provided
Monitor and record accidents	Report any faults in equipment
Act to prevent accidents occurring	Remove dangerous equipment from use

Manual handling regulations

All manual handling operations must be assessed. This means not only the moving of residents but also the moving of stores, laundry bags and other items. The Health and Safety Executive and the Health and Safety Commission have produced guidance to help reduce risks.

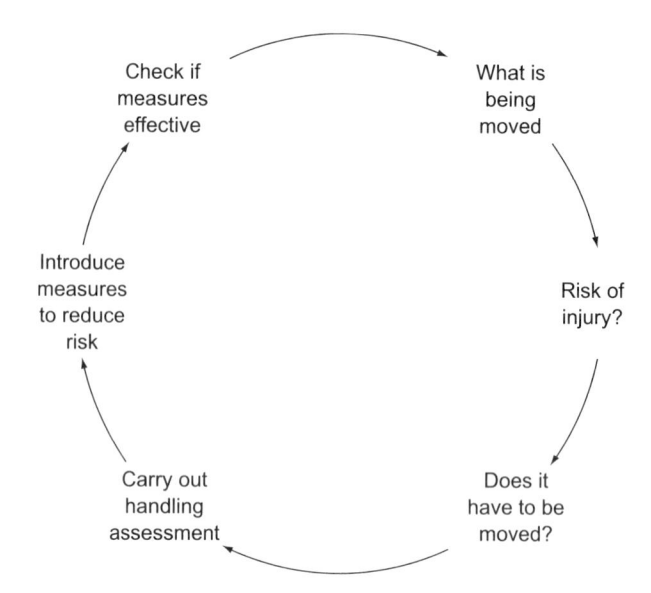

Figure 12.1 The risk assessment process. Reproduced with permission of Arjo UK.

The regulations are not specifically about people. People are different to objects. They have feelings and do unpredictable things. When you are moving people you will need to use a specific manual handling assessment. Every individual who requires manual handling should be assessed. The assessment should include the person's weight, factors affecting handling and methods to be used and equipment required to assist the person to move. This assessment should be recorded and kept with the resident's records. Each care home will have an assessment tool and this should be completed. When you have completed it you will have some idea of the level of assistance a person needs to perform specific tasks such as getting out of bed.

The employer should also carry out risk assessments (Fig. 12.1) to reduce the risk of injury when lifting or moving everyday items such as the boxes of books received from the library, soap powder and supplies. The assessment should include the weight of such items and where they are to be stored.

Responsibilities of the employer

Employers are obliged to take the following steps to reduce the incidence of back injury among staff:

- Eliminate manual handling wherever possible.
- Assess all manual handling tasks.

- Reduce the risk of injury where there is no alternative to lifting.
- Ensure that staff are physically capable of carrying out their duties – pregnant staff and staff who have had a baby within the last three months should be assessed separately from other staff.
- Ensure that all staff receive regular and appropriate training in moving and handling. This is normally part of the induction process. Ongoing training is incorporated within the home's training plan. Many homes employ staff who have received special training in moving and handling and are qualified to train staff. Sometimes smaller homes employ specially qualified trainers to carry out training sessions.
- Ensure that appropriate equipment is provided, maintained and monitored.
- Monitor and record all accidents and sickness – take action to prevent accidents recurring wherever possible.

Pregnant staff

Staff who are pregnant are less capable of lifting objects and are more at risk during any manual handling procedures. In pregnancy, the ligaments supporting the spine loosen and the pregnant member of staff is at greater risk of back injury than any other member of staff. Increasingly homes are carrying out risk assessments when a member of staff is pregnant and assessing the risks of the employee carrying out everyday tasks. Most homes forbid pregnant staff to lift everyday items such as stores or to manually move residents under any circumstances. This means that the pregnant member of staff does not lift boxes of dressing packs, stationery or any equipment, and does not lift a patient even in an emergency. Some homes prohibit pregnant staff from taking any part in manual handling. In a small home the employer may consider that it is not possible to have a member of staff on duty who is not able to take part in manual handling. If, for example, there are only two staff on duty and one of them is unable to assist residents to move, this would be unsafe. In these circumstances, the employer has a duty to find alternative work (at the same rate of pay) for the pregnant employee.

The employee has a duty to inform the employer as soon as she is aware of her pregnancy, so that steps can be taken to reduce the possible risk of injury to the member of staff, to other staff members and to residents.

Women returning to work after giving birth remain vulnerable to back injury for around six months after delivery as it takes time for muscles and ligaments to return to their pre-pregnancy state. Some employers now conduct risk assessments on staff who are returning to work less than six months after delivery. The employee may (depending on the risk assessment) not be able to undertake certain duties until she has fully recovered from the effects of pregnancy.

The Health and Safety Executive

If it is 'reasonably practical' for the employer to meet legal requirements and the employer fails to do so, the Health and Safety Executive can take action. Many residents enjoy showers but others prefer to bath. If a hoist is required to help dependent residents bath but the employer fails to provide one, the Health and Safety Executive could intervene. The Health and Safety Executive employs health and safety inspectors who visit and assess risks. The older person and staff would be at risk of injury if they attempted to lift the individual in and out of the bath. In such circumstances the Health and Safety Executive would serve a notice obliging the employer to supply equipment. The inspector specifies a period of time in which the employer must comply. The inspector will then return to ensure that the equipment has been supplied. If the employer fails to comply, he or she may be prosecuted under the Health and Safety at Work Act 1974. Employers who fail to comply can be imprisoned for up to two years and face unlimited fines.

Employee responsibilities

Employees have a duty under the legislation to take reasonable care of their own health and safety and those who may be affected by their omissions, and to cooperate with the employer. This means that employees:

- Have a duty to attend training sessions
- Should comply with moving and handling policies within the home
- Should not use manoeuvres designated as poor practice
- Should use equipment provided
- Should report any faults in equipment promptly
- Should remove dangerous equipment from use
- Should inform the employer of any risks identified
- Should inform the employer of any health problems that affect their ability to carry out their role.

How great is the risk of back injury?

Legislation states that employers should, so far as reasonably practical, avoid the need for employees to undertake any manual handling operations at work which involve the risk of their being injured.

But will it really hurt to lift a resident? Research suggests that staff working with older people are very much at risk of developing back pain and are more likely to suffer injury as a result of lifting. One survey discovered that 28% of nurses working on surgical wards in NHS hospitals suffered from back pain at least once a week. In elderly care wards 92% of staff suffered from regular back pain. Research has shown that before the use of hoists became widespread an elderly care nurse could lift a ton during a shift. Moving and handling regulations aim to make this a thing of the past.

Backs can be injured not only by lifting or by accidents; they can also be injured by the strain of lifting day in and day out for years. Repetitive movements, poor posture, prolonged stooping, awkward postures and sudden movements can also cause back injury and pain.

Wearing appropriate clothing

Uniforms should enable you to move freely. A uniform that restricts your ability to move freely can increase the risk of back injury. In the past female nursing staff wore traditional dresses with narrow skirts. These restrict movement and make it more difficult to move freely. In other countries such as the United States and Australia research has shown that nurses who wear tunics and trousers are much less likely to suffer from back injury. If dresses are worn these should have pleats to enable staff to move freely. Increasingly British healthcare staff are adopting practical uniforms to enable them to move easily and avoid the risk of injury.

Wearing appropriate footwear

Staff working with older people spend a lot of time on their feet and it's important to have appropriate footwear. Shoes should be flat – this increases the grip of the shoes on the ground and reduces the risk of you slipping. It also provides your feet with better support and prevents aching at the end of the day. Flat shoes are also quieter so you do not clump around and disturb residents. Shoes should have soles that grip the ground to reduce the risks of you slipping. The soles on some shoes can lose their grip within a matter of weeks. Your feet may spread by the end of the day. Lace-up shoes allow you to loosen the laces. You should not wear clogs or sandals as these can slip off.

Some homes allow staff to wear trainers. These may be black (to match uniforms) or white. Trainers are comfortable and safe working shoes but you should check whether these are permitted in your workplace before wearing them.

Moving and handling policies

Staff working with elderly people can, with the best of intentions, move and handle older people who with aids, instruction and encouragement could move themselves. This practice causes the older person to become more dependent on staff, reduces quality of life and increases staff workload.

Any resident who requires help to move should have a moving and handling assessment. It is good practice to complete a short assessment even on patients who do not require assistance. The assessment should indicate when the person requires help, what help is required and detail any aids that will be used. This assessment should be documented and referred to in the care plan. The assessment should be updated every six months, or sooner if the individual's needs change. Most homes now have printed risk assessment forms. This form should be simple and easy to fill in. The risk assessment should be carried out by a competent registered nurse or suitably qualified member of staff.

Care plans

The information from the manual handling assessment is used to draw up a plan of care to which staff should refer before handling. The care plan should specify:

- The equipment required to perform the task. Equipment falls into three categories:
    - Equipment to enable the person to move independently such as a slide board or a grab rail
    - Equipment to assist in the move such as a sliding sheet
    - Equipment to move the full weight of the person such as a hoist.
- The number of staff required to carry out the handling procedure.
- The handling procedure: The procedure for assisting a person to transfer from bed to chair will differ from that used to help the person transfer from chair to toilet. The care plan should give details of each handling procedure, e.g. bathing, using the toilet or moving from wheelchair to armchair.
- How the person can help with the transfer.
- Any difficulties or constraints, e.g. the person may be confused and need reassurance and time to enable safe moving and handling.
- Any other information that staff require.

Care plans should be reviewed regularly. If the person's abilities change and the methods of handling change these must be noted on the care plan.

Training

All staff should receive training in moving and handling before being required to move people.

Employers have a legal duty to provide training to enable staff to move people and objects and to avoid injury. The latest recommendations are that all staff receive classroom-based training on induction. The training required will depend on the previous level of training but should be between two and five days. Box 12.1 provides details of what should be included in training courses.

Training and supervision should continue in the home. Staff should receive regular refresher courses. A one-day update is required every two years; this can either be workplace- or classroom-based.

Box 12.1 Details of manual handling training courses

- The home's moving and handling policy
- Information about how the spine functions and how back pain is caused
- Principles of assessing risk and assessing the patient
- Assessing risk and assessing the patient
- How to teach the patient to move unaided
- The environment and equipment – known as ergonomics
- Handling aids
- Manual handling techniques
- General health awareness including awareness of good movement at work and at home
- Responsibilities for reporting risks and injuries

Training records

Employers now keep records of training as they may be needed for legal reasons. When you complete a training course your employer may ask you to sign a form stating that you have attended the course and are aware of the home's policies relating to moving and handling and assessment.

Principles of safe practice

Avoid manual handling whenever possible. When this is not possible plan carefully, prepare thoroughly, position thoughtfully and proceed cautiously. The aim is to achieve a safe system of work. Safe practice involves assessment, planning, preparation, positioning and proceeding.

Assessment

Before you move anything or anyone, assess. Use LITE to remind you of what to do.

- Load – What are you going to move?
- Individual (you) – Are you wearing appropriate clothing? Are you able to carry out this task? Are you fit enough to carry out this task? Are you physically able to carry out this task?
- Task – What are you going to do?
- Environment – Where are you doing it? Have you got enough room? Is it safe to do this here?

Planning

Before you move anything or anyone work out how you intend to do this. Check records and risk assessment. This may contain details of what you should do to minimise risks of injury. Ask for help if required.

Prepare

Do you need equipment? If so check that it is available and that you know how to use it. Prepare the equipment. Check the environment. You may need to move things. Make sure that if you are working with a partner or other team members that everyone is clear about what they are to do.

Position

Make sure that your feet are in a walking position, even if you are squatting. This provides you with a stable base and reduces the risk of injury. If you are lifting something keep the load close to your body. Bend your knees and make sure that your back is not twisting. Have your leading foot placed in the direction that you are moving. If you are working with a colleague ensure that you are both working together to the same rhythm and timing.

Proceed

Keep the object close to you throughout the movement. Do not twist as you move. Move weight from one foot to another and move your feet as you complete the procedure. Maintain a good posture at all times.

Equipment

The employer is required to provide a range of appropriate equipment to enable staff to safely handle people and loads such as soap powder, kitchen stores, etc. Care homes must provide appropriate equipment to enable the individual to be moved safely. Increasingly insurers demand evidence of risk assessment and details of staff training and equipment provided before agreeing to insure the home.

Using hoists and slings

Hoists can be used for a range of moving tasks. A range of hoists are available. We can work out which is the best hoist by examining the task, the person and the environment.

Mobile hoists

Mobile hoists are used to move a person who is unable to weight bear (Fig. 12.2). The hoist is brought to the person and the person is moved using a sling.

Mobile hoists can be manually operated or battery operated. Battery-operated hoists should be charged when not in use. Some mobile hoists can be folded for storage.

Mobile hoists are designed to move people of different weights. Most manufacturers make a small-based and a large-based hoist. Small-based hoists are designed to move people weighing 100–140 kg. Large-based hoists can move people weighing 160–250 kg. Small-based hoists are

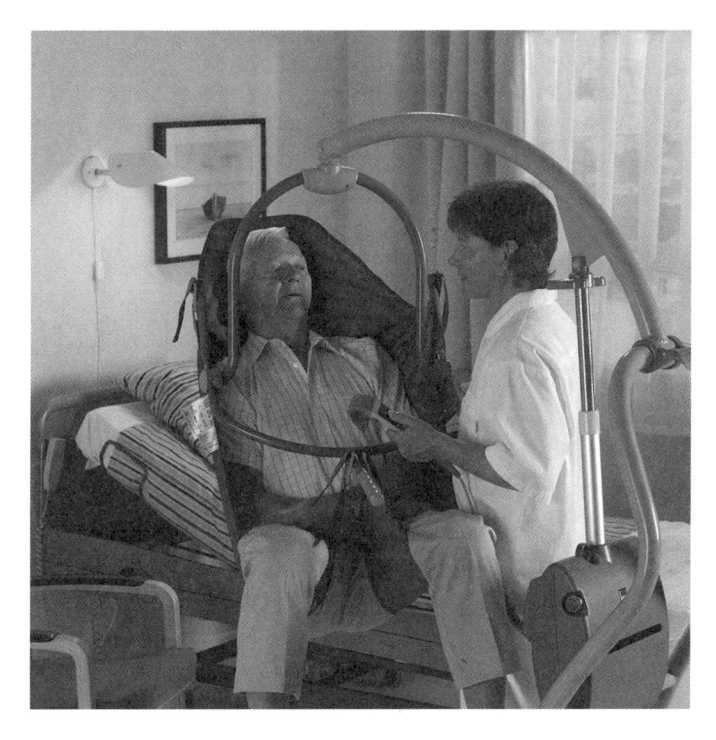

Figure 12.2 Using a mobile hoist and sling.

smaller, easier to manoeuvre and store and are less expensive. They are not suitable for people weighing more than 140 kg. Mobile hoists are flexible. You can use them for more than one person. They can be put away when not needed. They are relatively cheap. If lots of residents require a hoist to move, it is important to have sufficient hoists.

Standing hoists

Standing hoists are used for people who can take some weight through their legs (Fig. 12.3).

The hoist helps the person move from a seated to a standing position. It has a padded section that supports the person's knees while the person is being moved. It can be used to help a person regain the ability to stand and walk and to help the person to transfer. It is not suitable for moving a person long distances, unless it has a seat for this purpose.

Standing hoists tend to be bulky. It takes time to get used to manoeuvring them. They are not suitable for all residents. They do make a real difference to moving and handling and can help people regain or retain ability.

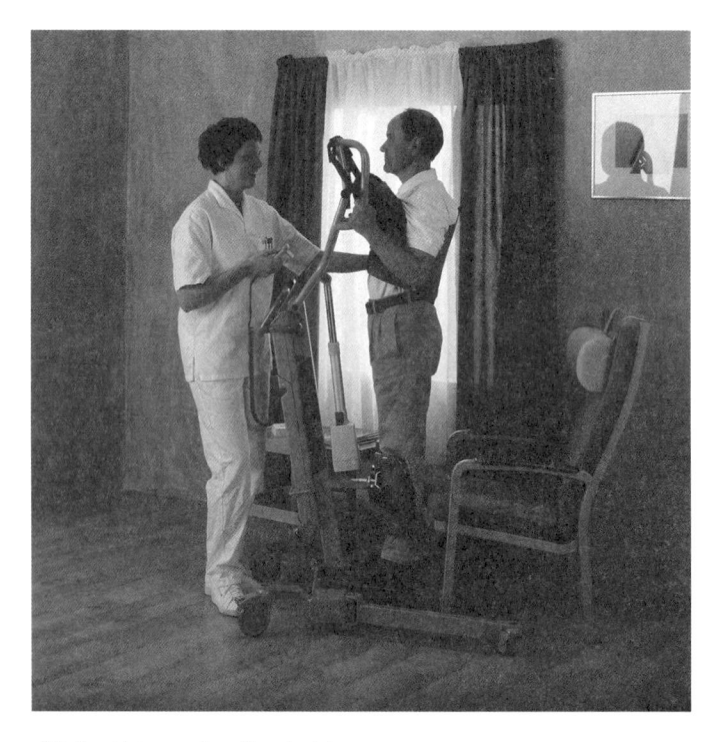

Figure 12.3 Using a standing hoist.

Bath hoists

Bath hoists are used to enable people to get in and out of the bath (Fig. 12.4). There are a range of bath hoists. Some such as the one shown are suitable for people who are reasonably mobile, while others are specifically designed for more disabled people.

Bath hoists are an essential piece of equipment and enable older people who could otherwise not bath to enjoy a bath.

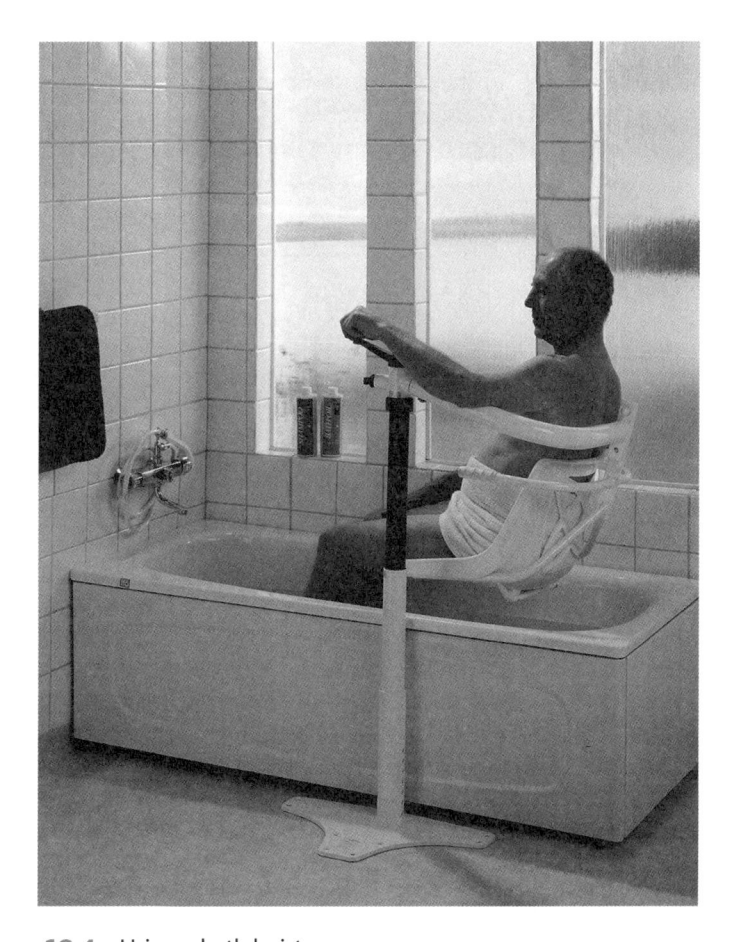

Figure 12.4 Using a bath hoist.

Tracking hoists

There are three parts to a tracking hoist.

1. The track: This can be straight, curved or have junctions like a railway track.
2. The power lifting unit: This can be permanently fixed to the track or it can be removable. The advantage of a fixed power unit is that you don't have to move it. They can be heavy. The disadvantage of a fixed unit is that you cannot move it. You are restricted to using the unit in the area covered by the track and the power unit. This usually means one room.
3. A sling is attached to the power unit to enable you to move the person.

Tracking hoists take up no floor space and are less intrusive than mobile hoists. They are less flexible than mobile hoists and can usually only be used for one person at a time. Tracking hoists are expensive and currently fairly unusual in care homes. As the price of technology falls they will no doubt be more widely used.

Why staff don't always use equipment

Despite the fact that employers provide hoists and have introduced no-lifting or safer lifting policies, staff continue to lift patients manually, risking the health of the patient, their own health and that of their colleagues. Research shows that there are a number of reasons why staff do not use hoists (Box 12.2).

If there are problems using the hoist you must inform a member of senior staff. The senior member of staff can organise training, work with you to explain to the older person and his or her family why the hoist is needed and arrange education so that staff can use equipment safely.

Box 12.2 Reasons why staff do not use equipment

- Insufficient room to move the hoist around
- The hoist will not fit in the toilet or bathroom
- The hoist is poorly maintained – the wheels may stick or staff may struggle to use it
- Staff have not been trained to use the hoist
- The resident (or relatives) do not like the hoist and do not understand why staff insist on using it
- Other staff do not use the hoist

Preparing for moving and handling

It is important to make sure that you have enough space to move. Move the equipment and furniture if necessary. If the person requires help to move you may find it easier to rearrange the furniture in the room. If the bed is against the wall and two staff are required to help move the person it makes sense to rearrange the furniture so that staff have access to both sides of the bed. Remember though that this is the person's home; obtain consent before moving furniture. If the person wants the bed in a particular position you may have to move the bed out to ensure access each time you help the person to move. Avoid moving people who can move independently. The person is at risk of becoming physically weaker and losing the ability to move independently. Ensure that you have enough people and the correct equipment to move the person.

Working with the person to be moved

It is important to work with the person who is to be moved. You need to obtain the consent and whenever possible the active participation of the person who is to be moved. Explain what you intend to do. Ask the person to cooperate. Explain what you wish the person to do and check that the person has understood.

Some individuals may be unconscious or may appear to be too confused to understand what you intend to do. It is still important to explain because we do not know what the individual understands and it is a matter of courtesy to explain. Sometimes the person who has limited ability to understand may be able to understand that you are going to do something just by hearing the tone of your voice. People who have limited ability to comprehend remain human and should be treated with the same dignity, respect and courtesy as those who are able to communicate.

Encouraging independence

It is important to encourage the older person to be as independent as possible. This has physical and psychological benefits. Sometimes the older person requires a little assistance to move. Aids can be used in such circumstances. Sometimes the older person may be able to use an aid independently; at other times the person will require assistance to use the aid.

Transferring

Many older people can be encouraged and helped to move around the home in wheelchairs. Although the older person has lost the ability to walk, she has retained independence and is not forced to rely on staff to move around. Moving a wheelchair around is fairly hard work and this exercise strengthens the muscles in the arms and chest. Many people who use wheelchairs can use these strong arm and chest muscles to transfer from wheelchair to chair, wheelchair to toilet or wheelchair to bed.

When transferring, the side of the wheelchair is normally removed. In some cases the individual is able to put some weight on their legs and slide into a chair while holding on to one side of the wheelchair and the arm of the chair. When transferring from wheelchair to toilet, grab rails can be used to pull the body up. The care assistant can, if required, pull down clothing. The person can then use the grab rails to pull themselves over and onto the toilet seat.

When transferring from bed to chair some patients use a special pole known as a 'monkey pole', which has a grip suspended from a chain. This grip helps the person to lift up and swing over into the chair. Using a monkey pole requires strong muscles and the ability to lift the arms above the head. Some people, especially those suffering from arthritis, are unable to use monkey poles.

They may find using a special board (known as a transfer board) easier. One end of the board is placed on the wheelchair and the other on the bed (usually this end is placed under the mattress). The care assistant remains with the person who uses the arms and, if possible, muscles in the lower body to wiggle along the board and into the bed or chair. The board is then removed. Some people are able to transfer independently without assistance or supervision.

Turning a person in bed

People who are unable to turn over in bed without help are at risk of developing pressure sores. Details on preventing pressure sores are given in Chapter 9. If the person is unable to turn over unaided you must turn the person. A range of equipment is available to enable you to slide and turn the patient.

Summary

In the past staff lifted people without considering how this practice could injure residents and staff. Now things are different. Before we move people or objects we must consider the safest and most sensible way to do this. In the past there were few aids to enable us to move people; now we have a large range of equipment and aids to enable us to move patients safely and to avoid risk of staff injury. Modern moving and handling techniques aim to encourage people, wherever possible, to move independently using aids and equipment when required. Modern techniques aim to avoid injury to patients and staff and to make homes and hospitals safer places for those who provide care and those who require it.

Key points

- Employers must ensure that they act to minimise risk of injury.
- Staff must comply with policies on moving and handling.
- Staff should be trained in moving and handling.
- Risk assessments should be carried out before moving and handling.
- The person who requires assistance should have this detailed on a care plan.
- The home must have a range of equipment to minimise the risks of injury.
- Your role in encouraging and enabling people to move around, assisting people to move and reporting any problems is of vital importance.

Portfolio preparation

Your assessor must have evidence that you can meet the performance criteria for this unit. Before beginning this unit, discuss assessment strategies with your assessor. Most of the evidence for this unit can be gained by direct observation of your work. This might include watching you assist a resident to get into bed or get up. This might be supplemented by questioning about the care plan and the reasons for using certain methods to assist the individual, and more general questions about moving and handling.

Products: This might include a copy of progress notes or a care plan on pressure area care that you have completed. It could be a note in a resident's notes giving details of any aids that the person uses or details of assistance that the person requires, detailed on a care plan. It could be a care plan that you have drawn up or contributed to on how you are contributing to reducing risk factors.

Witness testimony: This is a statement from a senior member of staff. It might be a statement detailing how you have met certain performance criteria.

Written work: You might be asked to write an account of how you helped a particular resident to move and the aids and techniques used. You might be asked to prepare a piece of work about the factors that increase the risk of back injury and how these can be avoided. You might be asked to write a case history about how you helped a resident use aids to move.

Your assessor may also use other methods to help you gain evidence for this unit. These may include:

- Verbal questioning
- Written questions.

Simulations can be used if it is not possible to obtain evidence by direct observation. Simulations can be used to assess your ability to use equipment for moving and handling.

Further information

BackCare
16 Elmtree Road
Teddington
Middlesex TW11 8ST
Helpline: 0845 130 2704
Website: http://www.backcare.org.uk

BackCare, the charity for healthier backs, produces information and publishes books on moving and handling and back care. Their website has details.

The GMB trade union has produced a leaflet, *Health and Safety in the Care Sector*. It is available free from Regional Health and Safety Officers or National Office or via the GMB website (www.gmb.org.uk/health&safety – look under health and safety documents).

The **Disabled Living Foundation** produces a wealth of information on moving and handling including information on how to choose equipment (www.dlf.org.uk/factsheets/pdf/Choosing_a_mobile_hoist.pdf).

Further reading

If you wish to learn more you can check if your college or local library has these books.

Health and Safety in Care Homes (£8.50) is available from HSE Books, PO Box 1999, Sudbury, Suffolk, CO10 2WA (telephone: 01787 881165).
Safer Handling of People in the Community (1999) is available from BackCare.
The Guide to the Handling of People, 5th edition, is available from BackCare.

Chapter Thirteen
Equality, Diversity, Rights and Responsibilities
HSC234
Ensure your own actions support the equality, diversity, rights and responsibilities of individuals

This unit consists of three elements:
HSC234a Respect the rights and interests of individuals
HSC234b Treat everyone equally and in ways that respect diversities and differences
HSC234c Act in ways that promote individuals' confidence in you and your organisation

This chapter

- Provides information about the older person's role in society
- Explains about the legal rights of a person living in a care home and their rights to healthcare and services
- Explains how a person's cultural background can affect expectations of healthcare
- Provides information about how to meet a person's cultural needs
- Explains the importance of treating all residents with dignity and respect
- Provides information on how you can support the older person to meet their cultural needs

Older people and society

In the past, it was unusual for people to live as long as they do now. At the beginning of the last century when old age pensions were introduced, few older people lived long enough to collect their pensions. During the twentieth century improved living conditions and improved medical care have resulted in people living longer than before (Fig. 13.1).

The number of people over the age of 85 rose from 70 000 at the beginning of the twentieth century to 1.2 million by the end of the century. Most people living in care homes are women. Statistics show that for every 77 women over the age of 85 years there are 23 men. Statistics also show that older men are less likely to be admitted to homes than women are. When men are admitted to homes, they require much greater levels of care than women.

There are several reasons for this. Women in the past tended to marry men who were on average five years older. When these men become ill and require care, their wives care for them for as long as possible. Research shows that these younger wives are well organised and obtain help from family members, district nurses and social services. The married older man is cared for at home for as long as possible. It is only when the older man's wife can no longer cope that he is admitted to care. Women still live on average five years longer than men and by the age of 70 two-thirds of all women are widowed or divorced. Half of the women over the age of 60 either had no children or have lived longer than their children. So women, because they live longer and married older men, are less likely to have anyone to care for them when they require help.

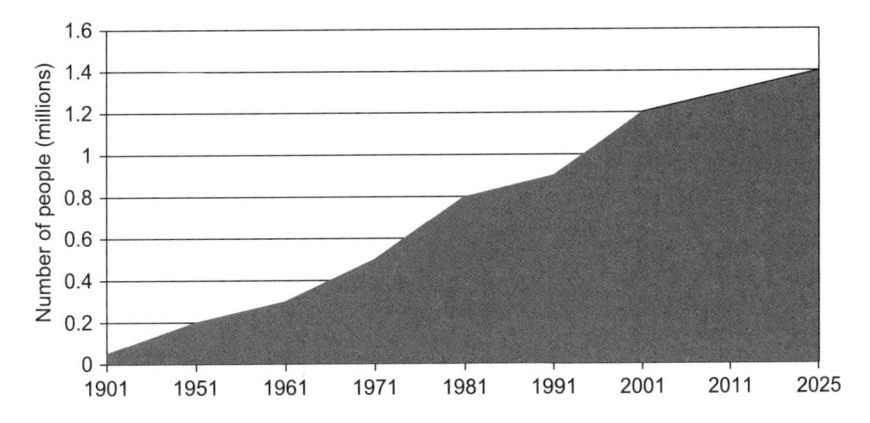

Figure 13.1 Rising numbers of people aged 85+.

Older people and their families

We often hear people complaining that families no longer care for old people in the way that they did in the past. In fact, fewer families cared for older people in the past because there were fewer older people. At the beginning of the century, families often lived under the same roof. The family might consist of grandparents, parents and children. In many cases, the family did not live together out of choice but because they could not afford separate homes. As people have become more prosperous, it has become rare for several generations to live under the same roof. Interestingly though, higher UK house prices seem to be reversing this trend.

Research shows that families still care for the older members of the family. This research confirms what many people often forget: older people have more experience and offer younger members of the family advice and support, while younger members of the family help with physical tasks which the older person may now find difficult.

There are seven million carers in the UK. Many have given up their own well-paid jobs to care for a member of their family.

Research shows that families do provide practical help and support for older people. Care assistants can help families remain involved when the person is admitted to a home. Some older people do not have any family and because they may not have help and support they are more likely to be admitted to a home.

The legal rights of a person living in a home

A person living in a home has the same legal rights as any other citizen. In some countries, such as the USA, there is a written constitution and every citizen is aware of his or her rights because these are written down. People being cared for in hospitals and homes have a series of basic rights that are legally binding. In the UK our legal system is older and has evolved over more than a thousand years. There is no legal declaration of each citizen's rights, but instead a series of Acts of Parliament and common law that define a person's rights.

People living in homes have not given up any of their rights when they enter the home. If the person wishes to leave the home, staff cannot forcibly detain the person except in special circumstances. If the person is at serious risk of injuring themselves or others then a doctor, social worker or police officer can exercise special powers to detain the person for a limited period. If this is the case, the person will be transferred to hospital or a specialist home for care by nurses specialising in caring for people with mental health needs. Consent must be obtained before care is carried out or medication is given. Forcing a person to bath against their will or forcing a person to take medication or have treatment is an offence. Sensitive care will involve working with the older person to meet needs, not imposing a regime on the individual.

Sometimes the older person is unable to consent to care because of confusion or illness. The person lacks what the legal system calls 'capacity'. This is the ability to make choices about different aspects of life and care. Capacity varies according to the decision being made. An older woman with dementia, for example, may no longer be able to be capable of handling her finances, however she is able to decide what she wishes to wear and eat. If an older person has soiled herself or is very dirty she may decline a bath. Staff have to persuade the person to bath because the person is not capable of understanding her need and staff have a duty to care for the person. New legislation (The Mental Capacity Act) is being introduced. This act provides staff with legal authority to provide healthcare that is in the person's best interests when the person is unable to consent. Although staff will still have to persuade the person to accept the care offered, the person providing care is providing that care legally.

Rights to healthcare and services

People living in care homes have the same rights to healthcare as people living in their own homes. Older people have the same right to choose their own GP as other adults. Some homes have a GP who visits on a regular basis and provides care for many of the older people living in the home. If the older person lives locally, her GP can continue to visit and offer medical care. Unfortunately, many older people admitted to homes are no longer in the area where their GP has agreed to provide care.

Right to medical services

GPs may be unable to care for people who have moved out of the area in which they practise because of the difficulty in travelling some distance to visit the older person in the home. In most homes, the older person moving out of the area to the home is asked if she wishes to receive medical care from the GP who visits the home. The person has the right to choose another GP in the local area if she wishes. In practice this can be difficult, as some GPs are reluctant to offer care to individuals living in homes. Some GPs state that older people living in homes require more care than older people living in their own homes, and they prefer not to offer this service. If an older person does not wish to have medical care provided by the home's GP, and a local GP cannot be found to offer care, then the older person, the family or the manager will have to contact the primary care trust, who will find a GP in these circumstances.

Right to specialist nursing services

People living in homes have the same right to see nurse specialists as people living in their own homes. Most people living in homes receive excellent specialist care from nurses specialising in areas such as diabetes, continence promotion, wound care and stoma care. However, it is difficult for specialists to visit the home because home visits are very time consuming. Specialist nurses are keen to work with nursing and care home staff to help them develop the skills to care for residents with specific needs. Some primary care trusts have study days where staff can learn to develop their skills in specific areas of practice. This enables specialists to concentrate on the most complex cases.

Right to therapy services

People living in homes are entitled to services such as chiropody and physiotherapy. Unfortunately, although the number of people living in homes has increased tenfold since the mid-1980s, the number of people employed to provide such services has not increased. Things have improved in the last few years; however, in some areas staff working in homes still find it difficult to obtain these services for residents. The local primary care trust has a responsibility to provide services for local people. If these services are not available, your manager can make senior members of the trust aware of the problem.

Right to continence aids

People who are incontinent are entitled to continence aids. The local primary care trust is responsible for supplying aids. The primary care trust may choose to do this in one of two ways. The primary care trust may assess the person and supply pads that are appropriate to the person's needs. Or the primary care trust may choose instead to pay the person an allowance that can be used to buy pads. VAT is no longer chargeable on incontinence pads. Disposable pads are normally supplied. If the person wishes to use washable, reusable pads (see Chapter 11 for details) then the person has a right to have these supplied instead.

Right to confidentiality

When an older person enters a home, care assistants get to know the person's innermost secrets. You may, because of the nature of the caring relationship, know more about the person's thoughts and feelings than even the person's family. People who confide their secrets and share their feelings with care assistants do so because they trust care assistants completely. You must guard those secrets well and maintain the person's trust.

In some homes and hospitals, sensitive information is bandied about. If a person suffers from diabetes this may be recorded on a label above the bed! In some homes charts giving details of the person's continence are displayed in corridors and lounge areas where other residents, relatives and even people delivering supplies can see them. This is unacceptable.

If the older person suffers from haemorrhoids (piles) she could be deeply embarrassed if staff mentioned this in front of another resident, even one who is sharing a room. Care assistants should be tactful and ensure that details of a personal nature are not discussed in front of others. This would not only be insensitive but also a breach of confidentiality. Confidentiality of information is dealt with in detail in Chapter 1.

Right to dignity and respect

All people have a right to be treated with dignity and respect. We all choose to work in a caring setting because we wish to care for people. Sometimes though something goes wrong and staff become insensitive to the person's need to be treated with dignity and respect. We have all heard of cases where people are placed on commodes in full view of others, or of cases where people are not dressed properly and care is poor.

Sometimes care assistants ask, 'What is acceptable and what isn't? How do I know if the care I am giving is good enough?' The answer to this is simple. If you would be happy to be treated in such a way, if you would be happy for your own mother to be treated in this way, then the care is acceptable. If you would not be happy to be treated as residents are treated, then the care is unacceptable.

Right to choose

Older people living in care homes have the same right to make choices as people living within their own homes. Unfortunately, it is much more difficult for people living within homes to exercise choice. People living in homes rely on staff to help them and many fear that if they complain they will be seen as 'trouble-makers' or 'moaners'. So many fit in and go along with the routine in the home. If older people do not make choices about how to lead their lives, they can quickly lose all sense of control over their own lives. They become disinterested in their surroundings, and physical and mental health deteriorates.

Research shows that in homes where staff work hard to enable older people to remain involved in decisions about their day-to-day life, staff and residents are more fulfilled. Regular meetings between residents and staff help older people remain involved. In some homes residents have formed residents' committees. These committees may plan recreational activities and in some homes they sit on panels to interview new members of staff.

Right to culturally sensitive care

We live in a multicultural society, yet few people from ethnic minority groups live in homes. There are thought to be two reasons for this. First, many people who came to this country to work are only now reaching the age when they may require care in homes. Second, care within homes is geared to the native population. Older people entering homes feel vulnerable and anxious. People who have difficulty in speaking English or who have a different diet or religion may feel terrified by the thought of entering a home. In some areas homes have been set up specially to cater for people from certain religious or ethnic groups. Special homes have been set up to meet the needs of people from Poland, Italy, Germany and Hong Kong. There are a number of homes that aim to care for people of different faiths. There are homes providing care for Sikhs, Jews, Muslims and people of other faiths.

From time to time, you may care for people from different cultures. If the person does not speak English, it can be difficult to communicate; further details on communication are given in Chapter 1. Care given should be appropriate to the person's needs. The person should, like all other residents, be treated in accordance with her culture and wishes. The diet should be appropriate to the person's culture; this is dealt with in detail in Chapter 7.

Right to worship

The person should be encouraged and helped to follow her chosen religion. People of different faiths celebrate special events. People of the Jewish faith celebrate the Passover. People of the Muslim faith celebrate Eid. People of the Hindu faith celebrate Diwali (the Hindu festival of light). People of different faiths should be encouraged to celebrate special festivals either with their family or with other residents in the home. With a little planning the home's calendar of celebrations can begin with New Year's Day and include St David's Day, St Patrick's Day, St George's Day and all the other celebrations within a year.

Spiritual needs

People of all ages find that spirituality and religion play an important part in their lives. Many older people enjoy watching the Sunday service on television and appreciate the effort that staff have made to ensure that the minister visits. Many, though, would prefer, given a choice, to attend church. There is a great difference between listening to a service and taking part in one. Wherever possible the staff at the home should help older people who wish to attend church services to do so. The local ministers of religion can often put staff in touch with active church members who will escort the individual to church. Church members can befriend older people new to the area and help involve them in all types of church activities.

People who are not of the Christian faith also enjoy participating in religious services. Ministers and members of the Jewish, Muslim, Hindu and other faiths can help arrange transport so that, wherever possible, the person can attend religious services.

Summary

Older people have the same rights as anyone else to be treated with dignity and respect and in a way that is appropriate to their cultural background. Ensuring that people are treated in this way at all times is vitally important. Many homes have policies that emphasise and reinforce the importance of this.

Key points

- People are living longer and 1.2 million people in the UK are now aged 85 and over.
- Older people have the same legal rights as other citizens.
- People living in care homes have the same rights to healthcare services as those living at home.
- It is important to support and enable people to remain involved in everyday life and to make decisions about the way they lead their lives.
- The person's decisions about how they wish to lead their life is influenced by their cultural and religious background.
- It is important to understand and respect the values of people of all cultures and backgrounds and to provide care that is sensitive to this.
- Your role in encouraging and enabling people to express their specific needs and assisting people to lead their lives in the way that they choose is of vital importance.

Portfolio preparation

Your assessor must have evidence that you can meet the performance criteria for this unit. Before beginning this unit, discuss assessment strategies with your assessor. Most of the evidence for this unit can be gained by direct observation of your work. This might include observing how your actions support and enable an older person to exercise choice or how you support the older person who wishes to fulfil spiritual needs.

Products: This might include a copy of progress notes or a care plan that you have completed. It could be a note in a resident's notes giving details of how you enable and support the person in exercising choice. It could be a care plan that you have drawn up or contributed to on how you are contributing to providing culturally sensitive care.

Witness testimony: This is a statement from a senior member of staff. It might be a statement detailing how you have met certain performance criteria.

Written work: Many homes have a philosophy of care and this usually includes a statement about equality. You might be asked to prepare one or two sides of A4 paper explaining how these aims are met within the home. Many homes also have an operations policy. This normally gives details of how the home is to be run in order to fulfil its stated aim or philosophy. Your assessor may want you to write a short passage on the difficulties staff face in putting such policies into practice and how you cope with these challenges. Check to see if your home has a policy on dignity and respect. Your assessor may want you to write a short passage on how this policy works in practice and how you cope with any problems that arise and enable residents to maintain dignity.

If your home cares for people from differing cultural backgrounds your assessor may question you or ask you to write about how cultural and spiritual needs are met, by:

- Verbal questioning
- Written questions.

Simulations can be used if it is not possible to obtain evidence by direct observation. Simulations can be used to assess your ability to use equipment for moving and handling.

Further reading

Chester R & Smith J (1996) *Acts of Faith*. Counsel and Care, London. This book investigates how older people of all faiths draw comfort and support from their local church.

Counsel and Care (1992) *Not Such Private Places*. Counsel and Care, London. This book examines issues relating to privacy and dignity in nursing and residential homes.

Chapter Fourteen
Negotiating Specific Environments
HSC235
Enable individuals to negotiate specific environments

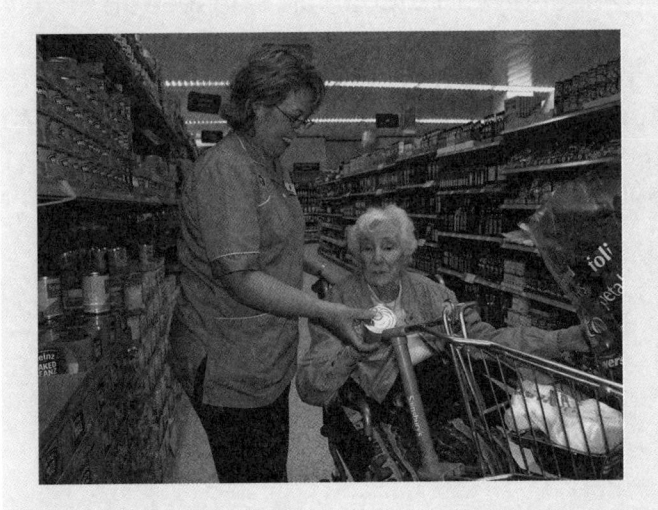

This unit consists of three elements:
HSC235a Support individuals to assess their ability to negotiate specific environments
HSC235b Support individuals to negotiate specific environments
HSC235c Observe and contribute to the evaluation of programmes

This chapter

- Provides information about the reasons why the older person might need support
- Explains how the older person might dread admission to a home and how you can support the individual who moves to a home
- Provides information on how you can support and keep in touch with a resident who has been admitted to hospital
- Provides information about how to support an older person having day surgery
- Provides information on how to support the older person attending an outpatient appointment
- Explains how you can support the person who is receiving rehabilitation or respite care

Why older people need support

Few of us have any idea how distressing and worrying it is to enter a home. For us the home is our place of work and it holds no terrors for us. If we are unhappy in the home, we can always leave. Some older people are admitted to homes from hospital. In most cases, the admission to hospital was because of a sudden illness or accident. In other cases, the older person may have been admitted to hospital because an existing condition, such as arthritis or Parkinson's disease, became much worse. When people go to hospital, they expect to have an operation or treatment, get better and go home. It can be a terrible shock for the older person to be told that she must leave hospital but cannot go home.

Most older people given a choice would avoid homes and would prefer to return to their own homes. People entering homes may have moved from their own home to hospital, had treatment and may have been moved to another ward before entering the home. The individual may dread the thought of another move and may worry about the staff. Will they be friendly and kind? Will I get the help I need? What is it going to be like?

You need to be aware of the fears and anxieties that people will experience when entering a home. A little time and trouble taken in getting to know the individual and offering support will help allay the person's fears.

Preparing for admission

Many homes encourage residents to bring items from home to make their room seem like home. Many older people have framed photographs of their families that they treasure. The individual's family can bring in framed photographs and pictures from home and these can be hung on hooks on walls. Ornaments brought from home can be placed around the room. The individual may have a favourite chair, cushions and footstool. These could be placed in the room. Some individuals may wish to bring in other items of furniture such as small tables, a bed, wardrobe, china cabinet or bureau. If the individual can bring treasured items to the home, it becomes more like moving home than being 'put in a home'. Some individuals may wish to bring bedspreads or bedcovers from home. Most homes have fully furnished rooms but there is no reason why this furniture cannot be stored so that the individual can bring in her own belongings.

Older people who become involved in planning the move to a home, and who can decide which items to bring with them, normally feel more positive about entering the home. Some homes do not allow people to bring in furniture and bedding because they fear that the fire officer will not allow this. In homes mattresses and all soft furnishings have to meet specific fire retardancy standards. These regulations and guidelines were introduced to make homes as safe as possible. They were not, however, introduced to prevent older people from bringing treasured items from home. Most fire officers, if asked about this, state that the home must purchase items that meet fire retardancy standards and that individuals may bring items from home that do not meet these standards.

It is important to prepare the room for the person's arrival. Make sure fresh water and a glass are supplied. Check that the bed is made neatly and there are towels available. If the room appears stuffy air it, remembering to close the window a few hours before the person is expected if it is cold outside. If it is cold, check that the heating is on. Make sure that the lights and the call bell work; if not, arrange repairs quickly. Check that the wardrobe has hangers in it and that the drawers and locker are clean. If possible, place a flowering plant or some flowers in the room. The person will find that the room is warm, comfortable and welcoming when she arrives. This makes a real difference; first impressions count. The impression you want to give is that the person is welcome and that you have taken the trouble to prepare for her arrival.

Admission to the home

Most older people who are admitted to a home from hospital are transferred to the home by ambulance. The individual may have waited either on the ward or in the hospital transport department for many hours before commencing the journey to the home. In some ambulances a number of people are transported at once so the journey may take some time. By the time the older person arrives at the home her bladder may be full to bursting and she may be tired, hungry, thirsty or in pain. You should be sensitive to these possibilities; now is not the time to introduce her to all the other residents or launch into lengthy admission procedures. Introducing yourself and helping the person to her room is best. When the person's immediate needs have been met, the admission procedures can begin. If the person is very tired, she may wish to rest for a few hours first.

On first name terms?

These days people often use first names even when addressing people they do not know well. The people admitted to homes come from a different generation. They were, in their youth, addressed by their title and surname in many situations and first names were used only by close friends and family. Some older people view the way we use first names now as refreshing and friendly; others may think it over-familiar or patronising. We address children by their first names but use titles and surnames as a mark of respect.

It is important to ask the individual how he or she wishes to be addressed and to use that form of address. The person who wishes to be addressed as Mrs Harley-Smith may in time ask staff to call her Ellen. Some older people, like younger people, dislike their names and use a nickname or a completely different first name. For example, Mrs Dorothy Mason may be called Anne by her friends. You should make a note in the care plan or inform senior staff of how the person prefers to be addressed.

Supporting the individual after admission

People entering the home normally require a lot of help and support in the first month after admission. It takes time for the person to settle in and discover how the home is run. Care should revolve around the individual. The individual, though, will need a little time and some guidance to develop a routine that suits his or her needs. Most people develop routines in their lives and people living in homes are no different. A routine offers structure to the day but should be flexible enough to enable the individual to enjoy life. The person entering the home has to learn a great deal: the names of the staff, mealtimes, arrangements for laundry, when activities take place. If the individual is given too much information at once, it can be difficult to remember it all. It is also difficult to decide which information is the most important. To the keen reader the location of the library books is very important, while to another individual that is of minor interest. Make sure that new residents and their families are aware that they can ask for information about the home.

Homes now produce information books that provide a great deal of information about the home. These are usually made up of loose-leaf sheets held in plastic sleeves in a ring binder. Information can be updated quickly and easily. Such information books are a requirement under the national minimum standards. Some homes have used this as an opportunity to prepare an information booklet that is truly useful to residents and helps the person to settle in. The new resident can read through the information book and find the information that is important to him or her. Some homes have produced a tape cassette giving information about the home for residents who are no longer able to read.

Dignity and privacy

One of the things many older people fear most on entering a home is the loss of dignity and privacy. At home the older person's privacy was protected by her front door; before anyone could enter, she had to open it. In homes disabilities may prevent the older person from locking her room door. One day perhaps we'll have the technology to lock and unlock doors using a handheld remote. If you are a parent you know how annoying it is to have people barging into your room without knocking. In some homes room doors are not even closed and the older person can be seen by anyone walking along the corridor. You should always knock and ask permission before entering a person's room.

Some residents, especially those living in nursing homes, are more disabled than others. Some disabled people depend on staff to get clothing from wardrobes and chests of drawers. You should always ask the person's permission before getting clothing and items out. Some residents do not always close bedroom doors before undressing. Others forget to close the toilet door before using the toilet. It is important to be alert to such problems and to protect the person's dignity at all times.

Sharing a room

Fifteen years ago, most people living in homes shared a room with one or two others. This was considered a great advance on geriatric hospitals where people were cared for in wards with an average of 21 beds. Now three quarters of all people living in nursing and residential homes have their own room. In some homes, residents do not have their own room but share the room with another person.

The individual may have been living alone for many years and may be very embarrassed about sharing a room with others. The individual may have developed a close friendship with her roommate. Whatever the circumstance you should be very careful to safeguard the person's privacy and dignity in such situations. In sharing rooms, each bed has bed curtains. These should be used to protect the person's privacy when she is washing, dressing, using a commode or bedpan, or wishes to have them drawn. If the room has a wash basin, this will also have curtains. These should be used to maintain the person's privacy when washing.

Hospital admission

People living in homes are more acutely ill than before and the number of people being readmitted to hospital from homes has risen rapidly. Older people living in residential homes are more likely to be readmitted to hospital than those living in nursing homes. There are three different types of admission: emergency admission, planned admission and day surgery.

Emergency admission

Emergency admissions are, of course, unplanned. The older person may have fallen and a fracture is suspected, or she may have become acutely ill and require hospital treatment. There is no time to prepare for the admission and the person who has settled into the home suddenly has to cope with the stress of going to hospital. The individual is often worried about her health and the prospect of leaving the home and going to hospital. If the person is very ill there is little time to prepare and often there is only time to prepare a toilet bag.

In emergencies, patients are taken to the accident and emergency department (A&E) where they are assessed and investigated and the doctors decide whether the person requires hospital treatment. If the person's GP has arranged the emergency admission, the GP will write a letter to the medical staff in A&E. Sometimes the staff at the home have called for an ambulance and the patient has not been seen by a GP. In these circumstances, the person in charge of the home will write a letter giving details of the person's medical history, the current problem and details of any medicines that the individual is taking.

It is good practice for staff from the home to escort a person requiring emergency treatment. In nursing homes, if the person is seriously ill a registered nurse will accompany the patient, provided that staffing levels allow this. In smaller homes and in residential homes, care assistants may accompany an acutely ill person to hospital. Each emergency ambulance is fully equipped and has two trained paramedical staff. Both are specially trained in caring for acutely ill people. Your role is to reassure and support the individual and to communicate with hospital staff on arrival at the hospital.

Hospital accident and emergency departments can be very busy. You should stay with the older person, accompany her to X-ray if required, explain procedures, and provide practical help and moral support. People are now seen, treated and discharged or admitted within four hours of arriving at accident and emergency departments. When the individual is admitted to the ward, you should remain until the person is settled in if possible. Find out as much as possible about the plan of treatment before leaving. If possible, try to get some indication of how long the person is expected to remain in hospital.

Keeping in touch

Approximately 10% of people living in homes have no close relatives or friends. Although it is important to keep in touch with all residents who are in hospital, those without family or friends may feel particularly alone and lost and require special support. A daily telephone call to check how the individual is progressing will help the person feel she is not forgotten. In most hospitals there are telephones by each bedside so it is usually possible to speak directly to the person unless she is very unwell. If possible visit the person in hospital, telephoning first to check whether she requires anything from home.

Many older people worry that if they become ill or require greater levels of care than before, the home will refuse to have them back. Residential homes do not normally employ registered nurses and employ fewer staff than nursing homes. In some cases if the older person becomes more disabled she may be unable to return to the residential home. Most nursing homes care for older people who require high levels of skilled care, but some are unable to care for people with very high dependency needs. If an individual is worried that she will be unable to return to the home, inform your manager. The manager can visit, discuss this with the person, and in the vast majority of cases set the person's mind at rest.

People returning to the home after a hospital stay may be weaker and less able to care for themselves than previously. It may take time for the individual to regain strength and ability after an illness. The person's room should be prepared ready for readmission and any get well cards from friends, relatives, residents and staff put in the room.

Planned admission

In the past older people in homes were seldom admitted to hospital for non-emergency treatment. Now, though, attitudes are more positive and medical staff are more aware that in some cases hospital treatment may improve an older person's quality of life. Planned hospital treatment is becoming more common. When non-emergency treatment is required, there is time to prepare and support the person. You should find out as much as possible about the treatment planned. Normally hospital and professional staff working in homes explain the treatment in detail; however, residents may wish to discuss treatment with you. You may need professional advice about planned treatment.

Day surgery

Day surgery is becoming very common. Now people who a few years ago would have remained in hospital for a few days after surgery are admitted in the morning and discharged home in the evening. It is possible to treat greater numbers of people on a day surgery basis. Many older people who develop cataracts find that instead of joining long waiting lists they can be treated quickly as day cases. People requiring day surgery are normally sent by their GP to see a specialist at the local hospital. If the specialist feels that the case is suitable, the person is placed on a day surgery waiting list. A short time before planned admission (usually a week) the person visits the day surgery unit for assessment and investigation, and professional staff give full details of the planned surgery and the care required afterwards. Most surgery units supply written patient information booklets.

On the day of the operation, if a general anaesthetic is required the person does not eat or drink. (The day surgery unit will supply instructions about eating and drinking.) Many cases of day surgery are carried out under local anaesthetic. The person is normally admitted to the ward in the morning, prepared for surgery, and taken to theatre. After the operation the patient usually rests for some time, nursing staff carry out routine post-operative checks and the doctor examines the patient before agreeing discharge if all is well.

It is policy in some homes that a member of staff accompanies the individual to hospital and remains at the hospital, providing support and practical help during the person's stay. If you are to escort a patient to day surgery and wish to watch the operation, discuss this with your manager. The nurse in charge of the day surgery unit can ask the surgeon if you can enter the theatre and observe the operation. Many surgeons explain the operation as they carry it out. Many older people become increasingly worried about day surgery as the day of the operation approaches. Knowing that a member of staff will be with them makes many people less anxious.

Outpatient visits

Visits to the hospital outpatient department may be required for a number of reasons:

- Following surgery at the hospital
- To check on an existing medical condition
- To consider if further treatment is required for a specific problem.

In some homes, all older people are escorted to outpatient appointments by a member of staff. In other homes, transport is arranged to hospital but the home does not provide an escort. In some cases, a member of the resident's family arranges to meet her at the hospital.

If you are asked to escort an older person to an outpatient appointment, make sure that you know the reason for the visit. Is it a routine check-up? Is it to discuss possible further treatment? The individual or your manager will have an appointment card giving details of which clinic to attend, the doctor to be seen and the time of the appointment. Senior staff at the home will ask you to bring a letter giving details of current medication and treatment.

If ambulance transport has been arranged it is important to bear in mind that ambulances can arrive very much earlier or later than ordered. Help the person to get ready in plenty of time. An early breakfast or lunch may be required. When transport arrives, it may be picking up a number of other people before going to the hospital. Ask the individual if she wishes to use the toilet before leaving. If it is cold outside make sure the individual's coat is at hand and help her to put it on before leaving.

You may find that you have to wait a few hours in the outpatient department before the patient is seen, so be prepared. Take some 20p pieces so that you can both have a cup of tea while waiting; most outpatient departments have vending machines. If you don't have a mobile phone take extra change so that you can telephone the home if there is a problem getting transport back. Take something to pass the time; perhaps magazines, the person's knitting or some playing cards. When the doctor or nurse sees the patient, check that you both understand the outcome of the visit. On returning to the home the individual may be feeling tired after the journey. Be sensitive to her needs and offer the person an opportunity to rest if she wishes. Inform the person in charge of the outcome of the visit and record this.

Rehabilitation

Greater numbers of older people are now admitted to homes so that they can fully recover from operation or illness and return home. If the individual is admitted to the home for a short stay, you will normally work with a range of other staff to help prepare the person for discharge home. Many staff, such as the physiotherapist and occupational therapist, and the GP will be working with the person to help her to regain the ability to care for herself at home. Your role is an important one. It is to work with the team. Recovering after a major illness is hard work, and there will be times when the older person feels low. You can offer encouragement and support at such times.

Respite care

There are seven million people caring for older people in their own homes in the UK. They care for relatives or friends who might otherwise require long-term care. For many years, carers have not received the help required to enable them to continue to care. Now respite care is becoming more available and homes will be caring for more people on a respite basis in the next few years.

Respite care is a planned period of care. The older person is admitted to the home for a short period, normally two weeks, so that the carer can have a break. This might be so that the carer can have a holiday or it might be part of a regular rolling programme of respite breaks. Caring for an older person at home without assistance is very hard work. Many carers find it difficult to do the things that we take for granted, such as go to the shops or visit friends. The aim of respite care is to enable carers to continue caring for longer periods by offering planned breaks.

In some homes a number of beds are booked as respite beds. The individual is booked in for certain weeks throughout the year. Many older people who are admitted for respite care for the first time worry that they will never return home. You should be sensitive to such fears and reassure individuals that this is a temporary admission. Many carers have developed ways of meeting the older person's needs at home and have developed a routine. It is important that staff obtain as much information as possible about the older person's normal care and routine and do not disrupt this. It may be easier for two members of staff to help the person onto the toilet, but if the carer and the older person live alone and have been managing, you will only make life more difficult when the older person returns home. If the person's bedroom at home is upstairs, staff should be careful to continue walking upstairs with the older person and not use the lift. If the older person loses the ability to walk upstairs, how will she cope at home?

During the period of respite care staff may be able to help organise services such as chiropody or suggest that aids such as grab rails may help the older person manage at home. Such suggestions and offers of help should be made sensitively as carers may feel that staff are critical of their ability to cope. Many older people and their carers benefit from regular respite care and find that the support of staff in the early days is vitally important.

Summary

The role of homes is changing rapidly. Now older people move from hospital to home and home to hospital more than ever before. Change is difficult to cope with at the best of times. Older people who have been ill or who have undergone recent surgery can feel very vulnerable and worried as they move between care environments. Care assistants who are aware of older people's worries can respond sensitively and help individuals adjust to changing circumstances.

Key points

- Older people, given a choice, would prefer to remain at home. The older person entering a home will require help and support when entering the home.
- People living in homes may require emergency or planned hospital treatment.
- If the older person is admitted to hospital it is important to keep in touch and if possible to visit.
- People requiring day surgery benefit from information and support, before, during and after surgery.
- Some older people attend outpatient appointments and may require support.
- If a person is admitted for respite care it is important to acknowledge fears and support the person and the carer.
- Your role in supporting and enabling people in different care settings is of vital importance.

📖 Portfolio preparation

Your assessor must have evidence that you can meet the performance criteria for this unit. Before beginning this unit discuss assessment strategies with your assessor. Most of the evidence for this unit can be gained by direct observation of your work. This might include observing how your actions support and enable an older person to settle in the home and to negotiate specific environments or how you support the older person when going out.

Products: This might include a copy of progress notes or a care plan care that you have completed. It could be a note in a resident's notes giving details of how you enable and support the person in attending an outpatient clinic or during day surgery. It could be a care plan that you have drawn up or contributed to on how you are aware of the person's hopes and aspirations and how you are supporting the person as she settles into the home.

Witness testimony: This is a statement from a senior member of staff. It might be a statement detailing how you have met certain performance criteria. This might be a statement detailing how you have helped support a resident moving to the home or a resident admitted for respite care.

Written work: You might be asked to prepare a piece of work about how you help residents to feel that the home is their home. You might be asked to write a case history on how you helped a resident settle in. You might be asked to outline how you use the home's policy on admission, any difficulties you have faced and how you have dealt with them.

Your assessor may also use other methods to help you gain evidence for this unit. These may include:

- Verbal questioning
- Written questions.

Simulations can be used if it is not possible to obtain evidence by direct observation.

Glossary

Alzheimer's disease A progressive disorder of the brain. It causes total disintegration of the personality and eventually the person loses the ability to reason and to carry out the activities of daily living. There is no known cure for this terminal disease.

anaemia A reduction in the number of red cells or the amount of haemoglobin (the substance in red blood cells which carries oxygen); causes of anaemia include poor diet and bleeding.

angina Lack of oxygen to the heart muscle caused by narrowing or blockage of the arteries supplying the heart with blood.

anomia Difficulty in finding words.

aphasia Inability to speak.

arthritis Pain, stiffness and sometimes inflammation of one or more joints.

asthma Narrowing of the bronchial tubes which allow air into the lungs. Caused by allergies including medication, dust and pollen. Treated with tablets and inhalers which help the bronchial tubes to relax and open, allowing air to pass freely into the lungs.

atonic colon The bowel becomes inactive and dependent on ever larger amounts of stimulant laxatives.

bladder dysreflexia *See* Overactive bladder.

capillaries Small blood vessels that carry oxygen and glucose to the tissues.

cataract The lens of the eye, which we look through in order to see clearly, becomes white, cloudy and milky in appearance. This affects the vision and can, depending on severity, lead to visual problems or blindness. Treatment is surgical. The cataract is removed and usually a contact lens is inserted into the eye to replace the lens which has been removed.

catheter (urinary) A tube which passes from the urethra to the bladder and is used to drain urine.

cellulitis Inflammation of tissue. This term is normally used to refer to an inflammation of the skin.

cerebrovascular accident A medical term for a stroke.

Colles fracture A fracture of the wrist.

constipation No bowel action for three days or more or passing very hard, dry stools which may resemble rabbit droppings.

decubitus ulcer A medical term for pressure sore.

deep vein thrombosis A clot which forms in the deep veins of the legs or pelvis. This clot can break off and travel around the body until it becomes stuck in an artery. This is known as a pulmonary embolus. People who are immobile are at risk of developing a deep vein thrombosis.

dementia *See* Alzheimer's disease *and* Multi-infarct dementia.

diabetes This is known as diabetes mellitus (sweet diabetes) because the urine contains sugar. This condition was first described by the ancient Greeks who diagnosed it by tasting the urine. The body is unable to use glucose (sugar) because of absence or shortage of insulin. Treatment is either by diet, so that the overweight diabetic loses weight and there is enough insulin to go round, or tablets to make the body produce more insulin, or insulin injections. Untreated diabetes leads to high levels of sugar in the blood. These high sugar levels can cause kidney damage, blindness and circulation problems.

dysarthria Difficulty in forming and articulating words.

dysphasia Difficulty in speaking or understanding words. *See* Expressive dysphasia *and* Receptive dysphasia.

elder abuse Mistreatment of an older person. It can be a single act or a long-term pattern of abuse.

electrolytes Balance of chemicals in the blood. These can become unbalanced because of disease, medication or poor diet.

expressive dysphasia General difficulty in expressing what a person wishes to say.

fracture A broken bone.

gastrostomy An opening from the stomach to the skin. This is created by a surgeon to enable nursing staff to feed people who are unable to swallow. A tube is placed into this opening and special liquid feeds are given.

glaucoma An eye condition which causes the pressure within the eye to become raised. There are a number of different types of glaucoma. Glaucoma can be treated medically or surgically. Untreated glaucoma can cause blindness.

gut transit time The length of time it takes food to move from mouth to anus.

hemianopia Loss of sight in half the visual field. This means that the person has 'blind spots' and visual difficulties.

hemiplegia Paralysis of one side of the body usually as the result of a stroke or injury to the brain.

incontinence The inability to 'hold on' to urine or faeces until a suitable place can be found to empty the bladder or bowel.

intravenous infusion This is commonly known as a 'drip'. Sterile fluid is given slowly into a vein.

ketones Substances which are produced within the body and removed in the urine when the body is burning fat. Seen in poorly controlled diabetics, people who have been vomiting and in starvation.

motor neurone disease A progressive degenerative condition. The neurones (nerve cells) degenerate leading to paralysis and eventually death. There is no known cure.

multi-infarct dementia Interruption of the blood supply to the brain by a small clot, causing tissue death. These small clots cause brain tissue to die and the person loses the ability to reason and function if treatment is not effective. Treatment, such as control of high blood pressure and giving a small dose of aspirin, aims to prevent clots forming in the circulation of the brain.

nasogastric tube A tube which goes down the nose and into the stomach. It is used to give fluids directly into the stomach when a person is unable to swallow, perhaps because of a stroke or motor neurone disease.

osteo-arthritis Arthritis of the hands, knees, hips and big toes.

osteoporosis Thinning and weakening of the bones which makes them fracture more easily.

overactive bladder The bladder muscle contracts before it is completely full. The person passes small amounts of urine frequently and may find it difficult to hold on until the toilet can be reached. This can be caused by strokes or Parkinson's disease.

overflow incontinence Difficulty in emptying the bladder completely caused by a blockage. Constipation, Parkinson's disease and an enlarged prostate are some of the causes of overflow incontinence.

Parkinson's disease A brain disorder caused by a reduction of a chemical, called dopamine, in the brain. It is a progressive disease and eventually the person loses the ability to carry out the activities of daily living. It causes difficulty in moving and speaking. In the early stages medication helps control symptoms.

penile sheath A condom-like device which fits over the penis and drains urine into a catheter bag.

pressure sore   An area of tissue which has died because unrelieved pressure has caused the circulation to the tissue to be cut off. Pressure sores can affect skin, fat, muscle and bone, depending on the severity.

pulmonary embolus   A clot which forms in the deep veins of the leg or pelvic veins, breaks off and travels to the heart. It can cause death by blocking a heart valve or the pulmonary artery. A smaller clot can damage lung tissue.

receptive dysphasia   Difficulty or inability to make sense of messages received by speech.

rheumatoid arthritis   An inflammatory disease of the joints. The synovial tissue that covers the joints becomes inflamed. This causes the affected joints to become hot, swollen and painful.

shearing forces   Damage to the capillary circulation caused by dragging or friction. The damage caused can lead to pressure sores developing.

specific gravity   A way of checking how concentrated urine is. This enables staff to discover if a person is not receiving enough fluid.

stoma   A stoma is an opening from the inside of the body to the outside. A colostomy is an opening created by a surgeon from the large bowel (colon) to the surface of the abdomen. An ileostomy is an opening from the small bowel (ileum) to the surface of the abdomen. Body waste which comes out of these stomas is collected in a bag.

stress incontinence   A leak of urine on moving, coughing or sneezing. Caused by weakness of the muscles in the pelvic floor.

stroke   An interruption of the blood supply to the brain caused by either bleeding or a clot. This leads to an area of tissue death and also bruising to brain tissue.

synovial fluid   A thick fluid that surrounds the end of the bone and the cartilage.

urethra   The tube that enables the bladder to discharge urine.

Index

abuse, 33, 92–104
   financial, 93–4
   medication, 44, 95–6
   neglect, 94–5
   physical abuse, 92–3
   preventing, 98–103
   profile abused person, 98
   sexual abuse, 94
   signs of, 93, 94, 95
accidents, 46–51
Action on Elder Abuse, 111
activities and interests, 133–44
   arts and crafts, 141
   exercise, 142
   games, 139
   gardening, 143–4
   knitting, 141
   music, 139–41
   outings, 144
   pets, 137–8, 144–6
   reading, 142–3
   sport, 141–2
   television and films, 143
activities of daily living, 117–18
admissions, 19–20, 315, 316, 317
   hospital, 318–22, 318–21
   records, 19
adult protection, 101, 102
after-shave, 255
Age Concern, 111
Age Exchange Reminiscence Centre, 148
ageing, 227–8
aggression, 109
airway obstruction, 56–7
Alzheimer's disease, 14–16
Alzheimer's Society, 112
ambulance, 60, 319, 321
anaemia, 159–60
antibiotics, 56, 206, 277
anti-inflammatory drugs, 178
aphasia, 7

arthritis, 48, 163, 176–9
The Arthritis and Rheumatism Council for
   Research (ARC), 192
assessment, 207, 270
assisted washes, 246–7
asthma, 58

back injury, 287, 289, 290, 292–3, 300
bacteria, 52, 54, 56
barrier creams, 214, 248
bath oils, 243
baths, 242–5
bed baths, 247–9
bedpans, 236, 241
bed rails, 50–51
bed sores, see pressure sores
bladder, 227–9, 261, 262
   function, 228, 262
   retraining, 237–8
bleeding, 59
bowel, 231–7, 279–81
Braden scale, 207, 209–12, 215
breathing, 58
breathing difficulties, 56–8
The British Colostomy Association, 283
bubble baths, 243
burns and scalds, 60–61

calories, 152
capillaries, 197–8
carbohydrates, 158
care plans, 22, 115–28, 292
care pathways, 128
Care Standards Act, 22
cataracts, 17
catheter bags, 276, 278
catheters, 275–9
cerebro-vascular accident, see stroke
chairs, 46–7
chest pain, 59
chewing, 166

chiropody, 252–3
choice, 87, 89, 169–70, 309–10
choking, 56–7
The Cinnamon Trust, 138, 147–8
circulation, 58–9
cleaning materials, 21
clothing, 58, 90, 91, 239
cognitive impairment, 133
colostomies, 153, 281–2
Coloplast, 222
Commission Social Care Inspection (CSCI), 78, 100–101, 103, 104
Commodes, 235, 241
communicating, 3–20, 25–6
   aids, 17–18
   physical disabilities, 14–15
   strokes, 6–8
Community Care Act, 22
computers, 23
confidentiality, 24–6, 308–309
confusion, 13–16, 104–108, 154, 167–8, 200–201, 270
Consent, 306–307
constipation, 234–5, 267, 280–81
continence, 226–8, 259–84, 308
continence advice helplines, 283
   Bard, 283
   Hollister, 283
The Continence Foundation, 283
Convatec, 222
cosmetics, 256
Counsel and Care, 112
culture, 310
cups, 155
cushions, pressure relieving, 217–19
cutlery, 167

day surgery, 320–21
deafness, 9–13
   conductive, 10
   sensory neural, 10–11
decubitus ulcers, *see* pressure sores
deep vein thrombosis, 183
dehydration, 151–4
dementia, 14–16, 107–110
   Alzheimer's disease, 14–16, 107–110
   multi–infarct, 107
dentures, 251
diabetes, 162–3, 201
Diabetes UK, 171–2
diarrhoea, 153, 279

diet, 157–62, 89, 90, 201
   diabetic, 162
   high-calorie, 164
   high-fibre, 164, 236
   Hindu, 166
   Jewish, 167
   Muslim, 166
   purée, 164–5
   reducing, 162
   vegetarian, 163
dietary supplements, 166
dietician, 166
dignity, 317–18, 309
Disabled Living Foundation, 302
duty of care, 39–40
dysarthria, 7
dysphasia, 6, 7

education, 44–5, 67–83
elbow protectors, 219
emergencies, 56–61
emergency admissions, 318–19
escorting residents, 319–22
exercise, 179, 189
eye tests, 183
eyesight, 49, 167, 170

faeces, 223, 235, 237
fainting, 58–9
falls, 49–50
families, 306
fire
   drill, 44
   exits, 45
   training, 44–5
   fire information, 45
fluids, 151, 156, 225–7, 235–6, 270, 277
   charts, 156
food and drink, 149–72
footwear, 47–8, 291
fractures, 48–9, 59–60, 181–2
furniture, 315–16

gastrostomy tube, 156
general practitioner, 307
gestures, 18
glasses, 7
gutter frames, 185

hair, 253–5
handling policies, 288–90

hand washing, 55
hazards, 33–4, 46–7,
health and safety, 33–63, 239–40
    regulations, 38–9, 40, 41, 42, 287–90
Health and Safety Executive, 62, 290
hearing, 9–13
    hearing aids, 11–12
    hearing tests, 11
Hearing Concern, 29
heel protectors, 219
hoists, 245, 295–8
Huntleigh Health Care, 222

ileostomies, 281–2
immobility, 199–200, 236
incontinence, 261–75
    drug therapy, 266
    functional, 268
    incontinence pads, 272–4
    overflow (underactive bladder), 266–7
    stress, 267–8
    urge (overactive bladder), 262–6
infection, 52–6
    chest, 183, 189, 229
    urine, 274–5, 276–8
    wound, 206

Johari Window, 68–71
journeys and visits, 189–90

Kellogg's, 172
kidneys, 225–7
Kylie bedsheets, 216

learning needs, 78–81
learning organisation, 67–8
lifting, 287–94
listening, 74–5
longevity, 305–306

manual handing regulations, 287–91
    employee responsibilities, 288, 290
    employer responsibilities, 288–9
mattresses and overlays, 214–17
medication, 17–18, 24, 38, 44, 236–7, 269
    analgesics, 177–8
    antibiotics, 63, 246, 279
    sedatives, 201
    sleeping tablets, 135, 269
Maslow's hierarchy needs, 87–9
memory, 14

minerals, 159–60
    calcium, 159
    cobalt, 159
    copper, 159
    iodine, 159
    iron, 159–160
    phosphorus, 160
    sodium, 160
    zinc, 160
missing residents, 45–6
mobility, 133, 173–93, 199–200, 270
money, 26
mouth care, 250, 251–2

nail care, 252–3
names, 89, 316–17
nasogastric tube, 155
National Association for Providers of
    Activities for Older People (NAPA),
    135, 147
national minimum standards, 122–3, 317
networks, 72–3
Norton scale, 207
nurse specialists, 22, 308
Nursing and Midwifery Council (NMC) 23,
    124
nursing models, 117
nutrition, *see* diet

osteo-arthritis, 176–8
osteoporosis, 48–9, 182
outpatient visits, 321–2
overweight, 98, 145, 156, 178, 181–2, 202, 226

pain, 49, 142, 144–6, 149–50, 181, 182, 210
parasites, 53
Parkinson's disease, 8–9
Parkinson's Disease Society, 29
passive movement, 189
penile (urinary) sheaths, 274
personal development plans, 78–81
pets, 138
Pets as Therapy (PAT), 147
physiotherapy, 308
pregnant staff, 43
pressure relieving aids, 214–19
pressure sores, 195–223
    development, 177–8
    gradings, 204–206
    preventing, 212–14
    risk, 198–203

pressure sores (*continued*)
  sites, 203–204
  treatment, 219–20
privacy, 219, 239, 245, 248, 317–18
Protection of Vulnerable Adults (POVA), 98–101
protein, 157, 158
Public Concern at Work, 112

quality of life, 50

razors, 225
records, 19–24, 51–2
  accidents, 45, 51–2
  money, 26
reflective practice, 75–7
rehabilitation, 322
relatives, 18–19, 24–6
respect, 309
respite care, 322–3
restraint, 50–51
rheumatoid arthritis, 178–9
rights, 302–13
risks, 34–7
role of care assistant, 82
routine, 90–91
Royal National Institute for Deaf People (RNID), 29–30
Royal National Institute for the Blind (RNIB), 193

safety, 32–8, 49–52
scalp, 254
security, 37–8
septicaemia, 206
shampoo, 253–5
shaving, 255
shoes, 45
shouting and screaming, 109
showers, 246
skin, 199–200, 210–12, 249, 279
sleep, 188, 189
Smith & Nephew, 222
soap, 243, 244
Social Services, 101
soiled linen, 280
speech, 6–9
  Parkinson's disease, 8–9
speech and language therapists, 17
spiritual needs, 310–11

splints, 189
staff training, *see* education
St John Ambulance, 61
stoma, 280–81
stroke, 5–8, 179–81
The Stroke Association, 192
swallowing, 166–7

talcum powder, 244, 247
Talley Group Ltd, 227
teeth, 250
thirst, 228
toe nails, 252–3
toilet, 238
tripods, 185–6
turning, 213–14

underweight, 202
uniforms, 291
urine, 225, 230–31, 261

values 73–4
valuables, 26–7
vegetarian, 163
Vegetarian Society, 172
vetting and barring, 101–102
viruses, 52–3
vision, 7, 17–18, 167, 168, 170, 182–3, 229, 238
vitamins, 160–62
  vitamin A, 160
  vitamin B, 160–61
  vitamin C, 161
  vitamin D, 161
  vitamin K, 162
vomit, 57, 156

walking, 134, 136, 183
  aids, 184–7
  sticks, 186
wandering, 14–15, 109
Waterlow scale, 207, 208, 215
wax (ear), 10
well-being, 87–9
wheelchairs, 187–8
  repairs, 188
  self-propelling, 187–8
  transferring, 188
Winslow Press, 148

Zimmer frames, 185